Rhinitis and Related Upper Respiratory Conditions

Jonathan A. Bernstein

Editor

Rhinitis and Related Upper Respiratory Conditions

A Clinical Guide

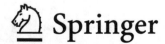 Springer

Editor
Jonathan A. Bernstein
Division of Immunology, Rheumatology and Allergy
Department of Internal Medicine
University of Cincinnati
Cincinnati, OH, USA

ISBN 978-3-030-09215-3   ISBN 978-3-319-75370-6   (eBook)
https://doi.org/10.1007/978-3-319-75370-6

Printed on acid-free paper

This Springer imprint is published by the registered company Springer International Publishing AG part of Springer Nature.
The registered company address is: Gewerbestrasse 11, 6330 Cham, Switzerland

I want to dedicate this book to my wife, Lisa, who has always been my greatest personal advocate. I also want to dedicate this book to all of my patients with chronic rhinitis who are continually teaching me about rhinitis and inspire me to find better approaches for medical management of their conditions.

Preface

Rhinitis is not a trivial disease. Patients suffering from chronic rhinitis experience significant impairment due to uncontrolled symptoms and comorbidities resulting in a diminished quality of life, which directly impacts work productivity and school performance. This results in significant direct and indirect costs to our health care system. Despite this, very little emphasis in medical curriculums is placed on educating health care providers about the proper evaluation and treatment of chronic rhinitis conditions. In fact, unless significant comorbid conditions such as sinusitis present as the primary complaint, the importance of the nose is often ignored.

It is important to recognize that humans are obligate nasal breathers, and the main purpose of the nose is to filter, humidify, and condition air going into the lungs. However, it is also a central reservoir for the paranasal sinuses and lacrimal eye ducts. It is also in close proximity to other structures such as the torus tubarius, which is the opening of the Eustachian tubes into the posterior pharynx. Thus, it is not surprising that patients with chronic rhinitis can present with a constellation of symptoms ranging from nasal congestion; anterior and/or posterior rhinorrhea; sneezing; itching of the eyes, ears, nose, and throat; conjunctivitis; sinus pressure; headaches; and ear plugging, pressure, and popping, which makes the diagnosis and treatment of these patients challenging. Oftentimes the presenting symptoms extend beyond the upper respiratory tract, such as cough, chest tightness, wheezing, shortness of breath, nausea, sleep disturbances, recurrent sinusitis, and bronchitis, further confounding the management of these patients. Failure to address the nasal pathology in treatment of suspected comorbidities such as sinusitis, asthma, headaches, sleep apnea, conjunctivitis, and Eustachian tube dysfunction can significantly impact clinical outcomes.

Although many books on rhinitis are available, this book is unique because it discusses clinical cases related to a spectrum of rhinitis conditions and comorbidities in different patient populations commonly encountered in different clinical settings. Topics span from pediatric, adult, geriatric, and occupational rhinitis to the spectrum of rhinitis subtypes and their complications. Several chapters address secondary causes of rhinitis such as drug-induced rhinitis, CSF leak, and systemic diseases manifesting as rhinitis. Each chapter, written by an expert in the field, is nested with clinical cases illustrating the typical patient presentation, their diagnostic work-up, and treatment. It is anticipated that health care providers will gain a better appreciation for the importance of correctly diagnosing rhinitis and for recognizing related comorbidities so their patients can benefit from optimal available therapies, which in turn will improve their clinical outcomes and quality of life and reduce health care cost expenditures.

Cincinnati, OH, USA   Jonathan A. Bernstein

Contents

Contributors

Abdullah Al-Bader Department of Otolaryngology-Head and Neck Surgery, University of Miami, Miami, FL, USA

Roua Azmeh Section of Allergy and Immunology; Division of Infectious Diseases, Allergy and Immunology; Department of Internal Medicine, Saint Louis University School of Medicine, St. Louis, MO, USA

Fuad M. Baroody Section of Otolaryngology, The University of Chicago Medicine and The Comer Children's Hospital, Chicago, IL, USA

Esther Barrionuevo Allergy Unity, IBIMA-Hospital Regional Universitario of Málaga-UMA, Malaga, Spain

Robert P. Baughman Department of Internal Medicine, University of Cincinnati Medical Center, Cincinnati, OH, USA

Jonathan A. Bernstein Division of Immunology, Rheumatology and Allergy, Department of Internal Medicine, University of Cincinnati, Cincinnati, OH, USA

Leonard Bielory Department of Medicine, RWJ Barnabas Robert Wood Johnson University Hospital, Springfield, NJ, USA

Gador Bogas Allergy Unity, IBIMA-Hospital Regional Universitario of Málaga-UMA, Malaga, Spain

Paloma Campo Allergy Unity, IBIMA-Hospital Regional Universitario of Málaga-UMA, Malaga, Spain

Tara F. Carr Department of Medicine, University of Arizona, Banner-University Medical Center-Tucson, Tucson, AZ, USA

Roy R. Casiano Department of Otolaryngology-Head and Neck Surgery, University of Miami, Miami, FL, USA

Timothy Craig Department of Medicine, Division of Pulmonary, Allergy and Critical Care Medicine, Penn State Health Hershey Medical Center, Hershey, PA, USA

Mark S. Dykewicz Section of Allergy and Immunology, Division of Infectious Diseases, Allergy and Immunology, Department of Internal Medicine, Saint Louis University Hospital, St Louis, MO, USA

Ibon Eguiluz-Gracia Allergy Unity, IBIMA-Hospital Regional Universitario of Málaga-UMA, Malaga, Spain

Lauren Fine Division of Pulmonology, Department of Allergy, Critical Care and Sleep Medicine, University of Miami, Miami, FL, USA

Wytske Fokkens Department of Otorhinolaryngology, Academic Medical Centre, Amsterdam, Netherlands

Justin C. Greiwe Division of Immunology/Allergy Section, Department of Internal Medicine, The University of Cincinnati College of Medicine, Cincinnati, OH, USA

Bernstein Allergy Group, Cincinnati, OH, USA

Daniel L. Hamilos Department of Rheumatology, Allergy & Immunology, Harvard Medical School, Massachusetts General Hospital, Boston, MA, USA

Reece Jones Department of Medicine, Division of Pulmonary, Allergy and Critical Care Medicine, Penn State Health Hershey Medical Center, Hershey, PA, USA

David A. Khan Department of Allergy and Immunology, UT Southwestern Medical Center, Dallas, TX, USA

Merin Elizabeth Kuruvilla Department of Allergy and Immunology, Emory University, Atlanta, GA, USA

David M. Lang Department of Allergy and Clinical Immunology, Cleveland Clinic, Cleveland, OH, USA

Elyse E. Lower Department of Internal Medicine, University of Cincinnati Medical Center, Cincinnati, OH, USA

Sharmilee M. Nyenhuis Division of Pulmonary, Critical Care, Sleep and Allergy, Department of Medicine, University of Illinois Hospital and Health Sciences System, Chicago, IL, USA

Deepa D. Patadia Department of Allergy and Clinical Immunology, Respiratory Institute, Cleveland Clinic, Cleveland, OH, USA

Jill A. Poole Department of Medicine, University of Nebraska Medical Center, Omaha, NE, USA

Benjamin T. Prince Division of Allergy and Immunology, Department of Pediatrics, Nationwide Children's Hospital, The Ohio State University College of Medicine, Columbus, OH, USA

Carmen Rondón Allergy Unity, IBIMA-Hospital Regional Universitario of Málaga-UMA, Malaga, Spain

Andrew C. Rorie Department of Medicine, University of Nebraska Medical Center, Omaha, NE, USA

Geetika Sabharwal Department of Allergy and Immunology, Penn State University, Hershey Medical Center, Hershey, PA, USA

María Salas Allergy Unity, IBIMA-Hospital Regional Universitario of Málaga-UMA, Malaga, Spain

Allen Seiden Department of Otolaryngology, Head and Neck Surgery, University of Cincinnati Academic Medical Center, Cincinnati, OH, USA

Martin A. Smith Department of Allergy and Clinical Immunology, Cleveland Clinic, Cleveland, OH, USA

Peter K. Smith Department of Clinical Medicine, Griffith University, Southport, QLD, Australia

Kristin Claire Sokol National Institute of Allergy and Infectious Diseases, National Institutes of Health, Bethesda, MD, USA

Pamela Tongchinsub Department of Medicine, University of Arizona, Banner-University Medical Center-Tucson, Tucson, AZ, USA

Maria J. Torres Allergy Unity, IBIMA-Hospital Regional Universitario of Málaga-UMA, Malaga, Spain

Chandra Vethody Department of Internal Medicine, University of Louisville, Louisville, KY, USA

Preeti Wagle University Asthma and Allergy Associates, Springfield, NJ, USA

Abbreviations

AAO-HNS	American Academy of Otolaryngology–Head and Neck Surgery
AHI	Apnea hypopnea index
AIT	Allergen immunotherapy
Anti-LT	Anti-leukotriene
AR	Allergic rhinitis
ARIA	Allergic rhinitis and its impact on asthma
BPAP	Bilevel positive airway pressure
BP	Blood pressure
CBC	Complete blood count
CT	Computed tomography
CPAP	Continuous positive airway pressure
COPD	Chronic obstructive pulmonary disease
EOMI	Extra ocular muscles intact
FEV1	Forced expiratory volume in 1 s
FVC	Forced vital capacity
GERD	Gastroesophageal reflux disease
IgE	Immunoglobulin E
INCS	Intranasal corticosteroid
LAR	Local allergic rhinitis
MI	Myocardial infarction
MR	Mixed rhinitis
NAR	Nonallergic rhinitis
OTC	Over the counter
OCP	Oral contraceptive pill
OSA	Obstructive sleep apnea
PAP	Positive airway pressure
PAR	Perennial allergic rhinitis
PSG	Polysomnography
PERRL	Pupils equal round reactive to light
SAR	Seasonal allergic rhinitis

SDB	Sleep-disorder breathing
SCIT	Subcutaneous allergen immunotherapy
SLIT	Sublingual allergen immunotherapy
SPT	Skin prick testing
TSH	Thyroid stimulating hormone
URI	Upper respiratory tract infection
VMR	Vasomotor rhinitis

Seasonal Allergic Rhinitis

Roua Azmeh and Mark S. Dykewicz

Case Presentation 1

Eric is a 30-year-old man who lives in the Midwestern US and presents with symptoms of sneezing, itchy eyes/nose/ears/throat, nasal congestion, clear rhinorrhea, and red, watery eyes. He says that he has had mild symptoms for as long as he can remember, but over the past few years they have become more severe. Symptoms typically occur in March through May and again in mid-August through October. He has tried several over-the-counter antihistamines, which used to completely control symptoms but over the past few seasons no longer provide enough relief. He has come to your office in April because he can no longer tolerate his symptoms.

Physical exam reveals conjunctival injection, dark circles under his eyes, a transverse nasal crease, pale and boggy nasal turbinates, and cobblestoning consistent with postnasal drainage in the oropharynx.

R. Azmeh · M. S. Dykewicz (✉)
Section of Allergy and Immunology, Division of Infectious Diseases, Allergy and Immunology, Department of Internal Medicine, Saint Louis University Hospital, St Louis, MO, USA
e-mail: dykewicz@slu.edu

Diagnosis/Assessment

The main diagnoses in the differential are seasonal allergic rhinitis (SAR), nonallergic rhinitis (NAR)—which may be episodic and mimic SAR but also be perennial—and recurrent upper respiratory tract infections (URI) [1, 2].

Allergic rhinitis (AR) is estimated to affect 10–30% of adults and 40% of children in the United States [3–6]. Worldwide, it is estimated to affect 10–20% of the population [1]. Seasonal allergic rhinitis symptoms can persist for weeks or months depending on the local geographic environment. Although allergic rhinitis is sometimes viewed as a trivial condition, it can cause significant impairment of patients' quality of life and result in missed school and work days as well as significant "presenteeism," i.e., working while ill with resultant productivity loss [1–3, 7]. According to a recent study of US pharmacy claims data between 2009 and 2014, patients with SAR had an average of 2.4 AR-related prescriptions costing $313 annually, and total AR-related costs of $643 annually [7]. SAR alone can cause significant sleep disturbances, fatigue, and cognitive impairment, but it also interacts with comorbid respiratory diseases such as asthma, sleep apnea, and sinusitis to make these conditions much more difficult to manage [2, 3, 8–11]. In a 2012 phone survey of randomly selected US households, respondents rated their mean work productivity

29% lower when allergy symptoms were at their worst [12] and 50% of respondents on a 2015 online survey reported impairment of daily activities or mood disturbances due to SAR symptoms [11].

Both SAR and NAR can cause similar symptoms and physical exam findings, and NAR often can have an apparent seasonal presentation due to symptoms induced by seasonal weather variation such as temperature and barometric pressure changes [3]. Frequently, SAR will cause nasal itching and conjunctival symptoms such as itching and redness, although an URI can cause some conjunctival symptoms as well. History of exposure to sick contacts with similar symptoms or presence of additional symptoms such as fever, myalgias, lymphadenopathy, or exudative pharyngitis increases the likelihood of an URI. Additionally, an URI typically is associated with a shorter duration of symptoms [2]. Though a history of symptoms occurring during the same season each year supports a diagnosis of SAR, as would a parental history of physician-diagnosed AR or younger age of onset, the only way to definitively distinguish SAR and NAR is through allergy testing. However, patients can be treated empirically upon initial presentation and have allergy testing completed if symptoms are not controlled [2].

He is found to have elevated serum-specific IgE levels to ash, birch, oak, and elm tree pollens as well as ragweed pollen. A diagnosis of SAR is made based on his sensitization and clinical symptoms in response to seasonal aeroallergen exposure.

Allergy testing is based on detecting specific IgE either through skin prick testing or in the blood. Of note, in order for skin prick testing to be performed, the patient must abstain from H1-antihistamine medications prior to the testing. The diagnosis of SAR requires both evidence of specific IgE to allergens and correlating symptoms, being mindful that IgE sensitization may be present in the absence of clinical symptoms [13]. In this patient's case, if he had evidence of specific IgE to tree, grass, and ragweed pollens, his spring and fall symptoms would support tree and ragweed allergy but not grass allergy.

Diagnosis of SAR does not typically require any imaging, though it can be used to evaluate for comorbid conditions such as chronic rhinosinusitis [2].

While allergic rhinitis and other allergic disorders may be associated with blood eosinophilia, the presence of peripheral eosinophilia does not add to the assessment of an uncomplicated patient; therefore complete blood count (CBC) is unnecessary for initial evaluation.

Patients with allergic rhinitis are at increased risk for asthma and should be evaluated to assure that they do not have comorbid asthma, which can be done with a thorough review of systems, a screening PEFR followed by spirometry and bronchospastic evaluation depending on clinical suspicion. Given that AR is a risk factor and asthma is frequently an insidious disease presenting without respiratory symptoms, consideration for screening these patients routinely for asthma should be given.

Management/Outcome

Once allergen sensitivities have been identified, one management strategy for SAR can be reduction of exposure by limiting time outdoors when the relevant aeroallergen is known to be present, although complete avoidance is not possible. When symptoms become more severe, pharmacotherapy is indicated, as in Eric's case. Given their over-the-counter status and ease of use, oral antihistamines are often chosen by patients as their first pharmacotherapy trial for rhinitis symptoms, sometimes before seeking medical attention. Additionally, some try over-the-counter oral cough and cold medications containing antihistamines and decongestants. Second-generation oral antihistamines (cetirizine, levocetirizine, fexofenadine, loratadine, and desloratadine) are generally better tolerated than first-generation agents that can be associated with anticholinergic and sedative side effects [1, 3]. These side effects are especially important to consider when recommending treatment for children or elderly patients who may be more susceptible to some of them. Some of the second-generation oral H1-antihistamines can be sedating (cetirizine and levocetirizine at recommended doses; loratadine and desloratadine at doses exceeding the recommended dose) so patients should be counseled appropriately [3]. No single second-generation oral H1-antihistamine has conclusively been shown to be overall more effective than another [3] and as a class they are typically not effective in treating NAR.

In this patient, an empiric trial of intranasal corticosteroid is appropriate as it is the most effective medication class for management of moderate persistent SAR and can also be effective in the treatment of NAR [2, 3]. Many formulations are now available over the counter. No differences in efficacy have been found among the different available intranasal corticosteroids despite differences in potency of the different corticosteroid moieties, although some patients may prefer different products based upon attributes such as type of delivery device (e.g., aqueous vs. aerosol), and perceived scent or taste [2, 3]. They can have local side effects such as epistaxis, nasal dryness/irritation, or rarely, nasal septal perforation

Intranasal antihistamines are another available treatment modality recommended as first-line therapy for mild persistent SAR by GINA guidelines and are currently available in the United States by prescription only. While intranasal corticosteroids are generally more effective than intranasal antihistamines as monotherapy, intranasal antihistamines have the advantage of faster onset of action (as early as 30 min as opposed to approximately 12 h [2, 14–20]). The combination of an intranasal corticosteroid and intranasal antihistamine is more effective than the use of either product alone [2, 3]. Products are available that combine an intranasal corticosteroid and intranasal antihistamine into a single spray bottle for patient convenience. Side effects of intranasal antihistamines may include an unpleasant taste perceived by some patients and sedation.

Oral anti-LT agents are not as effective as intranasal corticosteroids, and are not more effective than oral H1-antihistamines. A combination of oral anti-LT and oral antihistamine has not been consistently shown to be more effective than using either alone, but may be an alternative for patients who cannot tolerate nasal sprays [1–3]. Oral corticosteroids can be very effective in treating symptoms of allergic rhinitis. However, due to significant side effects with long-term use, they are best reserved for severe symptoms and should be limited to short courses. Use of parenteral sustained-acting corticosteroids is not recommended even for single administration due to higher risk of side effects such as adrenal suppression and injection site effects such as muscle atrophy and fat necrosis [1, 3].

Intranasal cromolyn sodium is another available therapy over the counter that reduces release of inflammatory mediators. If used as maintenance therapy for SAR, it should be dosed 3–4 times daily on a regular basis and when begun during active symptoms has an onset of action of 4–7 days [1, 3]. While it is less effective than an intranasal corticosteroid for maintenance therapy of SAR and has low efficacy in treating symptoms once they have begun, it can be quite effective in acutely preventing symptoms before exposure to allergens such as cats. It is often recommended for a patient to use prior to anticipated allergen exposure (as in patients with episodic environmental allergic rhinitis) as it typically provides 4–8 h of protection, and can be redosed every 4–8 h during short-term allergen exposure.

Other treatment modalities for SAR include intranasal and oral decongestants. Intranasal decongestants can cause rhinitis medicamentosa if used for more than a few days (though there is patient-to-patient variability [21–24]) but concomitant use of intranasal corticosteroids has been noted to help protect against this effect [25–29]. At this time, however, the Joint Task Force, Allergic Rhinitis and its Impact on Asthma (ARIA), and American Academy of Otolaryngology–Head and Neck Surgery (AAO-HNS) guideline recommendations are still to use intranasal decongestants only for an acute exacerbation rather than maintenance therapy [1, 3]. Intranasal corticosteroids can also be used to treat rhinitis medicamentosa if needed. Oral decongestants are more effective in treating nasal congestion than oral antihistamines or leukotriene antagonists but can also be associated with adverse effects such as insomnia, anorexia, palpitations, dry mouth, and hypertension and thus should be avoided in patients with cardiovascular disease, diabetes, or hyperthyroidism [1, 3]. They may have a role as "rescue" medication for some patients to use intermittently [1].

Clinical Pearls and Pitfalls

- SAR is a clinically burdensome and significant disease that is often underrecognized as a cause of decreased quality of life.
- Intranasal corticosteroids are the most effective monotherapy for treating SAR.
- Treatment of SAR, as for any disease, must be selected based on symptoms, patient age/comorbidities, and patient/family preferences.
- Not all combinations of pharmacotherapies provide additive benefit to monotherapies. The combination of an intranasal corticosteroid and intranasal antihistamine can provide greater relief than either monotherapy, in contrast to combination use of an oral antihistamine and intranasal corticosteroid which generally is not superior to intranasal corticosteroid monotherapy.
- Refer to an allergist for symptoms that are refractory to treatment, long-standing, severe enough to interfere with sleep/work, or if the patient wishes to determine specific sensitivities.

Case Presentation 2

Carrie is an 18-year-old girl who lives in the Midwest US and comes into clinic for evaluation of a history of seasonal rhinitis symptoms. These include sneezing, itchy eyes/nose/ears/throat, clear rhinorrhea, and frequent throat clearing, associated with red, watery eyes. Her symptoms initially were mild when she was about 10 years old, but they have gotten more pronounced over the years, and typically are bothersome in the late spring and fall months. It is currently May. Due to her severe symptoms, she has been given more and more medications over the years and is currently taking an oral antihistamine, intranasal corticosteroid, and intranasal antihistamine. With a recent change in insurance coverage, Carrie can no longer see her previous physician and she would like to decrease her reliance on medications. She asks about non-pharmacologic treatments including "allergy shots." Physical exam reveals no abnormalities.

Diagnosis/Assessment

The main diagnoses in the differential are SAR and NAR. The seasonal pattern of nasal symptoms including nasal itching in association with eye symptoms makes SAR more likely. Note that patients with SAR may have a completely normal exam if seen during a time they are typically asymptomatic.

For this patient who has had symptoms requiring multiple medications and who is also interested in allergen immunotherapy (AIT), allergy skin prick testing or serum-specific IgE level testing is warranted to determine sensitivities which must then be correlated to exposure-associated symptoms.

Management/Outcome

In addition to AIT, non-pharmacologic treatment options for SAR include allergen avoidance measures and topical saline solution, either as a nasal spray or in the form of nasal irrigation.

Reduction of tree/grass/weed pollen exposure includes keeping windows shut, staying indoors when possible, and showering and changing clothes after spending time outside during the relevant pollination season. Reduction of exposure to outdoor molds can be addressed by limiting outdoor activities and keeping windows shut when mold counts are high, and wearing a dust mask when digging around plants, mowing lawns, or picking up or raking leaves. Indoor mold exposure can be decreased in the home by focusing on decreasing sources of moisture such as high humidity, water leaks, or cold surfaces on which water can condensate. Visible mold can be destroyed with dilute bleach solution [3].

Topical saline solution has been shown to be less effective in treating rhinitis symptoms than intranasal corticosteroids, but some benefit has been shown [30]. The mechanism for this benefit is currently unknown, though several hypotheses have been proposed including physical removal of antigen/inflammatory mediators/mucus or enhancement of ciliary beating and mucus clearance.

As with treatment of many chronic illnesses, treatment of SAR can be managed with a step-up or step-down approach depending on symptom severity, patient preferences, and clinician judgment.

In this case, the most appropriate medication to taper off first is the one least likely contributing to rhinitis control, the oral antihistamine. There is little supporting evidence that the combination of an oral H1-antihistamine and intranasal corticosteroid achieves better rhinitis control than an intranasal corticosteroid alone. In Carrie's case, a trial off the intranasal antihistamine may be attempted next, as intranasal corticosteroids are the most effective medication class for management of SAR. If symptoms return while off the intranasal antihistamine, it can be restarted with a quick onset of action. It is unlikely she would be able to completely come off medication without allergen immunotherapy (AIT).

AIT is the only therapy available with the potential to modify the underlying disease and long-term course of AR. SCIT has been practiced in the United States since the early 1900s [31]. A 2012 telephone survey of US households showed some or full symptom relief in 74.9% of patients treated with SCIT [32]. SLIT became FDA approved in the United States for ragweed and certain grasses in 2014, and for house dust mites in 2017. To date there are no studies that have reported efficacy of SLIT to multiple allergens administered as a mixture [33], whereas multiallergen SCIT trials generally have demonstrated efficacy [31]. Because of this, SCIT currently is considered better suited for treating patients who are sensitive to multiple allergens. A recent pooled analysis showed that SLIT provided almost as much relief of nasal symptoms as intranasal corticosteroids and more relief than montelukast or desloratadine in the treatment of SAR [34]. AIT carries a risk of anaphylactic reaction and therefore must be administered by a physician comfortable with recognizing and treating anaphylaxis. For this reason, it is also contraindicated in patients with medical conditions that would decrease survival from an anaphylactic reaction such as certain cardiovascular or respiratory diseases and should be used cautiously in patients who are on beta-blockers (which interfere with the response to epinephrine should anaphylaxis occur) [31]. AIT is typically given for a 3- to 5-year course in order to achieve lasting response. Clinical reduction of symptoms can take up to 1 year from start of SCIT, but is typically noted during the first season of taking SLIT when started several months prior to the relevant pollen season.

For patients presenting with rhinorrhea only, another option for treatment can be an intranasal anticholinergic agent. For treatment of SAR it is not considered first-line and intranasal corticosteroid or intranasal antihistamine would be preferred, but for patients intolerant of those medications it can be an option. Intranasal anticholinergics (most widely used in the United States is ipratropium bromide) are effective in treating rhinorrhea but not effective in treating other rhinitis symptoms [1, 3]. The most common side effects reported with this medication are nasal dryness and mild epistaxis. For treatment of rhinorrhea, combination use with an intranasal corticosteroid is more effective than use of either drug alone [1, 3].

Clinical Pearls and Pitfalls

- Patients with SAR may have a completely normal exam if seen during a time they are typically asymptomatic.
- SAR management can be approached in a step-up or step-down approach.
- AIT is the only potentially disease-modifying therapy available for AR and can also improve comorbid respiratory diseases such as sinusitis, asthma, and obstructive sleep apnea.
- AIT is indicated not only for failure/intolerance of pharmacotherapy but also if patients prefer to decrease reliance on medication.

References

1. Brozek JL, Bousquet J, Baena-Cagnani CE, Bonini S, Canonica GW, Casale TB, et al., Global Allergy and Asthma European Network, Grading of Recommendations Assessment, Development and Evaluation Working Group. Allergic rhinitis and its impact on asthma (ARIA) guidelines: 2010 revision. J Allergy Clin Immunol. 2010;126(3): 466–76.
2. Seidman MD, Gurgel RK, Lin SY, Schwartz SR, Baroody FM, Bonner JR, et al., Guideline Otolaryngology Development Group. AAO-HNSF. Clinical practice guideline: allergic rhinitis. Otolaryngol Head Neck Surg. 2015:152(1 Suppl): S1–43.

3. Wallace DV, Dykewicz MS, Bernstein DI, Blessing-Moore J, Cox L, Khan DA, et al., Joint Task Force on Practice, American Academy of Allergy, Asthma & Immunology, American College of Allergy, Asthma and Immunology, Joint Council of Allergy, Asthma, and Immunology. The diagnosis and management of rhinitis: an updated practice parameter. J Allergy Clin Immunol. 2008;122(2 Suppl):S1–84.

4. Settipane RA, Schwindt C. Chapter 15: allergic rhinitis. Am J Rhinol Allergy. 2013;27(Suppl1):S52–5.

5. American College of Allergy, Asthma & Immunology. Allergy facts. http://acaai.org/news/facts-statistics/allergies. Accessed 1 Jan 2017.

6. Soni A. Allergic rhinitis: trends in use and expenditures, 2000 and 2005. Statistical brief no. 204. Bethesda, MD: Agency for Healthcare Research and Quality; 2008.

7. Lang K, Allen-Ramey F, Huang H, Rock M, Kaufman E, Dykewicz MS. Health care resource use and associated costs among patients with seasonal versus perennial allergic rhinitis. Allergy Asthma Proc. 2016;37(5):103–11.

8. Meltzer EO, Gross GN, Katial R, Storms WW. Allergic rhinitis substantially impacts patient quality of life: findings from the nasal allergy survey assessing limitations. J Fam Pract. 2012;61(2 Suppl):S5–S10.

9. Canonica GW, Bousquet J, Mullol J, Scadding GK, VIrchow JC. A survey of the burden of allergic rhinitis in Europe. Allergy. 2007;62(Suppl 85):17–25.

10. Leger D, Annesi-Maesano I, Carat F, Rugina M, Chanal I, Pribil C, et al. Allergic rhinitis and its consequences on quality of sleep: an unexplored area. Arch Intern Med. 2006;166(16):1744–8.

11. Meltzer EO, Farrar JR, Sennet C. Findings from an online survey assessing the burden and management of seasonal allergic rhinoconjunctivitis in US patients. J Allergy Clin Immunol Pract. 2017;5(3):779–789.e6. https://doi.org/10.1016/j.jaip.2016.10.010.

12. Bielory L, Skoner DP, Blaiss MS, Leatherman B, Dykewicz MS, Smith N, et al. Ocular and nasal allergy symptom burden in America: the allergies, immunotherapy, and RhinoconjunctivitiS (AIRS) surveys. Allergy Asthma Proc. 2014;35:211–8.

13. Carr TF, Saltoun CA. Chapter 2: skin testing in allergy. Allergy Asthma Proc. 2012;33(Suppl 1):S6–8.

14. Meltzer EO, Rickard KA, Westlund RE, Cook CK. Onset of therapeutic effect of fluticasone propionate aqueous nasal spray. Ann Allergy Asthma Immunol. 2001;86:286–91.

15. Day JH, Briscoe MP, Rafeiro E, Ellis AK, Pettersson E, Akerlund A. Onset of action of intranasal budesonide (Rhinocort aqua) in seasonal allergic rhinitis studied in a controlled exposure model. J Allergy Clin Immunol. 2000;105:489–94.

16. Berkowitz RB, Bernstein DI, LaForce C, Pedinoff AJ, Rooklin AR, Damaraju CR, et al. Onset of action of mometasone furoate nasal spray (NASONEX) in seasonal allergic rhinitis. Allergy. 1999;54:64–9.

17. Horak F, Zieglmayer UP, Zieglmayer R, Kavina A, Marschall K, Munzel U, et al. Azelastine nasal spray and desloratadine tablets in pollen-induced seasonal allergic rhinitis: a pharmacodynamic study of onset of action and efficacy. Curr Med Res Opin. 2006;22:151–7.

18. Patel P, Roland PS, Marple BF, Benninger PJ, Margalias H, Brubaker M, et al. An assessment of the onset and duration of action of olopatadine nasal spray. Otolaryngol Head Neck Surg. 2007;137:918–24.

19. Patel D, Garadi R, Brubaker M, Conroy JP, Kaji Y, Crenshaw K, et al. Onset and duration of action of nasal sprays in seasonal allergic rhinitis patients: olopatadine hydrochloride versus mometasone furoate monohydrate. Allergy Asthma Proc. 2007;28:592–9.

20. Patel P, D'Andrea C, Sacks HJ. Onset of action of azelastine nasal spray compared with mometasone nasal spray and placebo in subjects with seasonal allergic rhinitis evaluated in an environmental exposure chamber. Am J Rhinol. 2007;21:499–503.

21. Morris S, Eccles R, Martez SJ, Riker DK, Witek TJ. An evaluation of nasal response following different treatment regimes of oxymetazoline with reference to rebound congestion. Am J Rhinol. 1997;11:109–15.

22. Yoo JK, Seikaly H, Calhoun KH. Extended use of topical nasal decongestants. Laryngoscope. 1997;107:40–3.

23. Petruson B. Treatment with xylometazoline (Otrivin) nosedrops over a six-week period. Rhinology. 1981;19:167–72.

24. Watanabe H, Foo TH, Djazaeri B, Duncombe P, Mackay IS, Durham SR. Oxymetazoline nasal spray three times daily for four weeks in normal subjects is not associated with rebound congestion or tachyphylaxis. Rhinology. 2003;41:167–74.

25. Thongngarm T, Assanasen P, Pradubpongsa P, Tantilipikorn P. The effectiveness of oxymetazoline plus intranasal steroid in the treatment of chronic rhinitis: a randomised controlled trial. Asian Pac J Allergy Immunol. 2016;34:30–7.

26. Meltzer EO, Bernstein DI, Prenner BM, Berger WE, Shekar T, Teper AA. Mometasone furoate nasal spray plus oxymetazoline nasal spray: short-term efficacy and safety in seasonal allergic rhinitis. Am J Rhinol Allergy. 2013;27:102–8.

27. Baroody FM, Brown D, Gavanescu L, DeTineo M, Naclerio RM. Oxymetazoline adds to the effectiveness of fluticasone furoate in the treatment of perennial allergic rhinitis. J Allergy Clin Immunol. 2011;127:927–34.

28. Ferguson BJ, Paramaesvaran S, Rubinstein E. A study of the effect of nasal steroid sprays in perennial allergic rhinitis patients with rhinitis medicamentosa. Otolaryngol Head Neck Surg. 2001;125:253–60.

29. Vaidyanathan S, Williamson P, Clearie K, Khan F, Lipworth B. Fluticasone reverses oxymetazoline-induced tachyphylaxis of response and rebound congestion. Am J Respir Crit Care Med. 2010;182:19–24.

30. Spector SL, Toshener D, Gay I, Rosenman E. Beneficial effects of propylene and polyethylene glycol and saline in the treatment of perennial rhinitis. Clin Allergy. 1982;12:187–96.

31. Cox L, Nelson H, Lockey R, Calabria C, Chacko T, Finegold I, et al. Allergen immunotherapy: a practice parameter third update. J Allergy Clin Immunol. 2011;127(1 Suppl):S1–55.

32. Skoner DP, Blaiss MS, Dykewicz MS, Smith N, Leatherman B, Bielory L, Walstein N, Craig TJ, Allen-Ramey F. The allergies, immunotherapy, and RhinoconjunctivitiS (AIRS) survey: patients' experience with allergen immunotherapy. Allergy Asthma Proc. 2014;35:219–26.

33. Greenhawt M, Oppenheimer J, Nelson M, Nelson H, Lockey R, Lieberman P, et al. Sublingual immunotherapy: a focused allergen immunotherapy practice parameter update. Ann Allergy Asthma Immunol. 2017 Mar;118(3):276–282.e2.

34. Durham SR, Creticos PS, Nelson HS, Li Z, Kaur A, Meltzer EO, et al. Treatment effect of sublingual immunotherapy tablets and pharmacotherapies for seasonal and perennial allergic rhinits: pooled analyses. J Allergy Clin Immunol. 2016;138:1081–1088.e4.

Perennial Allergic Rhinitis

2

Martin A. Smith and David M. Lang

Case Presentation 1

Mr. G is a 42-year-old microbiologist, seen for further evaluation of chronic rhinoconjunctivitis. He developed chronic nasal/ocular symptoms in childhood that have been worse for 3 years. His symptoms have been perennial in nature, but worse in the fall. He has experienced prominent bilateral nasal congestion and clear anterior drainage; he also described ocular pruritus, but denied remarkable pruritus affecting nose, eyes, ears, or palate. Mr. G had remarkable worsening of rhinoconjunctivitis symptoms during vacations in Marco Island during the previous spring, and prior to this in Myrtle Beach in late September. He recalled undergoing skin testing in adolescence that showed remarkable reactions to molds and "dust."

His current medications include diphenhydramine, which he takes 2–3 times per week, on an as-needed basis. This has not been associated with subjective awareness of drowsiness. He also takes intranasal fluticasone on an as-needed basis.

He denied asthma, chronic urticaria/angioedema, atopic dermatitis, or remarkable adverse reaction following food consumption or allergic bee sting reactions.

His other medical problems include hypertension, for which he takes hydrochlorothiazide daily. He is a nonsmoker.

Mr. G resides in a 25-year-old home with air-conditioning. His bedroom floor is carpeted and his mattress is 5 years old. He uses a down/feather pillow and there are two cats in the home, which have access to the bedroom but elicit no symptoms with close contact.

On physical examination, Mr. G was pleasant and in no distress. Blood pressure was 113/69, pulse 74, temperature 37 °C (98.6 °F), and respiratory rate 14. Limited cutaneous examination disclosed no urticaria. Chest auscultation was clear during tidal breathing. Cardiac exam showed regular rate and rhythm. Ocular exam showed no scleral icterus or conjunctival erythema or suffusion. Intranasal inspection revealed bilateral mucous membrane congestion with clear secretions and no remarkable mucosal irregularity or polyps. Otoscopic findings were unremarkable. Oral cavity showed a modest amount of mucoid material in the posterior pharynx. The neck exam showed no definite thyromegaly or lymphadenopathy. Extremities revealed no cyanosis or clubbing. Abdominal exam was non-tender with normal bowel sounds and no visceromegaly.

Diagnosis/Assessment

Options for confirming or ruling out the presence of allergic potential to inhalant allergens, and

6

M. A. Smith · D. M. Lang (✉)
Department of Allergy and Clinical Immunology,
Cleveland Clinic, Cleveland, OH, USA
e-mail: smithm49@ccf.org; langd@ccf.org

© Springer International Publishing AG, part of Springer Nature 2018
J. A. Bernstein (ed.), *Rhinitis and Related Upper Respiratory Conditions*,
https://doi.org/10.1007/978-3-319-75370-6_2

confirming a diagnosis of IgE-mediated allergic rhinoconjunctivitis, were explained and understood. Mr. G was told that immediate hypersensitivity skin testing or in vitro testing to aeroallergens could be performed, and that the advantages of in vitro testing include its utility for patients who are unable to suspend antihistamine medications or who have extensive dermatitis, while skin testing offers the advantages of providing results at the time of service, greater sensitivity, and association with lower cost [1]. He expressed a desire to proceed with skin testing.

Accordingly, skin testing to inhalant allergens revealed remarkable wheal/flare reactions at percutaneous level to *Dermatophagoides farinae* and *Dermatophagoides pteronyssinus*. Intracutaneous testing revealed remarkable wheal/flare reactions to cockroach and grass pollen.

Upon further questioning, Mr. G denied any evidence of cockroach infestation in his current home, but related that he had resided in an apartment in New York City in the past, in which cockroach infestation was a recurrent problem. For this reason, wheal/flare reaction was attributed to this past exposure.

He was told that intracutaneous skin testing may be associated with poor specificity, and that the positive skin test to grass pollen, in the absence of a compatible history of relevant rhinoconjunctivitis symptoms during the summer months, does not imply that grass is a clinically relevant allergen in his case [2].

Management/Outcome

Mr. G was told based on his history and results of skin testing that his symptoms are due to perennial allergic rhinitis (PAR), which he was informed may be defined as an inflammation of the nasal mucous membranes caused by immunoglobuin (Ig) E-mediated allergic reaction to aeroallergens present on a year-round basis. The causes of PAR are summarized in Table 2.1.

He was told that PAR is a major cause of patient visits to physicians in the United States, frequently complicates management of other conditions (e.g., asthma, chronic sinusitis), and if

untreated or undertreated can lead to considerable morbidity—including missed work/school, sleep disruption, and impaired quality of life [1]. In many cases, PAR does not lead to absence from work or school, but entails fatigue and impaired cognition, concentration, and decision-making ability [3]. Reduced quality of performance at the workplace, which has been termed "presenteeism," contributes to the substantial productivity loss associated with allergic rhinitis. The economic burden of AR is substantial [4]. Allergic rhinitis is associated with significant impairment in quality of life—comparable to that observed in patients with diabetes, cardiovascular disease, musculoskeletal disorders, and psychosomatic disorders [3, 5]. The health-related quality of life in patients with PAR due to dust mite allergy is poorer than in patients with seasonal allergic rhinitis (SAR) associated with pollen allergy, but it is unclear whether this is due to symptom frequency, duration, or severity [6].

Mr. G was also made aware that the allergic response is biphasic. Individuals with the potential for IgE-mediated allergic responses to otherwise innocuous inhalant allergens, with sufficient exposure, generate allergen-specific IgE after T-cell release of interleukins 4 and 13, and B-cell "switching" to produce IgE antibody—thereby becoming "sensitized." The IgE-mediated reaction that underlies PAR results from exposure to the allergen to which sensitization has occurred, which cross-links at least two IgE antibodies bound to the high-affinity

Table 2.1 Major aeroallergens that cause perennial allergic rhinitis

Dust mites
• *Dermatophagoides farinae*
• *Dermatophagoides pteronyssinus*
Mold spores
• *Aspergillus* species
• *Cladosporium* species
• *Penicillium* species
Pests
• Cockroaches
• Mice/rats
Pets
• Cats
• Dogs
• Rodents (e.g., rabbits, hamsters)

IgE receptor on pre-sensitized effector cells: mast cells or basophils [7]. Importantly, the IgE-mediated response includes both early and late phases [1]. The early phase occurs promptly, and spans approximately 1 h. The late phase characteristically begins in 3–6 h, peaks at 6–8 h, and wanes in 12–24 h. Almost half of the subjects when studied in laboratory settings exhibit this "dual" response [7, 8]. The symptoms of the early phase generally include sneezing, pruritus, and clear rhinorrhea; symptoms of the late phase may be similar, but usually the late phase entails more prominent congestion [1, 8]. The late phase is promoted by factors generated in the early phase, which encourage release of inflammatory mediators as well as activation and recruitment of cells to the nasal mucosa [1, 7, 8]. While histamine appears to be the major mediator of the early phase, the late phase is more closely associated with other mediators, chemokines, and cytokines that have both inflammatory and pro-inflammatory effects leading to recruitment of effector cells such as eosinophils and basophils. During a clinically relevant exposure in a sensitized individual, aeroallergens enter the nasal passages on a continual basis; for this reason, it is frequently difficult to separate the early and late phases of the allergic response in the real-world setting. Mr. G was made aware that in many cases of PAR, based on the chronic nature of aeroallergen exposure in individuals with dust mite allergy, affected individuals experience a perpetual late-phase response [1, 9].

Mr. G. was informed that in most areas of the United States, and the world, dust mites are a major source of allergens in the indoor environment [10]. In a study [11] carried out in eight geographic locations in the United States, most homes were found to be co-inhabited with *Dermatophagoides farinae* and *Dermatophagoides pteronyssinus*. One species typically predominates in each home; however, the pattern of which dust mite predominated varied substantially in each geographic area. For this reason, skin testing is generally performed with both *Dermatophagoides farinae* and *Dermatophagoides pteronyssinus*. He was informed that mite bodies and feces are the principal causes of sensitization and symptoms in affected individuals [12]. Allergens in mite feces are enzymes that derive from the mite's digestive tract. Dust mite allergen is commonly found in mattresses, bedding, rugs, upholstered furniture, stuffed animals, and clothing. The allergen is carried on particles that are much heavier than animal allergens, which do not remain airborne for long periods. The most substantial exposure to dust mite allergens occurs in association with exposure to bedding during sleep [12].

Mr. G was educated regarding the importance of dust mite avoidance measures, including but not limited to mattress and box spring encasement and washing bedding frequently in hot cycle [1, 12]. In a lengthy conversation in which an emotional attachment to his cats was acknowledged [13], he was told that this exposure may be a factor leading to an increase in the population of dust mites in his bedroom; accordingly, he was advised to restrict his two cats from the bedroom and to consider a HEPA filter in the bedroom and main activity room which can filter the room's air approximately four times per hour.

He was instructed to take a second-generation antihistamine on an as-needed basis, to supplant reliance on diphenhydramine, a sedating first-generation antihistamine. Evidence indicating that sedative effects from an agent such as diphenhydramine may occur without subjective awareness [14] was reviewed. He also was advised to use an intranasal corticosteroid on a regular basis, two sprays in each nostril daily, which he was told is the first drug of choice for treating allergic rhinitis [1]. He was also told to suspend use should local irritation or epistaxis occur.

At return visit in 8 weeks, Mr. G described improvement in rhinitis symptoms, but described incomplete relief of nasal congestion. He was told that use of an intranasal antihistamine would be preferred compared with an oral second-generation antihistamine for relief of congestion [15]. He was made aware of recent evidence demonstrating that combination treatment with an intranasal corticosteroid and intranasal antihistamine is associated with superior efficacy compared with an intranasal corticosteroid alone [16]. However, this was associated with only modest improvement. He was told that montelukast 10 mg taken daily may also be efficacious for allergic rhinitis [17] and agreed to take this daily. Montelukast was suspended after several weeks due to lack of evident benefit.

At return visit 5 months after initial visit, Mr. G described congestion and rhinorrhea in association with temperature change and exposure to irritants. He reported that he had implemented indoor avoidance measures for dust mites, including encasement of mattress and box spring and restoring hardwood floors after removal of carpets, and that he also had been restricting his cats from his bedroom.

Due to poor control of his symptoms, despite avoidance measures and regular use of medications, the option of initiating allergen immunotherapy was discussed. Mr. G was made aware that there is high-quality evidence supporting the therapeutic utility of subcutaneous allergen immunotherapy (SCIT) for management of patients with allergic rhinitis allergic to dust mites [18]. He was also made aware of recent data [19, 20] supporting the efficacy and safety of sublingual immunotherapy (SLIT), and was told SLIT may have a better safety profile compared with SCIT based on a lower risk for anaphylaxis, and would have the advantage of at-home administration and less time commitment [21]. He indicated a desire to initiate SLIT for dust mite allergy which was recently approved by the FDA in the United States.

Case Presentation 2

Ms. J.N. is a 22-year-old nurse, referred for allergy/immunology consultation for evaluation and management of a 2-year course of PAR. She described symptoms of anterior rhinorrhea; sneezing; pruritus affecting nose, eyes, and palate; nasal congestion; and hyposmia. Symptoms started shortly after she moved in with her grandparents, who have a cat. Her grandparents' home is a Tudor-style house, built in the 1920s, with mostly hardwood floors, poor air circulation, and several throw rugs. She denied a history of atopic dermatitis, asthma, nasal/sinus polyps, or frequent/recurrent sinusitis. She reported no remarkable

adverse reactions to medications, food, or stinging insects. She related that symptoms slightly improve during the day, while at work, and then worsen shortly after her return home. Symptoms have been present year-round without seasonal variation, and have been provoked by visiting homes where dogs reside. She has a brother with SAR and asthma. For the past year she has been taking loratadine 10 mg daily as needed, with minimal relief of her symptoms. Physical exam was remarkable for pale boggy nasal turbinates and mild conjunctival suffusion.

Diagnosis/Assessment

Options to confirm a diagnosis of PAR were explained and understood. Ms. J.N. expressed a desire to proceed with immediate hypersensitivity skin testing to locally prevalent and potentially relevant aeroallergens. This revealed wheal/flare reactions of 7/35 mm to cat dander and 7/26 mm to dog dander, and her histamine control was 9/40 mm with a negative control of 0/0 mm. Intradermal testing revealed no remarkable wheal/flare reactions.

She was told that these findings correlate with her history of PAR, and are consistent with IgE-mediated allergy to cat (*Fel d I*) and dog (*Can f I*).

Management/Outcome

Ms. J.N. was informed that treatment options for patients with PAR due to pet danders include avoidance, pharmacotherapy, and, in properly selected cases, allergen immunotherapy. Ms. J.N. was counseled that complete avoidance of exposure is ideal, but is often difficult to achieve.

According to a 2011 report by the American Veterinary Medical Academy (AMVA), more than six of ten pet owners considered their pets to be family members [22]. This emotional bond often makes it difficult for patients to adhere to a recommendation to eliminate a pet from their home. In a study [23] that evaluated compliance with the recommendation to implement avoidance measures, approximately 300 patients with allergic rhinoconjunctivitis and asthma underwent percutaneous skin testing. For patients in whom sensitization to animal danders was found, avoidance measures, including removing pets from the home and preventing indirect exposures, were recommended. Patients were then seen for follow-up on two occasions, 3–5 and 6–9 months after skin testing. At follow-up appointments, patients were asked if they had adhered to recommendations. At the first and second follow-up appointments, 92% and 88% of patients, respectively, still maintained the pets in their home. Of the six patients who no longer had the pets in their home, only two did so due to the medical recommendation. Of the other four patients, three pets went missing and one pet had died. In the same follow-up, two patients actually had procured a new pet to which they tested positive.

We told Ms. J.N. that even if she did not live in a household with a cat or a dog, she may still be exposed to pet dander in the community and due to passive transfer on shoes and clothing into the home. Data were shared from a Polish study [24] in which *Fel d I* and *Can f I* levels were measured in 17 cars, 14 classrooms, and 19 houses in a large metropolitan area. Air and dust samples were analyzed for cat and dog allergens, via a double-monoclonal ELISA assay. Air sampling is the preferred method to measure cat allergen, as the relationship between airborne and settled dust concentrations of cat allergens is not well defined. The study findings showed that significant levels of pet allergens present in homes of pet owners are transferred to their cars and to their school classrooms. This potentially places others at risk of exposure to pet allergens. Upholstered furniture appears to act as a significant reservoir for the allergen.

Ms. J.N. was told that there is reassuring evidence showing that even if the cat remains in her home, her level of allergen exposure can be reduced significantly by implementing several measures. A study done in the early 1990s [25] showed that repeated weekly washing of pet cats, increasing air circulation, and decreasing soft furnishings each can contribute to significantly reducing the level of *Fel d I* in a household.

Airborne measurements of *Fel d I* were measured by a cascade impactor and a monoclonal antibody-based immunometric assay. After a cat entered a clean room, *Fel d I* increased to 90 ng/m³ within half an hour. After the cat was washed weekly, the *Fel d I* level in the room only increased to 7 ng/m³ in half an hour. A qualitative difference in *Fel d I* was also observed, as there was a statistically significant reduction in smaller particles (defined as ≤2.5 microns), from 9.5 ng/m³ to ≤0.4 ng/m³. When a cat was maintained for 20 h a day in the same room, changing the rate of ventilation and amount of soft furnishings also affected airborne levels of cat allergen. Low ventilation, soft furnishings, and carpets were all found to be associated with a statistically significant increase in the level of *Fel d I* after 1 h. A carpet accumulates cat allergen at a rate 100 times that of a polished floor.

The above data were explained to Ms. J.N. She was also told that after a cat is removed from a home, the average time for cat dander to be significantly reduced may be as long as 24 weeks [26].

Ms. J.N. stated that she may wish to acquire a dog in the future. For this reason, avoidance measures for dogs were also discussed, including the utility of washing the dog [27].

She was encouraged to adhere to recommendations displayed in Table 2.2 [28].

Ms. J.N. was told that patients with PAR may have episodic or persistent rhinitis. As the vast majority of pet dander allergic patients will be exposed to *Fel d I* continuously (and *Can f I*, if she were to acquire a dog), she was told that she may expect to have persistent rather than episodic rhinitis. We pointed out to Ms. J.N. that even if the cat were to be removed from her home, she will likely

Table 2.2 Methods to reduce pet allergen in the home

Restrict pets from the bedroom
Use of HEPA (high-efficiency particulate air) filters in rooms
Minimize soft furnishings (including carpets, couches, and curtains)
Vacuum weekly (preferably with a HEPA filter-enabled vacuum)
Wash dogs biweekly and cats weekly
Consider improving ventilation system

still experience episodic symptoms up to 6 months later due to slow dissipation of indoor cat allergen as well as when visiting other homes where cats or dogs reside. Ms. J.N. was informed that her clothing may be a significant source of dispersing allergen into the community and to the hospital where she works [29]. Similarly, other pet owners also shed levels of pet danders from their clothing, such that cat and dog may be regarded as "community allergens." For the above reasons, she was advised to take medication on a daily basis.

Considering her current home environment, she will have persistent exposure *to Fel d I*, and thus persistent PAR symptoms. She was told that the single most effective medication would be an intranasal corticosteroid [30]. She was told that intranasal corticosteroids have been reported to be more effective than a combination of oral antihistamines and leukotriene inhibitors [31]. There are intranasal corticosteroids introduced more recently, formulated as "dry" nasal aerosols, which may be preferred by some patients who have an aversion to aqueous sprays. An industry-sponsored study demonstrated an increased retention of the dry nasal spray in nasal cavity, but these newer formulations have not been convincingly shown to be clinically superior to aqueous sprays [32].

Ms. J.N. questioned why there are so many different types of intranasal corticosteroid sprays. She was informed that all intranasal corticosteroids are hydrocortisone derivatives, but differ in chemical structure (bioavailability and lipophilic properties). According to their bioavailability, intranasal corticosteroids can be divided into first- or second-generation glucocorticoids, as described in Table 2.3 [33].

The lower the bioavailability, the lower the risk of systemic side effects. Thus, theoretically, the second-generation sprays, with lower bioavailability, may be preferable, particularly if she decides to become pregnant in the future. We reassured Ms. J.N. that since such limited systemic absorption occurs with second-generation intranasal corticosteroids, in the pediatric population, growth suppression has not been demonstrated at recommended dosing [34]. Several of the second-generation intranasal corticosteroids contain either furoate or propionate ester side chains, and are thus highly lipophilic. This lipophilic

Table 2.3 Intranasal steroid spray classification

First-generation glucocorticoids	Second-generation glucocorticoids
Beclomethasone	Ciclesonide
Budesonide	Fluticasone furoate
Flunisolide	Fluticasone propionate
Triamcinolone	Mometasone furoate

property allows the medication to be readily absorbed across the lipophilic phospholipid cell membranes found in the nasal mucosa [35].

She was made aware of common adverse effects, including nasal irritation, bleeding, and rare case reports of septal perforation. We instructed her on proper intranasal device technique, which includes spraying away from the septum [36].

Ms. J.N. was invited to participate in medical decision-making by expressing her values and preferences, and agreed to begin regular use of an intranasal corticosteroid, two sprays in each nostril daily.

Ms. J.N. agreed to return for a follow-up visit in 6 weeks.

Upon her return, Ms. J.N. related that her symptoms had improved. She had implemented recommended avoidance measures, and reported that she noted substantial improvement after restricting the cat from her bedroom, and removing upholstered armchairs that were next to her bed. During weekends, she supplemented the intranasal corticosteroid with oral cetirizine 10 mg/day. She asked whether additional measures could be employed.

She was told that the addition of a daily second-generation antihistamine to the intranasal corticosteroid is one of several steps that can be employed to improve symptom control. She was told to use a combination of the intranasal corticosteroid with an intranasal antihistamine [16]. Ms. J.N. was also made aware of the efficacy and safety of intranasal cromolyn, which can be purchased over the counter [37].

Lastly we discussed that she may consider intranasal saline rinsing, which has been shown to improve the quality of life of patients with PAR as an adjunctive therapy. Postulated mechanisms include washing allergen and inflammatory mediators from the nasal cavity and improving nasal ciliary function [38].

Ms. J.N. inquired whether she could acquire a "hypoallergenic dog," and if this would worsen her symptoms. She was told that the term "hypoallergenic" has been popularized in recent years, but that such animals have not been shown to produce less allergen. She was made aware of a recent study that investigated the levels of *Can f I* in homes. There was no statistically significant difference between "hypoallergenic" dogs and "non-hypoallergenic" dogs with regard to the levels of detectable dog allergen. *Can f I* levels did not appear to be influenced by dog weight or variables such as time spent indoors [39].

Clinical Pearls and Pitfalls

- PAR can lead to considerable morbidity—including missed work/school, sleep disruption, and impaired quality of life.
- Allergy to dust mites and pet danders is a major cause of PAR.
- Dust mite avoidance measures include keeping windows closed and dehumidification via air-conditioning, mattress and box spring encasement, and washing bedding frequently in hot cycle.
- For PAR due to pet allergy, removing the pet from the home is recommended and ideal, but the overwhelming majority of patients will not adhere to this recommendation due to their unconditional emotional attachment to pets.
- Several easy-to-implement measures can significantly reduce levels of pet dander in homes. These include increasing ventilation, limiting soft furnishings and carpets, and using HEPA filters and HEPA filter-enabled vacuum cleaners. Restricting pets from the bedroom and washing cats or dogs have also shown to be helpful.

References

1. Nelson HS, Oppenheimer J, Buchmeier A, Kordash TR, Freshwater LL. An assessment of the role of intradermal skin testing in the diagnosis of clinically relevant allergy to timothy grass. J Allergy Clin Immunol. 1996;97(6):1193–201.

2. Wallace DV, Dykewicz MS, Bernstein DI, Blessing-Moore J, Cox L, Khan DA, et al. The diagnosis and management of rhinitis: an updated practice parameter. J Allergy Clin Immunol. 2008;122(2 Suppl):S1–S84.

3. Fineman S. The burden of allergic rhinitis: beyond dollars and cents. Ann Allergy Asthma Immunol. 2002;88:2–7.

4. Crystal-Peters J, Crown WH, Goetzel RZ, Schutt DC. The cost of productivity losses associated with allergic rhinitis. Am J Manag Care. 2000;6:373–8.

5. Moock J, Kohlmann T. Comparing preference based quality of life measures: results from rehabilitation patients with musculoskeletal, cardiovascular, or psychosomatic disorders. Qual Life Res. 2008;17:485–95.

6. Linneberg A, Petersen KD, Hahn-Petersen J, Hammerby E, Serup-Hansen N, Boxall N. Burden of allergic respiratory disease: a systematic review. Clin Mol Allergy. 2016;14:1–14.

7. Pelikan Z. Late and delayed responses of the nasal mucosa to allergen challenge. Ann Allergy. 1978;41:37–47.

8. Naclerio R. Pathophysiology of perennial allergic rhinitis. Allergy. 1997;52:7–13.

9. Milanese M, Ricca V, Canonica GW, Ciprandi G. Eosinophils, specific hyperreactivity and occurrence of late phase reaction in allergic rhinitis. Eur Ann Allergy Clin Immunol. 2005;37(1):7–10.

10. Eggleston P, Wood R. Environmental allergen avoidance: an overview. J Allergy Clin Immunol. 2001;107:S403–5.

11. Arlian LG, Bernstein D, Bernstein IL, Friedman S, Grant A, Lieberman P, et al. Prevalence of dust mites in the homes of people with asthma living in eight different geographic areas of the United States. J Allergy Clin Immunol. 1992;90:292–300.

12. Arlian LG, Platts-Mills TAE. The biology of dust mites and the remediation of mite allergens in allergic disease. J Allergy Clin Immunol. 2001;107:S406–13.

13. Fitzgerald F. The therapeutic value of pets. West J Med. 1986;144:103–5.

14. Weiler J, Bloomfield JR, Woodworth GG. Effects of fexofenadine, diphenhydramine, and alcohol on driving performance. A randomized, placebo-controlled trial in the Iowa driving simulator. Ann Intern Med. 2000;132(5):354–63.

15. LaForce C, Corren J, Wheeler W, Berger W. Efficacy of azelastine nasal spray in seasonal allergic rhinitis patients who remain symptomatic after treatment with fexofenadine. Ann Allergy Asthma Immunol. 2004;93:154–9.

16. Carr W, Bernstein J, Lieberman P, Meltzer E, Bachert C, Price D, et al. A novel intranasal therapy of azelastine with fluticasone for the treatment of allergic rhinitis. J Allergy Clin Immunol. 2012;129(5):1282–9.

17. Patel P, Philip G, Yang W, Call R, Horak F, LaForce C, et al. Randomized, double-blind, placebo-controlled study of montelukast for treating perennial allergic rhinitis. Ann Allergy Asthma Immunol. 2005;95:551–7.

18. Cox L, Nelson H, Lockey R, Calabria C, Chacko T, Finegold I, et al. Allergen immunotherapy: a practice parameter third update. J Allergy Clin Immunol. 2011;127:S1–55.
19. Klimek L, Mosbech H, Zieglmayer P, Rehm D, Stage BS, Demoly P. SQ house dust mite (HDM) SLIT-tablet provides clinical improvement in HDM-induced allergic rhinitis. Expert Rev Clin Immunol. 2016;12(4):369–77.
20. Demoly P, Emminger W, Rehm D, Backer V, Tommerup L, Kleine-Tebbe J. Effective treatment of house dust mite-induced allergic rhinitis with 2 doses of the SQ HDM SLIT-tablet: results from a randomized, double-blind, placebo-controlled phase III trial. J Allergy Clin Immunol. 2016;137(2):444–51.
21. Cox L, Compalati E, Kundig T, Larche M. New directions in immunotherapy. Curr Allergy Asthma Rep. 2013;13(2):178–95.
22. American Veterinary Medical Association. U.S. Pet ownership & demographics sourcebook. Schaumburg, IL: American Veterinary Medical Association; 2012.
23. Sánchez J. Pet avoidance in allergy cases: is it possible to implement it? Biomedica. 2015;35:357–62.
24. Niesler A, Ścigała G, Łudzeń-Izbińska B. Cat (*Fel d 1*) and dog (*Can f 1*) allergen levels in cars, dwellings and schools. Aerobiologia. 2016;32:571.
25. De Blay F, Chapman MD, Platts-Mills TA. Airborne cat allergen (*Fel d I*). Environmental control with the cat in situ. Am Rev Respir Dis. 1991;143(6):1334–9.
26. Wood RA, Chapman MD, Adkinson NF Jr, Eggleston PA. The effect of cat removal on allergen content in household-dust samples. J Allergy Clin Immunol. 1989;83(4):730–4.
27. Hodson T, Custovic A, Simpson A, Chapman M, Woodcock A, Green R. Washing the dog reduces dog allergen levels, but the dog needs to be washed twice a week. J Allergy Clin Immunol. 1999;103(4):581–5.
28. Sublett JL. Effectiveness of air filters and air cleaners in allergic respiratory diseases: a review of the recent literature. Curr Allergy Asthma Rep. 2011;11(5):395–402. https://doi.org/10.1007/s11882-011-0208-5.
29. Almqvist C, Larsson PH, Egmar AC, Hedren M, Malmberg P, Wickman M. School as a risk environment for children allergic to cats and a site for transfer of cat allergen to homes. J Allergy Clin Immunol. 1999;103:1012–7.
30. Pullerits T, Praks L, Ristioja V, Lotvall J. Comparison of a nasal glucocorticoid, antileukotriene, and a combination of antileukotriene and antihistamine in the treatment of seasonal allergic rhinitis. J Allergy Clin Immunol. 2002;109:949–55.
31. Di Lorenzo G, Pacor ML, Pellitteri ME, Morici G, Di Gregoli A, Lo Bianco C, et al. Randomized placebo-controlled trial comparing fluticasone aqueous nasal spray in mono-therapy, fluticasone plus cetirizine, fluticasone plus montelukast and cetirizine plus montelukast for seasonal allergic rhinitis. Clin Exp Allergy. 2004;34:259–67.
32. Leach CL, Kuehl PJ, Chand R, McDonald JD. Nasal deposition of HFA-beclomethasone, aqueous fluticasone propionate and aqueous mometasone furoate in allergic rhinitis patients. J Aerosol Med Pulm Drug Deliv. 2015;28(5):334–40.
33. Chong LY, Head K, Hopkins C, Philpott C, Burton MJ, Schilder AG. Different types of intranasal steroids for chronic rhinosinusitis. Cochrane Database Syst Rev. 2016;4:CD011993.
34. Allen DB, Meltzer EO, Lemanske RF Jr, Philpot EE, Faris MA, Kral KM, et al. No growth suppression in children treated with the maximum recommended dose of fluticasone propionate aqueous nasal spray for one year. Allergy Asthma Proc. 2002;23(6):407–13.
35. Derendorf H, Meltzer EO. Molecular and clinical pharmacology of intranasal corticosteroids: clinical and therapeutic implications. Allergy. 2008;63:1292–300.
36. Schoezel EP, Menzel ML. Nasal sprays and perforation of the nasal septum. JAMA. 1985;253:2046.
37. Welsh PW, Stricker WE, Chu CP, Naessens JM, Reese ME, Reed CE, et al. Efficacy of beclomethasone nasal solution, flunisolide, and cromolyn in relieving symptoms of ragweed allergy. Mayo Clin Proc. 1987;62(2):125–34.
38. Harvey R, Hannan SA, Badia L, Scadding G. Nasal saline irrigations for the symptoms of chronic rhinosinusitis. Cochrane Database Syst Rev. 2007;18:3.
39. Nicholas CE, Wegienka GR, Havstad SL, Zoratti EM, Ownby DR, Johnson CC. Dog allergen levels in homes with hypoallergenic compared with nonhypoallergenic dogs. Am J Rhinol Allergy. 2011;25(4):252–6.

Nonallergic Vasomotor Rhinitis

3

Justin C. Greiwe

Chronic rhinitis is a ubiquitous condition leading to considerable economic impact in the United States with significant ramifications on patient quality of life. Classically, chronic rhinitis is divided into three main clinical phenotypes: allergic rhinitis (AR), infectious rhinitis, and nonallergic rhinitis (NAR) [1]. Around half of adult chronic rhinitis patients (20–70%) are not sensitized to aeroallergens and therefore largely suffer from NAR [1–3]. There are at least eight recognized NAR subphenotypes that are clinically relevant and include nonallergic rhinopathy, nonallergic rhinitis with eosinophilia, drug-induced rhinitis, gustatory rhinitis, hormone-induced rhinitis, senile rhinitis, atrophic rhinitis, and cerebral spinal fluid leak manifesting as rhinorrhea [4]. A number of rhinitis conditions were omitted from this list as they are not always nonallergic in nature and include mixed rhinitis, localized AR or entopic rhinitis, rhinosinusitis with and without polyps, and occupational rhinitis. These conditions will be discussed in other chapters throughout the book. The focus of this chapter is on the most common NAR subtype, nonallergic vasomotor rhinitis (NAVMR). The cases presented below highlight important concepts related to the diagnosis and treatment of NAVMR.

Case Presentation 1

A 60-year-old female with a history of chronic cough and upper respiratory symptoms presents to the office for a second opinion. She has been managed by an otolaryngologist (ENT), who is currently treating her symptoms with fluticasone two sprays each nostril when symptomatic, montelukast 10 mg daily, and cetirizine 10 mg daily with little improvement and occasional epistaxis. Symptoms began in her early 40s, and there is no family history of allergies on either parent's side. Her symptoms include excessive postnasal drainage (PND), nasal congestion, facial pressure, throat itching, and cough. No sneezing or other nasal, eye, or ear symptoms were reported. Symptoms are perennial in nature but seem to worsen during the change in seasons, particularly spring and fall. Triggers include weather changes, perfumes, house cleaners, and cigarette smoke. She has four dogs and four cats at home with access to the bedroom but denies symptoms around them. Around 10 years ago she was placed on allergen immunotherapy for 2 years. The patient seemed to think that allergy shots helped her symptoms but did not receive them consis-

No funding was required for this research. Conflict of interest: speaker for Mylan Pharmaceutical.

J. C. Greiwe (✉)
Division of Immunology/Allergy Section, Department of Internal Medicine, The University of Cincinnati College of Medicine, Cincinnati, OH, USA

Bernstein Allergy Group, Cincinnati, OH, USA
e-mail: jgreiwe@bernsteincrc.com

Table 3.1 Distinguishing features of nonallergic rhinitis and allergic rhinitis[a]

Nonallergic rhinitis	Allergic rhinitis

• Onset of symptoms later in life, more common after age 20
• No indication of familial pattern
• More common in females
• Perennial symptoms with very little seasonal variation
• Negative aeroallergen skin testing and/or serum sIgE testing
• Broad range of irritant triggers
• Symptoms include
  – Nasal congestion
  – Postnasal drainage with or without cough
  – Infrequent eye complaints
  – Minimal itching
• Physical examination (more variable)
  – Nasal mucosa can be normal with increased clear watery secretions, may be erythematous or atrophic
	• Usually presents in childhood
	• Persuasive family history of atopy (asthma, rhinitis, and atopic dermatitis)
	• Affects females and males equally
	• Most have seasonal exacerbation of symptoms
	• Positive aeroallergen skin testing and/or serum sIgE testing
	• Aeroallergen triggers
	• Symptoms include
	  – Congestion, sneezing, rhinorrhea, and nasal itch
	  – Ocular conjunctivitis, watering, and itch
	• Physical examination
	  – Nasal mucosa edematous, pale, and boggy
	  – Allergic shiners (dark areas under the eyes)

[a]Adapted from [21]

tently and therefore never achieved maintenance dosing. Skin testing using end-point dilution technique was completed recently by ENT that showed extensive seasonal and indoor sensitivities to dust mite, cat, dog, mold, trees, grasses, and weeds. Skin testing was positive to soy, wheat, mustard, milk, and peanut as well. These later tests were applied without a stated history of immediate food reactions. The patient had a history of exercise-induced asthma as a child, but has had no issues with asthma as an adult. She denies acid reflux symptoms. Physical examination revealed a nasal mucosa that is erythematous with evidence of cobblestoning in the posterior pharynx consistent with chronic PND. Her lung and heart exams were unremarkable. Two weeks later, the patient returned for skin prick testing (SPT) to aeroallergens off antihistamines. She had a positive histamine control, but all seasonal and perennial aeroallergens tested were negative. Pulmonary function testing and exhaled nitric oxide (eNO) were completed as well, and both were normal.

Diagnosis/Assessment

Symptoms/Triggers
This case highlights the importance of using clinical characteristics to help distinguish between rhinitis phenotypes. While patients with AR and NAR frequently present with similar symptoms, there are certain clinical features that can help differentiate between these two conditions (Table 3.1). NAR patients are more often female and tend to develop symptoms later in life (after age 20). Symptoms are typically perennial in nature with a broad range of irritant triggers; however, NAR patients regularly blame pollens for any seasonal worsening they experience. These variations are, of course, not pollen related but rather caused by changes in temperature, humidity, barometric pressure, or possibly outdoor air pollutants causing acute worsening of perennial symptoms. Unlike NAR, AR usually presents in childhood often with a family history of atopy (asthma, rhinitis, and atopic dermatitis). Most patients have seasonal exacerbation of symptoms to various aeroallergen triggers.

One of the most common complaints of NAR is excessive PND, especially in older patients, which can lead to a chronic cough. Frequently chronic cough is the most bothersome presenting symptom leading many to seek care. Differentiating PND-induced cough from asthma and/or gastroesophageal reflux (GERD) is an important first step in evaluating these patients. In this example the patient's main complaint focuses on excessive PND, which is likely contributing to cough as pulmonary function/eNO testing was normal, and there were no stated GERD symptoms. It is important to emphasize that a provocation test, like a methacholine challenge, may be necessary to definitively rule out airway hyper-responsiveness consistent with cough variant asthma and/or empiric therapeutic treatment with a proton pump inhibitor may be warranted to exclude asymptomatic GERD as a cause of the cough. Although not pathognomonic, the patient did not exhibit sneezing attacks or eye itching and watering. These symptoms paired with the patient's gender, age, and triggers that include perfumes, house cleaners, and cigarette smoke should steer the clinician toward NAR as the likely diagnosis. Of course, negative skin testing to aeroallergens is necessary for confirmation. A stipulation to this diagnosis is the possibility of local AR which will be discussed in a later chapter. These patients have clinical presentations similar to patients with AR and respond in kind to medications recommended to treat this rhinitis subtype.

Testing

SPT and/or serum-specific IgE (sIgE) tests are essential tools for distinguishing between AR and NAR. The defined sensitivity of SPT compared with sIgE immunoassays can vary with technique; however the simplicity, low cost, and high sensitivity make SPT preferable to in vitro testing for determining the presence of sIgE in patients with rhinitis [5, 6]. There are clinical scenarios where in vitro testing is preferred however, including patients who cannot discontinue medications (i.e., antihistamines), dermatographism, extensive dermatitis, uncooperative patients, or when there is a high risk of an adverse outcome (i.e., severe, poorly controlled asthma or pregnancy). As with all tests, positive results should be correlated with the patient's history and physical exam to confirm their clinical relevance [7]. While SPT is useful for confirming suspicion of aeroallergen triggers by identifying the offending allergens, it can also be used as an effective tool to demonstrate nonreactivity. Many patients are convinced that they have allergic triggers so negative SPT in the presence of a positive histamine and negative saline control provides objective evidence that aeroallergens are not contributing, and would lead the clinician in a different direction with respect to questioning the patient about nonallergic triggers. Often patients may have well-defined nonallergic triggers but also a few allergic triggers confirmed by testing consistent with a diagnosis of mixed rhinitis to be discussed in a later chapter. An initial screening battery for inhalant allergens should be representative of the antigens patients are exposed to in their geographic area and workplace environment. Panels of 40 or more inhalant allergens, and panels that automatically include foods, are excessive, unnecessary, and should raise a white flag about the accuracy of the initial evaluation. The goal of testing is to identify antigens to which patients are symptomatically reactive. Unfortunately, there is no single method of performing in vivo or in vitro testing, with several different techniques and devices available. Each technique has a different level of sensitivity and specificity. This, combined with differences in test interpretation and documentation, can lead to impressive inconsistencies in results. Furthermore, positive tests in the absence of clinical reactivity upon exposure do not necessarily confirm the presence of a clinical allergy, adding more complexity to an already confusing medical picture.

Skin testing using the end-point dilution technique is commonly used among otolaryngologists for the diagnosis of allergy. This approach is prone to false-positive reactions and therefore not used by allergy specialists. Instead, most allergists rely on prick/puncture followed by standard intracutaneous testing with a single weight/volume dilution, otherwise known as modified quantitative testing (MQT), which has been shown to be a safe, cost-effective, and accurate way of diagnosing allergic disease [8–10]. The applicability of intracutaneous testing needs to be taken in context. Negative SPT followed by a positive intracutaneous test has a low-positive predictive value for the presence of symptoms upon allergen exposure [11]. Positive intracutaneous testing to both cat and grass allergens, for example, has been shown to add little to diagnostic accuracy [12, 13]. False positives can be attributed to a number of causes including intracutaneous bleeding resulting in a hematoma that is falsely interpreted as a positive reaction or the effect of naturally occurring histamine, endotoxins, and other skin irritants in inhalant extracts [14].

Nasal provocation testing can be considered in cases of local AR or when sIgE testing is inconclusive (i.e., when testing is negative in patients with a high suspicion of having AR). While nasal challenges are considered the gold standard in diagnosing occupational rhinitis, provocation testing is not used routinely in clinical practice due to lack of standardization, and is mainly used in research settings [1]. Work is ongoing to develop more practical ways for clinicians to reliably diagnose local AR in their office.

Allergy testing seems like a simple way to differentiate between NAR and AR; however significant variations in test results are not uncommon. As this case demonstrates, discrepancies often arise between providers and across subspecialties. Recognition of these inconsistencies allows the clinician to look at previous testing objectively, and not jump to conclusions based on inaccurate data. The above concepts underscore the importance of a comprehensive past medical history in order to correlate positive testing with the patient's reaction history.

Monitoring Control

Once the appropriate diagnosis has been obtained, continued follow-up is encouraged as NAR is a chronic condition that needs to be regularly reassessed. To date there are very few validated tools to help evaluate NAR control nor are there consensus treatment algorithms for NAR. However, it is possible to extrapolate a stepwise treatment algorithm proposed by Papadopoulos et al. for AR to NAR based on symptom control [1]. The algorithm includes four control medication steps that build on each other depending on treatment response. The first step includes one of the following medications: an oral antihistamine, intranasal antihistamine, intranasal cromolyn/nedocromil, or leukotriene receptor antagonist. However, for NAR, using a second-generation oral antihistamine, intranasal cromolyn or nedocromil sodium or a leukotriene antagonist would not be indicated as the pathomechanisms for NAR do not involve the need to stabilize mast cell membranes, block histamine, or block leukotriene receptors. A better first-line treatment approach for NAR would

be to select either a nasal corticosteroid, a nasal antihistamine, or possibly a first-generation H1-antihistamine dosed at bedtime to take advantage of the anticholinergic effects that help to reduce drainage and their sedating side effects, respectively. Steps two through four build on this regimen by using an intranasal corticosteroid and intranasal antihistamine in combination with a first-generation H1-antihistamine at bedtime and saline rinses. In contrast to AR, allergen immunotherapy is not recommended for NAR but may be effective for mixed rhinitis [15]. Step four involves referring to a specialist with expertise in medical management of chronic rhinitis conditions and most notably NAR. This may require referral to an otolaryngology specialist for sinus surgery. Regardless of the rhinitis subtype, assessment of control is based on three control criteria [1]:

1. Symptoms: congestion, rhinorrhea, sneezing, pruritus, and PND
2. Quality of life: impairment in sleep or daily activities
3. Objective measures: peak nasal inspiratory flow, rhinomanometry, or close-mouth test which instructs patient to close mouth and breathe solely through nose for 30 s

Loss of control is considered when patients experience worsening of the above criteria or require increased use of rescue medications including oral or intranasal decongestants, intranasal anticholinergics, and oral corticosteroids. Stepping-up therapy should be considered if there is any concern for deteriorating control but only after rhinitis comorbidities liked asthma, sinusitis, and obstructive sleep apnea have been evaluated and appropriately treated.

Management/Outcome

Patient Education

There are a number of factors to consider when managing patients with NAR. Since NAR is a perennial condition that often requires year-round treatment, patients need a clear understanding of their disease so they better appreciate the importance of regular medication use. Patient education, therefore, is the first step toward better control with a focus on trigger avoidance and safety/efficacy of pertinent medications. While exposure to certain environmental triggers like weather shifts cannot be prevented, avoidance of chemicals, odors, and noxious irritants in the home and workplace can be successful in reducing trigger exposures to varying degrees. Disease-triggering factors should be directed to the specific rhinitis phenotype as much as possible (i.e., abstaining from certain outdoor cold weather activities that can lead to skier's nose and avoiding certain drugs that can lead to drug-induced rhinitis). Medication adherence should also be addressed as patient compliance is essential to improving control. Treatment failure is often due to poor communication between the physician and patient. Candidly addressing patient concerns about medication side effects and long-term use, as well as providing clear instructions on proper administration technique, will significantly improve adherence and outcomes. For example, discussing common side effects like nose bleeds with nasal sprays, elevated blood pressure with oral decongestants, azelastine's bitter taste, and somnolence sometimes associated with first-generation H1 antihistamines need to be discussed [16]. In the present case, we reviewed negative SPT results with the patient and discussed the difference between allergic and NAR. The concept of NAR is often difficult to comprehend as many patients frame their disease in relation to classic allergic triggers, interpreting nonallergic as not being allergic rather than having a condition called NAR. A detailed explanation is often required to clarify any misconceptions, reinforce the relevance of this diagnosis, and stress the clinical value of daily treatment with appropriate medications. In this case, pertinent triggers were discussed, including strong scents/odors and weather shifts during the spring and fall seasons. In addition, proper technique for nasal spray administration was reviewed to reduce the incidence of epistaxis and improve compliance.

Treatment

Despite appropriate avoidance measures, medication administration technique, and compliance, chronic rhinitis can be challenging to treat. Poor clinical outcomes occur when physicians take a "one-size-fits-all" approach, treating everyone with chronic rhinitis as if they have AR. Patients often have tried and failed multiple over-the-counter (OTC) and prescription therapies prior to seeking out specialist care, and many patients are frustrated with their current regimen. In fact, nearly 1/3 of allergy sufferers are not fully satisfied with their current prescription allergy medications [17]. In addition, pharmacotherapy may have different indications and effectiveness depending on the rhinitis phenotype.

In this case fluticasone, montelukast, and cetirizine were discontinued due to poor efficacy, which is consistent with the patient's negative aeroallergen testing as these medications are either less effective (i.e., fluticasone) or not effective (i.e., montelukast and second-generation antihistamines) in NAR. The patient was instead started on azelastine 0.1% two sprays each nostril twice daily as well as OTC first-generation antihistamine, chlorpheniramine maleate 4 mg tablet, nightly in conjunction with sinus rinses twice daily.

Azelastine nasal spray is a second-generation intranasal antihistamine approved for the treatment of both seasonal AR and NAR with H1-receptor binding significantly greater than both chlorpheniramine and hydroxyzine. Azelastine has a wide range of pharmacologic effects on chemical mediators of inflammation including leukotrienes, kinins, and platelet-activating factor in addition to downregulating intercellular adhesion molecule-1 expression and transient potential receptor vanillyl 1 (TRPV1) [18, 19]. This medication was chosen for its effects on congestion and PND, good safety profile, and rapid onset of action. For even greater efficacy, azelastine nasal spray can be combined with fluticasone propionate nasal spray, which has been shown to be more effective than either agent alone [20].

Case Presentation 2

A 72-year-old male presents to the office with a history of chronic, recurrent sinusitis, increased fatigue, and a concern for food allergy. According to the patient he gets around five to six sinus infections per year requiring antibiotics. He was evaluated by an otolaryngologist who recommended surgery. Currently, he has a severe frontal and retro-orbital headache as well as nasal congestion and is requesting antibiotics for what he considers to be a sinus infection. He has never had a computerized tomography (CT) scan of the sinuses. His chronic rhinitis symptoms include nasal congestion, PND, sinus pressure headaches, and excessive rhinorrhea that are perennial in nature with no seasonal variation. He has no eye itching or sneezing. His symptoms are triggered when going into his musty basement at home and he's concerned about mold allergy. The patient also has concerns about a number of foods since he experiences increased rhinorrhea every time he eats, especially with spicy foods. In addition to his nasal and sinus symptoms, the patient has chronic fatigue and poor cognitive functioning, which has impacted his overall quality of life.

Diagnosis/Assessment

Whereas AR requires symptoms on exposure to a sensitizing aeroallergen confirmed by SPT and/or serum sIgE, there are no conclusive tests available for the diagnosis of NAR. Instead, NAR is a diagnosis of exclusion based on the patient's history, nonatopic status, and triggers that often include increased symptoms in response to odorants and irritants in the absence of a specific etiology (i.e., infectious, immunologic, structural, hormonal) [21]. Before in vivo or in vitro testing is attempted, there are a number of recognizable clinical and epidemiological features of NAR that help distinguish this condition from AR. For example, a number of studies have confirmed that NAR more commonly occurs in females later in life (>20 years), and there is typically no well-defined family history of physician-diagnosed allergies. Furthermore, symptoms usually are perennial rather than seasonal, although patients often report seasonality due to confusion between temperature and barometric changes with pollination. Although symptoms alone are not useful for differentiating NAR from AR, patients with NAR typically present with nasal congestion, anterior or posterior rhinorrhea, recurring headaches, Eustachian tube dysfunction, and decreased olfaction. Often triggered by perfumes and fragrances that poorly respond to conventional treatments used for management of AR such as second-generation antihistamines, leukotriene receptor antagonists, and intranasal corticosteroids [22–24]. Complicating the diagnosis of NAR further is the observation that 30–50% of patients with chronic rhinitis might have an overlap of NAR and AR referred to as mixed rhinitis [22]. For this patient, his history is very suggestive of NAR but SPT or serum sIgE testing is necessary to rule out atopy. Furthermore, his reactions to eating are classic for a diagnosis of gustatory rhinitis and therefore food testing is not indicated. A more detailed synopsis of the differential diagnosis for chronic rhinitis is summarized in Table 3.2.

Diagnostic Imaging

While imaging is rarely part of the initial diagnostic workup for acute rhinitis associated with sinusitis, in cases presenting with chronic rhinitis with recurrent sinusitis, a CT scan without contrast of the sinuses may be appropriate to exclude structural issues, especially if the patient has been unresponsive to OTC and/or prescription medications. Sinus CT without contrast is preferred over magnetic resonance imaging (MRI) due to better resolution of mucosal disease and sinus ostial occlusion [25]. However, although MRI doesn't display the bony anatomy as well as CT, it is considered better at evaluating the mucosa and distinguishing between bacterial-viral inflammatory disease and fungal concretions [26]. Sinus plain films are inappropriate because they fail to provide an accurate representation of the extent of disease with poor visualization of pertinent sinus anatomy and the paranasal sinus perimeter [27]. Minimizing the number of CT

Table 3.2 Differential diagnosis of chronic rhinitis[a]

- Allergic rhinitis (seasonal/perennial)
- Nonallergic rhinitis and various subtypes
  - Nonallergic vasomotor rhinitis/nonallergic rhinopathy (also known as irritant-induced rhinitis, and idiopathic rhinitis)
  - Nonallergic rhinitis with eosinophilia
  - Drug-induced rhinitis (i.e., rhinitis medicamentosa)
  - Hormonal induced rhinitis
  - Atrophic rhinitis
  - Senile rhinitis
  - Gustatory rhinitis (rhinorrhea associated with eating)
  - Cerebral spinal fluid leak manifesting as rhinorrhea
- Mixed rhinitis
- Infectious rhinitis (viral, bacterial, and chronic rhinosinusitis)
- Episodic rhinitis
- Occupational rhinitis
- Localized AR or entopic rhinitis
- Rhinosinusitis with and without polyps
- Aspirin intolerance (aspirin triad)
- Drug-induced rhinitis
  - Rhinitis medicamentosa (decongestants)
  - Beta-blockers
  - Birth control pills
  - Antihypertensives
- Rhinitis secondary to:
  - Pregnancy
  - Hypothyroidism
  - Horner's syndrome
  - Wegener's granulomatosis
  - Sarcoidosis
  - Relapsing polychondritis
  - Sjögren's syndrome
  - Midline granuloma
- Structural conditions causing rhinitis:
  - Foreign body
  - Nasal polyps
  - Nasal septal deviation (intranasal cocaine, septal surgery)
  - Enlarged tonsils and adenoids
  - Nasal tumors
  - Cerebral spinal fluid rhinorrhea
  - Choanal atresia
  - Hypertrophic turbinates

[a]Adapted from [21]

scans performed in patients with chronic rhinosinusitis is recommended, especially in children, due to the concern for cumulative radiation exposure over time. In this case, the patient was receiving recurrent courses of antibiotics and had been recommended for surgery; therefore, obtaining a CT scan of the sinuses to demonstrate the presence or absence of sinus pathology is appropriate. A CT sinus performed for this patient while actively symptomatic revealed no structural abnormalities, providing objective guidance for future management while negating the need for overusing antibiotics in the future.

Comorbidities

Assessment of chronic rhinitis comorbidities is often an overlooked aspect of a comprehensive NAR evaluation. Asthma, sinusitis, and obstructive sleep apnea syndrome (OSAS) can be associated with both AR and NAR. An estimated 10–40% of chronic rhinitis patients suffer from asthma [1]. Failure to recognize and treat chronic rhinitis appropriately can lead to worsening control and severity of these conditions [28–34]. For example, asthma is linked to chronic rhinitis by common epidemiologic, physiologic, and pathologic mechanisms as demonstrated by the hypothesis that both asthma and rhinitis are manifestations of the same disease that affects the entire airways [7, 35]. Recognizing this relationship is important as many patients do not readily report lower respiratory symptoms such as wheezing, chest tightness, or shortness of breath. Therefore, screening patients with a peak expiratory flow rate and, if decreased, with spirometry pre- and post-bronchodilators (and exhaled nitric oxide (eNO) if appropriate and available) should be incorporated into the workup in order to exclude asthma. Furthermore, if the patient manifests clinical signs of OSAS such as snoring, apnea spells, hypersomnolence during the day, headaches, and irritability, a sleep apnea study should be considered [7]. The patient in this case presented with a history concerning for chronic rhinitis, but also complained of chronic fatigue, headaches, poor cognitive functioning, and impaired quality of life. A sleep study was ordered that confirmed the diagnosis of moderate OSAS. In addition, SPT to aeroallergens was negative making a diagnosis of NAR more likely. Continuous positive airway pressure (CPAP) treatment in combination with more directed treatment of his NAR led to dramatic improvement in daytime functioning, and a resolution of chronic fatigue resulting in improved quality of life.

Treatment and Management/ Outcome

Chronic rhinitis that is more difficult to treat frequently is associated with a NAR component or is actually NAR. There are many treatment nuances that should be differentiated in the management of NAR compared to AR. In treating NAR, second-generation H1-antihistamines are ineffective because histamine is not the major mediator driving symptoms and these agents have little or no anticholinergic effects, which are useful for reducing PND. In addition, leukotriene-modifying agents have no role in the management of NAR for similar reasons. Frequently, nasal corticosteroids, which are now OTC and recommended as first-line treatment for AR, are often used by physicians to treat chronic rhinitis but are only partially effective and sometimes completely ineffective at controlling symptoms. Combination treatment with fluticasone and azelastine has proven to be very effective rather than using either agent alone in the management of AR. Although there are no definitive studies, clinical experience has found that this combination is also very effective for many patients with NAR. Both of these agents have been individually studied and found effective in the treatment of NAR through different mechanistic pathways. Azelastine has recently been demonstrated to desensitize TRPV1 similar to capsaicin [19, 36]. Fluticasone has been shown to increase degradation of neuropeptides. Furthermore, the combination of azelastine and fluticasone (Dymista™) has been found to be effective in reducing cold-induced rhinitis by reducing substance P and altering biologic pathways involved in ciliogenesis, epithelial barrier function, and mucus production [37].

In this case Dymista™ was started given his incomplete response to fluticasone. While currently only approved for the treatment of seasonal AR, Dymista™ is an effective nasal spray as demonstrated by a number of clinical trials. Symptoms in these studies were scored using a reflective total nasal symptom score (rTNSS) which included nasal congestion, rhinorrhea, nasal itching, and sneezing. Dymista™ demonstrated a rapid onset of action (within 30 min), lower spray volume compared to component devices, and impressive improvements in rTNSS relative to commercially available generic fluticasone propionate (90%) and azelastine (196%) [38–40]. Another single-blind, crossover study randomized AR patients into three treatment groups using nasal provocation testing and acoustic rhinometry to gauge symptom response and found that combined therapy with azelastine plus budesonide offered more substantial therapeutic benefits than either of the medications by themselves [41].

Ipratropium bromide nasal spray is an effective adjuvant in an NAR regimen, especially if the chief complaint is rhinorrhea. A number of studies have examined the safety and efficacy of this anticholinergic nasal spray with impressive results. There was improvement in patient quality of life, reduction in the need for other medications, significant reduction in rhinorrhea, and no drug-related serious or systemic anticholinergic adverse events [42–44]. It is important to note that there were minimal effects on duration or severity of PND, congestion, or sneezing in these studies. However, given the gustatory rhinitis component to his NAR, starting ipratropium bromide 0.03% nasal spray 1–2 puffs each nostril before each meal would be appropriate to lessen or stop his eating-induced rhinorrhea. Additional pharmacologic options for the treatment of NAR are detailed in Table 3.3.

Table 3.3 Summary of pharmacologic options for the treatment of nonallergic rhinitis

Nasal spray options
• Intranasal corticosteroids (i.e., fluticasone)
– Not as effective in NAR without eosinophils
• Intranasal antihistamines (i.e., azelastine)
• Intranasal corticosteroid in combination with intranasal antihistamine (i.e., Dymista™)
• Intranasal oxymetazoline short term as monotherapy
• Intranasal corticosteroid in combination with intranasal oxymetazoline [45–47]
– For maintenance therapy, especially useful when congestion is the main complaint
• Nasal irrigation with saline solution
– As monotherapy or combined with betadine and N-acetylcysteine
• Intranasal anticholinergic agents (i.e., ipratropium bromide)
• Intranasal capsaicin (i.e., sinus buster™)
• Intranasal lactoferrin
Oral medication options
• Oral first-generation sedating antihistamines (i.e., chlorpheniramine)
– Typically dosed at night to reduce drainage
• Oral anticholinergic agents (i.e., methscopolamine)
• Oral decongestant (i.e., pseudoephedrine)

Conclusion

As demonstrated by these patients, chronic rhinitis can present with a wide range of signs and symptoms, so correct diagnosis and treatment require a thorough understanding of the various phenotypes and sub-phenotypes as well as an appreciation for proper testing modalities and interpretation. A comprehensive clinical history detailing family history, age of symptom onset, allergic and/or nonallergic triggers, seasonality, pertinent comorbidities, and response to treatment are all important components of an appropriate evaluation. Continual reassessment of symptomatic control, compliance with treatment, and ensuring proper medication administration technique should be standard of care since NAR is typically a chronic condition. Ultimately, NAR is an overlooked and underappreciated syndrome. A better understating of the pathogenesis, prevalence, and economic impact of this condition is needed to bring attention to NAR and its impact on patients and the healthcare system.

Clinical Pearls and Pitfalls

- Onset of symptoms later in life (more common after age 20) with no evidence of a family history of physician-diagnosed allergies.
- More common in females.
- Perennial symptoms with very little seasonal variation and a broad range of irritant triggers including changes in temperature, humidity, barometric pressure, strong scents/odors, pollutants, and chemicals.
- Negative aeroallergen skin testing and/or serum sIgE testing.
- Symptoms most commonly include nasal congestion and postnasal drainage with or without cough. Infrequent eye complaints and minimal itching noted.
- Unlike AR, pure NAR does not seem to be as responsive to second-generation H1-antagonists, leukotriene-modifying agents, or allergen immunotherapy. These patients also have an incomplete or no response to nasal corticosteroids as monotherapy.
- NAR responds better to topical nasal antihistamines, a combination of nasal corticosteroids and nasal antihistamines, nasal saline rinses, and oral first-generation H1-antagonists because of their anticholinergic effect.

References

1. Papadopoulos NG, Bernstein JA, Demoly P, Dykewicz M, Fokkens W, Hellings PW, et al. Phenotypes and endotypes of rhinitis and their impact on management: a PRACTALL report. Allergy. 2015;70(5):474–94.
2. Molgaard E, Thomsen SF, Lund T, Pedersen L, Nolte H, Backer V. Differences between allergic and nonallergic rhinitis in a large sample of adolescents and adults. Allergy. 2007;62:1033–7.
3. Settipane RA, Charnock DR. Epidemiology of rhinitis: allergic and non-allergic. Clin Allergy Immunol. 2007;19:23–34.
4. Kaliner MA. Classification of non-allergic rhinitis syndromes with a focus on vasomotor rhinitis, proposed to be known henceforth as non-allergic rhinopathy. World Allergy Organ J. 2009;2:98–101.
5. Chong Neto HJ, Rosario NA. Studying specific IgE: in vivo or in vitro. Allergol Immunopathol (Madr). 2009;37(1):31–5.

6. Chinoy B, Yee E, Bahna SL. Skin testing versus radio-allergosorbent testing for indoor allergens. Clin Mol Allergy. 2005;3(1):4.

7. Wallace DV, Dykewicz MS, Bernstein DI, Blessing-Moore J, Cox L, Khan DA, et al. The diagnosis and management of rhinitis: an updated practice parameter. J Allergy Clin Immunol. 2008;122:S1–S84.

8. Peltier J, Ryan MW. Comparison of intradermal dilutional testing, skin prick testing, and modified quantitative testing for common allergens. Otolaryngol Head Neck Surg. 2007;137(2):246–9.

9. Lewis AF, Franzese C, Stringer SP. Diagnostic evaluation of inhalant allergies: a cost-effectiveness analysis. Am J Rhinol. 2008;22(3):246–52.

10. Shah SB, Emanuel IA. Cost analysis of employing multi-test allergy screening to guide serial endpoint titration (SET) testing versus SET alone. Otolaryngol Head Neck Surg. 2003;129(1):1–4.

11. Calabria CW, Hagan L. The role of intradermal skin testing in inhalant allergy. Ann Allergy Asthma Immunol. 2008;101(4):337–47.

12. Nelson HS, Oppenheimer J, Buchmeier A, Kordash TR, Freshwater LL. An assessment of the role of intradermal skin testing in the diagnosis of clinically relevant allergy to timothy grass. J Allergy Clin Immunol. 1996;97:1193.

13. Wood RA, Phipatanakul W, Hamilton RG, Eggleston PA. A comparison of skin prick tests, intradermal skin tests, and RASTs in the diagnosis of cat allergy. J Allergy Clin Immunol. 1999;103:773.

14. Williams PB, Nolte H, Dolen WK, Koepke JW, Selner JC. The histamine content of allergen extracts. J Allergy Clin Immunol. 1992;89:738.

15. Smith AM, Rezvani M, Bernstein JA. Is response to allergen immunotherapy a good phenotypic marker for differentiating between allergic rhinitis and mixed rhinitis? Allergy Asthma Proc. 2011;32(1):49–54.

16. Greiwe J, Bernstein JA. Combination therapy in allergic rhinitis: what works and what does not work. Am J Rhinol Allergy. 2016;30(6):391–6.

17. Asthma and Allergy Foundation of America. http://www.prnewswire.com/news-releases/new-survey-suggests-patients-want-fast-long-relief-of-allergy-symptoms-55421087.html. Accessed 30 Jan 2015.

18. Bernstein JA. Azelastine hydrochloride: a review of pharmacology, pharmacokinetics, clinical efficacy and tolerability. Curr Med Res Opin. 2007;23(10):2441–52.

19. Singh U, Bernstein JA, Haar L, Luther K, Jones WK. Azelastine desensitization of transient receptor potential vanilloid 1: a potential mechanism explaining its therapeutic effect in non-allergic rhinitis. Am J Rhinol Allergy. 2014;28(3):215–24.

20. Brandt D, Bernstein JA. Patient-reported symptoms induced by allergic and non-allergic triggers in randomized controlled trials of MP-Azeflu (Dymista) in seasonal allergic rhinitis (SAR) patients. Ann Allergy Asthma Immunol. 2006;96(4):526–32.

21. Greiwe J, Bernstein JA. Non-allergic rhinitis: diagnosis. Immunol Allergy Clin N Am. 2016;36(2):289–303.

22. Settipane RA, Lieberman P. Update on non-allergic rhinitis. Ann Allergy Asthma Immunol. 2001;86:494–507.

23. Di Lorenzo G, Pacor ML, Amodio E, Leto-Barone MS, La Piana S, D'Alcamo A, et al. Differences and similarities between allergic and non-allergic rhinitis in a large sample of adult patients with rhinitis symptoms. Int Arch Allergy Immunol. 2011;155(3):263–70.

24. Brandt D, Bernstein JA. Questionnaire evaluation and risk factor identification for non-allergic vasomotor rhinitis. Ann Allergy Asthma Immunol. 2006;96:526–32.

25. Hamilos DL. Chronic rhinosinusitis: clinical manifestations, pathophysiology, and diagnosis. In: Post TW, editor. UpToDate. Waltham, MA: UpToDate. Accessed 5 Jan 2017.

26. Meltzer EO, Hamilos DL. Rhinosinusitis diagnosis and management for the clinician: a synopsis of recent consensus guidelines. Mayo Clin Proc. 2011;86(5):427–43. https://doi.org/10.4065/mcp.2010.0392.

27. Meltzer EO, Hamilos DL, Hadley JA, Lanza DC, Marple BF, Nicklas RA, et al. Rhinosinusitis: establishing definitions for clinical research and patient care. J Allergy Clin Immunol. 2004;114:155.

28. Crystal-Peters J, Neslusan C, Crown WH, Torres A. Treating allergic rhinitis in patients with comorbid asthma: the risk of asthma-related hospitalizations and emergency department visits. J Allergy Clin Immunol. 2002;109:57–62.

29. Price D, Zhang Q, Kocevar VS, Yin DD, Thomas M. Effect of a concomitant diagnosis of allergic rhinitis on asthma-related health care use by adults. Clin Exp Allergy. 2005;35:282–7.

30. Ponte EV, Franco R, Nascimento HF, Souza-Machado A, Cunha S, Barreto ML, et al. Lack of control of severe asthma is associated with co-existence of moderate to-severe rhinitis. Allergy. 2008;63:564–9.

31. Bresciani M, Paradis L, Des Roches A, Vernhet H, Vachier I, Godard P, et al. Rhinosinusitis in severe asthma. J Allergy Clin Immunol. 2001;107:73–80.

32. Muliol J, Maurer M, Bousquet J. Sleep and allergic rhinitis. J Investig Allergol Clin Immunol. 2008;18:415–9.

33. Kiely JL, Nolan P, McNicholas WT. Intranasal corticosteroid therapy for obstructive sleep apnoea in patients with co-existing rhinitis. Thorax. 2004;59:50–5.

34. Ramos RT, da Cunha Daltro CH, Gregorio PB, de Freitas Souza LS, de Andrade NA, de Souza Andrade Filho A, et al. OSAS in children: clinical and polysomnographic respiratory profile. Braz J Otorhinolaryngol. 2006;72:355–61.

35. Cruz AA, Popov T, Pawankar R, AnnesiMaesano I, Fokkens W, Kemp J, et al. Common characteristics of upper and lower airways in rhinitis and asthma: ARIA update, in collaboration with GA(2)LEN. Allergy. 2007;62:1–41.

36. Van Gerven L, Alpizar YA, Steelant B, et al. Enhanced chemosensory sensitivity in patients with idiopathic

rhinitis and its reversal by nasal capsaicin treatment. J Allergy Clin Immunol. 2017;140(2):437–446.e2.

37. Singh U, Bernstein JA, Lorentz H, et al. A pilot study investigating clinical responses and biological pathways of azelastine/fluticasone in non-allergic vasomotor rhinitis before and after cold dry air provocation. Int Arch Allergy Immunol. 2017;173(3):153–64.

38. Hampel FC, Ratner PH, Van Bavel J, Amar NJ, Daftary P, Wheeler W, et al. Double-blind, placebo-controlled study of azelastine and fluticasone in a single nasal spray delivery device. Ann Allergy Asthma Immunol. 2010;105:168–73.

39. Carr W, Bernstein J, Lieberman P, Meltzer E, Bachert C, Price D, et al. A novel intranasal therapy of azelastine with fluticasone for the treatment of allergic rhinitis. J Allergy Clin Immunol. 2012;129:1282–9.

40. Meltzer EO, LaForce C, Ratner P, Price D, Ginsberg D, Carr W. MP 29-02 (a novel intranasal formulation of azelastine hydrochloride and fluticasone propionate) in the treatment of seasonal allergic rhinitis: a randomized, double-blind, placebo-controlled trial of efficacy and safety. Allergy Asthma Proc. 2012;33:324–32.

41. Fabbri NZ, Abib-Jr E, de Lima Zollner R. Azelastine and budesonide (nasal sprays): effect of combination therapy monitored by acoustic rhinometry and clinical symptom score in the treatment of allergic rhinitis. Allergy Rhinol (Providence). 2014;5(2):78–86.

42. Grossman J, Banov C, Boggs P, Bronsky EA, Dockhorn RJ, Druce H, et al. Use of ipratropium bromide nasal spray in chronic treatment of non-allergic perennial rhinitis, alone and in combination with other perennial rhinitis medications. J Allergy Clin Immunol. 1995;95(5 Pt 2):1123–7.

43. Georgitis JW, Banov C, Boggs PB, Dockhorn R, Grossman J, Tinkelman D, et al. Ipratropium bromide nasal spray in non-allergic rhinitis: efficacy, nasal cytological response and patient evaluation on quality of life. Clin Exp Allergy. 1994;24(11):1049–55.

44. Meltzer EO, Orgel HA, Bronsky EA, Findlay SR, Georgitis JW, Grossman J, et al. Ipratropium bromide aqueous nasal spray for patients with perennial allergic rhinitis: a study of its effect on their symptoms, quality of life, and nasal cytology. J Allergy Clin Immunol. 1992;90(2):242–9.

45. Baroody FM, Brown D, Gavanescu L, DeTineo M, Naclerio RM. Oxymetazoline adds to the effectiveness of fluticasone furoate in the treatment of perennial allergic rhinitis. J Allergy Clin Immunol. 2011;127:927–34.

46. Meltzer EO, Bernstein DI, Prenner BM, Berger WE, Shekar T, Teper AA. Mometasone furoate nasal spray plus oxymetazoline nasal spray: short-term efficacy and safety in seasonal allergic rhinitis. Am J Rhinol Allergy. 2013;27:102–8.

47. Kirtsreesakul V, Khanuengkitkong T, Ruttanaphol S. Does oxymetazoline increase the efficacy of nasal steroids in treating nasal polyposis? Am J Rhinol Allergy. 2016;30:195–200.

Mixed Rhinitis

4

Chandra Vethody and Jonathan A. Bernstein

Case Presentation 1

A 37-year-old Caucasian female with a history of seasonal allergic rhinitis (AR) since childhood presents with progressive worsening of nasal congestion, rhinorrhea, sneezing, and postnasal drip for the past 2 years. Her allergy symptoms are typically worse every spring and fall, controlled with an over-the-counter non-sedating H1-antihistamine. More recently, over the past 6 years she has noticed increased symptoms triggered by a spectrum of odorants and irritants, specifically fragrances, perfumes, fabric softeners, detergents, and gasoline fumes. She started to avoid using perfumes and hairsprays over the last 6 months, which seemed to reduce her rhinorrhea.

When she was a child she remembers being evaluated by an allergist for allergies and was told that she was allergic "to everything." She began allergen immunotherapy but only continued them for approximately 1 year as her family relocated to another city for work and they never pursued follow-up care for her condition as her symptoms

C. Vethody
Department of Internal Medicine, University of Louisville, Louisville, KY, USA

J. A. Bernstein (✉)
Division of Immunology, Rheumatology and Allergy, Department of Internal Medicine, University of Cincinnati, Cincinnati, OH, USA
e-mail: Jonathan.Bernstein@uc.edu

seemed to be controlled with medications during the season. She currently lives with her husband, who smokes but does so outdoors, but she is still bothered by tertiary smoke exposure from his clothes. More recently, she has been waking up at night two to three times a week choking and coughing from postnasal drainage. Her symptoms have worsened to the point where she is now unable to sleep at night, resulting in severe fatigue during the day. She has no history of asthma or recurrent sinus infections and is taking no other medications. She has no clinical signs or symptoms consistent with obstructive sleep apnea. She works on her family farm and lives in an old farmhouse heated by a wood-burning stove without air-conditioning.

On physical examination her nasal cavity shows enlarged turbinates with beefy red nasal mucosa and scant thick secretions greater on the right than left side.

Examination of her auditory canal revealed retracted tympanic membranes bilaterally, and her posterior pharynx revealed cobblestoning consistent with chronic postnasal drainage. Her lung and cardiovascular examinations were unremarkable.

Skin prick testing revealed sensitization to trees and ragweed, which correlated to her seasonal allergies. Initial treatment recommendations were to start a nasal corticosteroid spray and to continue use of an over-the-counter non-sedating H1-antihistamine on a daily basis. She now returns to the office feeling no better after taking this treatment regimen for 2 months.

Discussion

This case illustrates a patient presenting with mixed rhinitis (MR). Her history of seasonal allergic rhinitis (SAR) as a child has progressed in adulthood to a more complex condition that is unresponsive to conventional medications used to treat allergic rhinitis. Her symptoms are now predominantly triggered by a spectrum of odorants and noxious irritants. The diagnosis of AR versus nonallergic rhinitis (NAR) cannot be made based on symptoms alone, as sneezing, rhinorrhea, nasal congestion (anterior or posterior), and nasal itching can be present in patients with either condition [1]. A previous study investigated olfactory thresholds between patients with AR, MR, and NAR responses using an automated olfactometer using a single staircase paradigm. They found no difference in olfactory threshold responses between groups, indicating that overactive olfaction didn't account for the aberrant olfaction manifested by patients with NAR and MR [1].

Mechanistically, AR is IgE mediated, meaning patients exhibit specific IgE antibody responses in direct response to perennial and/or seasonal allergens and their symptoms are directly related to exposure to these sensitizing aeroallergen(s). In contrast, as discussed in Chap. 3 (Nonallergic Vasomotor Rhinitis) the most common subtype of this category is vasomotor rhinitis, which is likely neurogenic in origin [2]. The likely mechanism, in part, involves activation of TRP receptors in the nose by mechanical, osmotic, temperature, or chemical triggers that activate nociceptive fibers, resulting in depolarization and release of neuropeptides (i.e., substance P, calcitonin gene-related peptide, neurokinins …) as well as sending impulses through the CNS that results in overactivity of the parasympathetic nervous system, resulting in vasodilation and increased mucus production manifesting as nasal congestion and posterior or anterior rhinorrhea [2]. It is still unclear how NAR and AR biologic pathways interface, but neuropeptides released can cause direct activation of mast cells, which can thus synergistically enhance clinical symptoms [3]. Regardless, understanding that separate pathways are at play in this pathway can help clinicians and

patients better understand why medications approved to treat AR have an incomplete or no effect on the above patient.

Since the symptoms of AR and MR overlap, it is important to distinguish between these conditions by taking a thorough history and conducting a careful physical examination. Whereas a diagnosis of AR is more likely to begin early in life (i.e., childhood or adolescence) and is associated with a family history of allergies in either or both parent, NAR more commonly manifests later in the third or fourth decade of life and there is a poor family history of atopy. Furthermore, patients with AR may have evidence of the "allergic march," which is associated with other atopic disorders such as atopic dermatitis, food allergy, and asthma. Allergic rhinitis patients often have seasonal symptoms that are worse outdoors that improve indoors and/or symptoms in specific response to furry pets (i.e., cats greater than dogs), whereas NAR patients may have symptoms related to temperature or barometric pressure changes and frequently in response to noxious odorants and chemical irritants. Due to ambiguity of some close-ended questions, it is important to phrase questions correctly to ensure that the patient's responses reflect the intent of the question. For example, asking about seasonality of symptoms can be mistakenly misconstrued as seasonal allergies, when in fact they actually represent changes in barometric or temperature changes. Brandt et al. previously found that patients with no family history of atopy, adult onset of upper respiratory symptoms (>35 years), no seasonality of symptoms or worsening of symptoms around cats and other furry pets, and worsening of symptoms by fragrances/perfumes had 98% likelihood of having nonallergic vasomotor rhinitis, before allergen testing. However, not all NAR patients endorse these triggers, which could be due to a lack of exposure opportunity or poor recognition of hidden triggers in their surrounding environment. Therefore, an absence of characteristic nonallergic triggers should not exclude a diagnosis of NAR [4]. Thus, when patients exhibit both allergic and nonallergic triggers and/or a poor response to medications designed to treat allergic rhinitis (i.e., intranasal corticosteroids with or without second-generation H1-antihistamines), a diagnosis of mixed rhinitis should be considered [5].

A more recent study compared how diagnoses of AR, NAR, and MR subtypes using physician diagnostic criteria correlated with diagnosis using an irritant index questionnaire that quantifies the severity of rhinitis symptoms in response to 21 nonallergic triggers in conjunction with specific IgE testing [6]. It was found that a significant number of patients originally categorized as AR by physician history that didn't quantify the magnitude of symptoms in response to nonallergic triggers in conjunction with specific IgE testing were reclassified as MR based on irritant index questionnaire responses in conjunction with specific IgE testing [6]. These patients were referred to as AR with a high irritant burden (a.k.a. mixed rhinitis) [6]. Interestingly, it was also found that those patients with high irritant burden AR and high-burden NAR (i.e., VMR) were more likely to have a physician diagnosis of asthma as well as a greater magnitude and severity of self-reported rhinitis symptoms compared to those reclassified as low-burden AR or NAR patients [6]. Thus, in the patient above, it is clear that based on her history of symptoms in response to the nonspecific irritants along with symptoms that seem to be exacerbated during the spring, her clinical diagnosis is suggestive for MR.

On physical examination, swollen turbinates with pale mucosa are suggestive of AR, whereas perennial AR or VMR typically has more erythematous beefy red turbinates. However, it should be noted that physical examination alone, like symptoms, is not able to reliably differentiate between AR, MR, and VMR.

The diagnosis of MR requires evidence of sensitization to aeroallergens confirmed by allergen skin prick or serologic testing. However, negative testing does not completely rule out AR or MR due to the presence of possible localized mucosal specific IgE levels referred to as local allergic rhinitis (LAR) or *entopic rhinitis* [7]. Local allergic rhinitis refers to a localized nasal allergic response in the absence of systemic atopy characterized by local mucosal production of IgE antibodies [7]. Characteristics of LAR such as younger age of symptom onset and family history of atopy that are more consistent with AR can help differentiate this condition from NAR. However, lack of response to medications designed to treat AR is a fairly good indicator that the patient more likely has at least a NAR component to their chronic rhinitis condition. Diagnosis of LAR is confirmed by a nasal aeroallergen provocation test to the suspected allergen and favorable response to medications used to treat AR, unlike what is observed in NAR or MR [7]. Figure 4.1 summarizes the algorithmic approach for diagnosing AR, NAR, and LAR [8].

Nasal cytology can also be used to differentiate chronic rhinitis subtypes, especially the rhinitis subtype, nonallergic rhinitis with eosinophil syndrome or NARES [9, 10]. Nasal cytology has also been used to characterize NAR with increased mast cell and NAR with increased neutrophils [9, 10]. Despite its ability to differentiate these chronic rhinitis subtypes and their differential responses to treatment, nasal cytology cannot be easily performed in a clinical setting and is technically difficult to reproduce making this testing less practical.

In summary, diagnosis of MR requires a careful history to elicit inciting triggers and diagnostic testing to assess the patient's allergic status. These patients have some sensitizations that account for some but not all of their clinical symptoms. Typically, they also notice increased congestion, drainage with or without sinus pressure/headaches, and ear popping/plugging in response to chemicals, odorants, and changing or extreme weather conditions. Incomplete treatment response to medications designed to treat AR is an important clinical clue that a more complex form of chronic rhinitis exists.

Case Presentation 2

A 45-year-old female with a past medical history of AR confirmed by SPT and high serum IgE levels in the past currently treated with intranasal fluticasone daily and cetirizine 10 mg once daily and allergic asthma and chronic idiopathic hives treated with omalizumab presented to the office for follow-up of progressively worsening rhinitis symptoms.

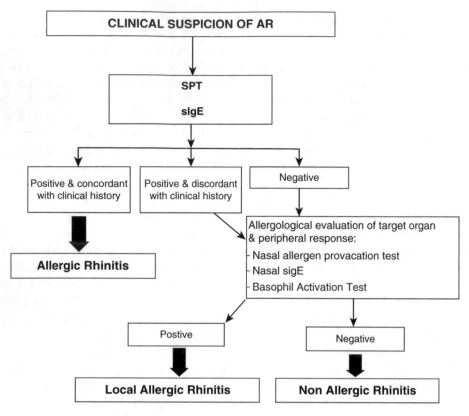

Fig. 4.1 Algorithmic approach to the diagnosis of AR, MR, and LAR. Reprinted from Campo P, Rondón C, Gould HJ, Barrionuevo E, Gevaert P, Blanca M. Local IgE in non-allergic rhinitis. Clin Exp Allergy, 2015. 45(5): 872–881, with permission from John Wiley and Sons

She reports decreased control of her sneezing, postnasal drip, and itchy nose on the above medications over the last several years. She reports occasional cough but denies any chest tightness or dyspnea. Lately, she has also noticed increasing rhinorrhea and nasal obstruction when she went on a ski trip to Colorado and has been reacting in a similar fashion to strong perfumes and potpourris.

Her last allergy testing was 10 years ago, which confirmed sensitivity to most seasonal and perennial aeroallergens including cats, dogs, and dust mites. She had been treated with allergen immunotherapy (AIT) at that time for 3 years with some improvement in her symptoms, but she still required daily medications. She reports good control of her asthma and hives. She has no recurrent sinus infections, evidence of obstructive sleep apnea, or headaches.

Physical examination shows bilateral hypertrophied turbinates with cobblestoning consistent with postnasal drainage. Her chest exam was clear to percussion and auscultation. Spirometry was normal.

Discussion

Her history of irritant exposure and weather changes worsening her symptoms indicates that she may have a nonallergic rhinitis component to her rhinitis. Furthermore, she has not responded to first-line therapy, which included a nasal corticosteroid spray indicated for mild-to-moderate AR [11]. Thus, it is reasonable to suspect that her symptoms are not completely due to AR or LAR, which typically respond well to nasal corticosteroids with or without oral H1-antihistamines. Also of note, previous treatment with AIT only elicited partial improvement of her clinical symptoms. The next steps would be to ensure that she was adherent to previous rhinitis medications and to reassess her allergic status to determine if she is sensitized to seasonal and/or perennial aeroallergens.

Skin prick testing does indeed indicate sensitization to dust mite, box elder tree, timothy grass, short ragweed, and cat. However, the testing didn't correlate with her history, as she denies any seasonality to her symptoms and doesn't notice symptoms when she is around cats. This could be the result of persistent tolerance from previous AIT and/or omalizumab, which blocks peripheral IgE and down-regulates high-affinity IgE receptors on mast cells, thereby stabilizing mast cell membranes. Although omalizumab has not been extensively studied or FDA approved for AR, it is plausible that similar pathomechanistic targets implicated for asthma and chronic idiopathic urticaria may also be involved in AR [12].

Treatment of MR requires using combination therapies effective for AR and MR. As discussed, neurogenic pathways are involved in MR similar to NAR, resulting in overactivity of the parasympathetic nervous system [2]. Thus, in contrast to AR, in which therapies target specific biologic pathways, treatment of the NAR component of MR is primarily symptomatic due to the paucity of medications approved to treat this condition. Exceptions are medications such as capsaicin and azelastine, which can bind to and down-regulate TRPV1 receptors, and both have been found to be effective in the management of NAR [3, 13, 14]. Over-the-counter intranasal capsaicin sprays have been shown to be effective in reducing nasal congestion, sinus pressure, headache, and pain in less than a minute; however, their half-lives are short and therefore require frequent dosing [15]. Similarly, intranasal antihistamines have been found to be effective in treating NAR [13]. Intranasal azelastine efficacy may be in part due to its effects on downregulation of TRPV1 receptors, anticholinergic activity, and inhibition of neuropeptides like substance P released when nociceptive nerve fibers are depolarized [3]. The combination of intranasal corticosteroids and intranasal antihistamines approved for AR has also been recently studied for NAR [16, 17]. A study investigating the effect of azelastine/fluticasone combination therapy in an environmental control chamber after exposure to cold dry air found that there was an objective reduction in nasal congestion measured as minimum cross-sectional area ($p < 0.05$) by acoustic rhinometry, reduced cough count ($p < 0.05$), and decreased substance P ($p < 0.01$) [16]. The reduced substance P correlated strongly with reduced cough.

Furthermore, gene targets for differentially expressed miRNAs enriched for biological pathways regulating epithelial ciliogenesis and cell integrity were down-regulated in the azelastine/fluticasone-treated group compared to placebo [16]. Because both fluticasone and azelastine have been studied for AR and NAR and found to be effective, it is plausible that they will be similarly effective for the treatment of MR [13, 18].

Ipratropium bromide is effective in alleviating anterior and posterior rhinorrhea in NAR and has been used in MR to control postnasal drainage with some effect [19]. Using this topical agent is preferable in older patients who may be more susceptible to the anticholinergic effects of oral anticholinergic agents. Other therapies that can be useful in VMR include nasal irrigation with saline [20], oral first-generation H1-antihistamines, and systemic anticholinergics like methscopolamine or glycopyrrolate due to their anticholinergic effects [5]. These latter two agents should be reserved for patients with copious amounts of postnasal drainage not controlled with topical therapy and/or simple first-generation antihistamines like chlorpheniramine or diphenhydramine at bedtime. Medications like leukotriene receptor antagonists, although approved for AR, have no effect on NAR and are generally not found to be very effective in MR patients [5].

Allergen immunotherapy has been studied limitedly in MR compared to AR in a historical pre- and posttreatment study design [21]. Both MR and AR groups experienced reduced episodes of acute sinusitis and a significant decrease in the mean number of rhinitis medications after AIT ($p < 0.001$); however, the reduction in number of medications was significantly greater for the AR group (1.24 ± 1.09) compared to the MR group (2.09 ± 1.55) ($p = 0.0023$) [21]. This study suggests that the benefits of AIT are likely on the AR component in MR, since the MR group required more medications after a 5-year course than the AR group [21].

Nasal congestion continues to be a prominent and difficult-to-treat symptom of chronic rhinitis. Recently there have been several studies that suggest that oxymetazoline, a topical nasal decongestant, can be used for an extended period (2 weeks) of time when it is used in conjunction with an intranasal corticosteroid [22–24]. In our experience, this has been a very useful approach for treating patients with refractory congestion who have no other structural or systemic explanation for this persistent symptom.

In summary, successful treatment of MR first requires recognition that there is a nonallergic component associated with AR, making it a "difficult-to-treat rhinitis" condition. Once this is determined, tailoring treatment using a wide range of medications is required based on the patient's tolerance of medications, severity of symptoms, comorbidities like sinusitis, cost, and their preference. These cases require medication management with ongoing follow-up to ensure optimum clinical outcomes.

Clinical Pearls and Pitfalls

Pitfalls

- Mixed rhinitis is a relatively common form of chronic rhinitis that can be misdiagnosed, especially in a primary care setting as AR and NAR symptoms can overlap.
- Correct diagnosis of MR requires a careful clinical history with focus on elements such as family history of atopy, symptoms in response to irritants, odorants and weather changes, and previous responses to medications in conjunction with allergy testing to assess for atopy.
- Conventional therapies for AR like systemic oral non-sedating H1-antihistamines and intranasal corticosteroids are less effective for MR, so additional medications are typically required.

Pearls

- A thorough history, physical examination, skin prick testing, or serum-specific IgE levels are essential for distinguishing between AR, MR, and NAR.
- A negative skin or serologic test does not exclude AR, as testing can be negative for LAR, which requires confirmation by nasal

allergen bronchoprovocation and measurement of nasal specific IgE.

- Rhinorrhea and nasal obstruction that occur in response to nonspecific odor and irritants or weather changes in conjunction with a positive aeroallergen skin or serologic testing that correlates with symptoms during exposure confirm a diagnosis of MR.
- MR is treated most commonly with intranasal antihistamines (i.e., azelastine), intranasal ipratropium bromide, and medications that can control congestion and drainage. Tailoring therapy to the patient's needs and preferences is essential for a successful management plan.

References

1. Rezvani M, Brandt D, Bernstein JA, Hastings L, Willwerth J. Investigation of olfactory threshold responses in chronic rhinitis subtypes. Ann Allergy Asthma Immunol. 2007;99(6):571–2.
2. Bernstein JA, Singh U. Neural abnormalities in nonallergic rhinitis. Curr Allergy Asthma Rep. 2015;15(4):18.
3. Singh U, Bernstein JA, Haar L, Luther K, Jones WK. Azelastine desensitization of transient receptor potential vanilloid 1: a potential mechanism explaining its therapeutic effect in nonallergic rhinitis. Am J Rhinol Allergy. 2014;28(3):215–24.
4. Brandt D, Bernstein JA. Questionnaire diagnosis of nonallergic rhinitis. Clin Allergy Immunol. 2007;19:55–67.
5. Bernstein JA, Rezvani M. Mixed rhinitis: a new subclass of chronic rhinitis? In: Kaliner M, editor. Curent review of rhinitis. 2nd ed. Philadelphia: Current Medicine; 2006. p. 69–78.
6. Bernstein JA, Levin LS, Al-Shuik E, Martin VT. Clinical characteristics of chronic rhinitis patients with high vs low irritant trigger burdens. Ann Allergy Asthma Immunol. 2012;109(3):173–8.
7. Campo P, Salas M, Blanca-López N, Rondón C. Local allergic rhinitis. Immunol Allergy Clin N Am. 2016;36(2):321–32.
8. Campo P, Rondón C, Gould HJ, Barrionuevo E, Gevaert P, Blanca M. Local IgE in non-allergic rhinitis. Clin Exp Allergy. 2015;45(5):872–81.
9. Gelardi M, Iannuzzi L, Tafuri S, Passalacqua G, Quaranta N. Allergic and non-allergic rhinitis: relationship with nasal polyposis, asthma and family history. Acta Otorhinolaryngol Ital. 2014;34(1):36–41.
10. Gelardi M, Fiorella ML, Russo C, Fiorella R, Ciprandi G. Role of nasal cytology. Int J Immunopathol Pharmacol. 2010;23(1 Suppl):45–9.

11. Wallace DV, Dykewicz MS, Bernstein DI, Blessing-Moore J, Cox L, Khan DA, et al. The diagnosis and management of rhinitis: an updated practice parameter. J Allergy Clin Immunol. 2008;122(2 Suppl):S1–84.

12. Stokes J. Anti-IgE treatment for disorders other than asthma. Front Med (Lausanne). 2017;4:152.

13. Banov CH, Lieberman P, Vasomotor Rhinitis Study Groups. Vasomotor rhinitis study, efficacy of azelastine nasal spray in the treatment of vasomotor (perennial nonallergic) rhinitis. Ann Allergy Asthma Immunol. 2001;86(1):28–35.

14. Singh U, Bernstein JA. Intranasal capsaicin in management of nonallergic (vasomotor) rhinitis. Prog Drug Res. 2014;68:147–70.

15. Bernstein JA, Davis BP, Picard JK, Cooper JP, Zheng S, Levin LS. A randomized, double-blind, parallel trial comparing capsaicin nasal spray with placebo in subjects with a significant component of nonallergic rhinitis. Ann Allergy Asthma Immunol. 2011;107(2):171–8.

16. Singh U, Bernstein JA, Lorentz H, Sadoway T, Nelson V, Patel P, et al. A pilot study investigating clinical responses and biological pathways of Azelastine/fluticasone in nonallergic vasomotor rhinitis before and after cold dry air provocation. Int Arch Allergy Immunol. 2017;173(3):153–64.

17. Lieberman P, Meltzer EO, LaForce CF, Darter AL, Tort MJ. Two-week comparison study of olopatadine hydrochloride nasal spray 0.6% versus azelastine hydrochloride nasal spray 0.1% in patients with vasomotor rhinitis. Allergy Asthma Proc. 2011;32(2):151–8.

18. Meltzer EO. The treatment of vasomotor rhinitis with intranasal corticosteroids. World Allergy Organ J. 2009;2(8):166–79.

19. Georgitis JW, Banov C, Boggs PB, Dockhorn R, Grossman J, Tinkelman D, et al. Ipratropium bromide nasal spray in non-allergic rhinitis: efficacy, nasal cytological response and patient evaluation on quality of life. Clin Exp Allergy. 1994;24(11):1049–55.

20. Lin L, Lu Q, Tang XY, Dai F, Wei JJ. Nasal irrigation for the treatment of vasomotor rhinitis: a pilot study. Zhonghua Er Bi Yan Hou Tou Jing Wai Ke Za Zhi. 2017;52(6):446–52.

21. Smith AM, Rezvani M, Bernstein JA. Is response to allergen immunotherapy a good phenotypic marker for differentiating between allergic rhinitis and mixed rhinitis? Allergy Asthma Proc. 2011;32(1):49–54.

22. Baroody FM, Brown D, Gavanescu L, DeTineo M, Naclerio RM. Oxymetazoline adds to the effectiveness of fluticasone furoate in the treatment of perennial allergic rhinitis. J Allergy Clin Immunol. 2011;127(4):927–34.

23. Meltzer EO, Bernstein DI, Prenner BM, Berger WE, Shekar T, Teper AA. Mometasone furoate nasal spray plus oxymetazoline nasal spray: short-term efficacy and safety in seasonal allergic rhinitis. Am J Rhinol Allergy. 2013;27(2):102–8.

24. Vaidyanathan S, Williamson P, Clearie K, Khan F, Lipworth B. Fluticasone reverses oxymetazoline-induced tachyphylaxis of response and rebound congestion. Am J Respir Crit Care Med. 2010;182(1):19–24.

Local Allergic Rhinitis

Carmen Rondón, Ibon Eguiluz-Gracia,
Gador Bogas, Esther Barrionuevo, María Salas,
Maria J. Torres, and Paloma Campo

Introduction

Rhinitis is an inflammatory disorder of the nasal mucosa clinically defined by two or more symptoms of nasal itching, sneezing, anterior or posterior rhinorrhea, and nasal blockage [1]. When the symptoms are present at least 1 h daily and last longer than 2 weeks rhinitis is considered chronic [2]. The lifetime prevalence rates of acute rhinitis and chronic rhinitis are 100% and >20%, respectively, which explains the considerable financial burden that the condition imposes to healthcare systems [3]. Moreover, chronic rhinitis negatively affects work and school performance and has been related to learning disabilities in children [4], and to an impairment in quality of life greater than that of arterial hypertension [5]. Chronic rhinitis is often associated with sinusitis, conjunctivitis, and asthma which further amplifies its impact [6]. Nevertheless the condition has been historically trivialized and only in recent years it has gained significant attention.

Several classifications have been proposed for chronic rhinitis based on different parameters such as pathophysiology, pattern of symptoms, or trigger eliciting rhinitis [2]. One easy classification divides the disorder into allergic rhinitis (AR) and nonallergic rhinitis (NAR). AR is the most frequent form of chronic rhinitis [7], and constitutes a homogenous phenotype with known pathophysiology defined by IgE sensitization to environmental allergens [6]. Conversely, NAR comprises a highly heterogeneous group of diseases where immune-mediated inflammation is not always apparent [8]. The individuals suffering from all NAR phenotypes show negative IgE sensitization tests, namely skin prick test (SPT) and serum-specific IgE (sIgE) [7]. Nonallergic rhinitis with eosinophilia syndrome (NARES) patients displays an eosinophilic infiltration of the nasal mucosa, together with perennial nasal symptoms [9]. Other phenotypes of NAR such as idiopathic or gustatory rhinitis are probably mediated by neurogenic stimuli affecting mucus-secreting glands, with very little if any involvement of immunologic responses [10, 11]. Cyclic variations of sexual hormones can also trigger congestive rhinitis in women by affecting the nasal vasculature perhaps through activation of nociceptive fibers and release of neuropeptides [12]. Atrophy of the nasal mucosa (especially the glands) and bacterial outgrowth elicit a rhinitis phenotype in the elderly with significant crusting and purulent discharge [13]. Other rhinitis categories do not properly fit in the allergic/nonallergic dichotomy. Occupational rhinitis is caused by factors in the work environment and can be driven by both allergic mechanisms [14], or by irritant

C. Rondón (✉) · I. Eguiluz-Gracia · G. Bogas
E. Barrionuevo · M. Salas · M. J. Torres · P. Campo
Allergy Unity, IBIMA-Hospital Regional
Universitario of Málaga-UMA, ARADyAL, Málaga,
Spain

© Springer International Publishing AG, part of Springer Nature 2018
J. A. Bernstein (ed.), *Rhinitis and Related Upper Respiratory Conditions*,
https://doi.org/10.1007/978-3-319-75370-6_5

agents [15]. Similarly, drug-induced rhinitis can arise from inflammatory or neurogenic mechanisms after the intake of medications [16]. The excessive local administration of decongestant sprays (either sympathicomimetics or imidazolines) is responsible for rhinitis medicamentosa due to rebound nasal congestion [17].

Chronic rhinosinusitis (CRS) is a differentiated disorder defined by the inflammation of the mucosa lining the nasal cavity and paranasal sinuses [18]. Chronic rhinosinusitis pathophysiology has been related to an altered immune response to bacterial or fungal products in the nose and sinuses [19] and can be divided into two groups: CRS with nasal polyps (CRSwNP) and CRS without nasal polyps [18]. Patients with nasal polyps in Europe usually display an eosinophilic inflammation of the upper airways, which makes their inflammatory pattern similar to NARES [19]. On the other hand, in Asian and some North American populations, neutrophilic polyps are more frequent [20]. Moreover, it is not uncommon that nasal polyps with eosinophilia coexist in the same patient with clinically relevant IgE sensitization to allergens [18, 21].

Allergic rhinitis is driven by reexposure to seasonal or perennial allergens in IgE-sensitized individuals [1]. Allergic rhinitis patients are by definition positive for at least one of the two tests to measure IgE sensitization: SPT and/or serum sIgE [6]. Nevertheless a significant proportion of nonallergic subjects also displays positivity for either test, demonstrating that the correlation of symptoms with allergen exposure is crucial for the interpretation of IgE sensitization [22]. A nasal allergen provocation test (NAPT) can help determine the clinical relevance of IgE sensitization in this setting [23]. Interestingly, some patients with seasonal or perennial rhinitis symptoms display positive NAPT with negative SPT and serum sIgE. This disease phenotype has been termed local allergic rhinitis (LAR) [24, 25]. This disorder does not properly fit into any of the above-mentioned classifications of chronic rhinitis. Studies have demonstrated that LAR patients have a type 2 and eosinophil-dominated nasal inflammatory response [26, 27], which could lead erroneously to their classification in the NARES

phenotype [2]. However, LAR patients share many clinical features and laboratory findings with AR individuals, including the reactivity to NAPT [28], and the presence of allergen-specific IgE in the nasal secretions [29]. Epidemiological studies have demonstrated that LAR is a moderate-to-severe condition that tends to worsen over time [30], and similarly to AR is often associated to asthma and conjunctivitis [31]. Local allergic rhinitis is not an initial state of AR, as studies have shown that the long-term conversion to systemic atopy is comparable between LAR subjects and the general population [30].

In this chapter the recent advances in LAR research will be described, with special focus on epidemiology, pathophysiology, diagnostic approach, and treatment.

Epidemiology

Clinical and epidemiological studies have demonstrated that LAR is an underdiagnosed entity that may affect individuals from different countries, ethnic groups, and age ranges [26, 27, 31–38]. Although a prevalence study in the general population is lacking, studies from different geographical areas have shown that LAR can be present in more than 47% of patients previously diagnosed of NAR or NARES [27, 37, 39–41], and in 25.7% of individuals with rhinitis symptoms referred for evaluation to allergy clinics [31].

Local allergic rhinitis patients can display seasonal or perennial symptoms, with persistent or intermittent patterns. Data available to date identify a few allergens as symptom triggers in most LAR individuals. They include house dust mite (HDM), grass and olive tree pollens [26, 27, 32, 42–45], and molds [31, 33]. Nevertheless, it is not studied whether other less common allergens can also elicit symptoms.

Available studies identify *D. pteronyssinus* as the main agent inducing nasal reactivity in both young adults and elderly patients with AR or LAR. Interestingly, reactivity to *Alternaria* was frequent in LAR subjects, whereas sensitization to animal dander was typical of AR individuals [31–33].

Local allergic rhinitis and AR patients share many demographic and clinical features. The prototypical LAR patient is a young nonsmoking woman, with severe or moderate rhinitis and persistent/perennial symptoms which are frequently associated with conjunctivitis and asthma. Nasal itching and watery rhinorrhea are the most frequent complaints and house dust is the most frequent trigger eliciting rhinitis [31].

Although LAR is more frequent in young adults [31], data from different studies show that children [31, 34, 46, 47] and elderly individuals [33] may also be affected.

The prevalence of LAR in elderly rhinitis patients (21%) is slightly lower than in young adults, as demonstrated in a study performed in 219 rhinitis patients [33]. In this study *D. pteronyssinus* was the main allergen in both AR and LAR elderly individuals and, similar to young adults, most LAR patients were women with persistent and perennial rhinitis [31]. However some differences between young adults and elderly subjects with LAR were observed. Older LAR patients were more frequently current or former smokers, had more commonly a family history of atopy, and suffered from milder rhinitis symptoms as compared with young adults with LAR [33].

Nevertheless significant differences in the prevalence of LAR and the demographic features of LAR patients might exist between distinct geographical areas, as environmental factors can influence the development and progression of the disease. In this regard, several aspects remain to be elucidated: Are the differences in LAR prevalence related to variations in the allergen exposure or allergenic load between geographical areas with distinct climates? Do environmental factors such as air pollution, temperature, or humidity influence more the onset of LAR than the onset of ("systemic") AR? [48].

A significant research effort is warranted during the upcoming years to address these and other questions. Of note, recent data have shed some light into the influence of environmental allergenic load on LAR development [48]. This study found a high proportion of LAR among subjects with rhinitis symptoms in two different geographical areas both with high allergenic load of two unrelated allergens: grass pollen and HDM. This study demonstrates that LAR is not exclusively limited to areas with low/moderate allergenic load [46, 49].

All of these observations indicate that LAR is often under- or misdiagnosed. In this regard, there is an urgent need to determine the prevalence and incidence of LAR by performing large multicenter population studies, both in adults and children, which take into account environmental factors such as pollution, and which use consensus procedures for LAR diagnosis.

Local Allergic Rhinitis in Pediatric Population

Allergic rhinitis is a frequent disease in the pediatric population that causes severe and disturbing symptoms affecting daily activities, school performance, and sleep. In addition, AR is associated with cognitive impairment and physical complications during childhood. Allergic rhinitis may often coexist with other diseases involving the skin and mucous membranes such as conjunctivitis, asthma, otitis media, and atopic dermatitis, or with systemic disorders such as food allergy. Typical symptoms and signs of AR are summarized in Table 5.1. AR prevalence in the Western population is ~20–40%, and the disease is nowadays considered a major public health problem that is on the rise [50]. Prospective studies show that AR prevalence rises from 3.4% at 4 years of age to >30% at age 18 [51]. Patients with typical rhinitis symptoms and no evidence of systemic atopy (negative SPT/serum sIgE) have been usually classified in the NAR phenotype. However, studies performed in the last decade demonstrate that the proper classification of patients with nasal symptoms and absent systemic IgE sensitization requires the evaluation of the target organ (the nasal mucosa) by means of a specific test such as NAPT [48].

The onset of nasal symptoms occurs during childhood in a significant proportion of LAR individuals. Recently, some authors have suggested that childhood LAR is merely the initial step of adult AR [52]. However, currently there is no experimental data supporting the conversion of LAR into AR. On the contrary, it has been demonstrated that in adults LAR is a stable condition that does not evolve to AR over time [30, 53].

Studies analyzing LAR in pediatric populations are still scarce (Table 5.2), include only a limited number of children, and report a wide prevalence ranging from 0 to 66.6%. In a study performed by Fuiano et al., in 36 individuals with ages ranging from 4 to 18 years NAPT with Alternaria was performed, and 64% of patients displayed positive responses [54]. Another study in Thailand with 25 NAR children between the ages 8 and 18 years did not find any positive responses to HDM nasal provocation [55]. More recent studies in children from distinct geographical areas have found NAPT reactivity to different allergens ranging from 25 to 66.6%.

These findings illustrate that LAR is an important condition that should be included in the differential diagnosis in children with presumed NAR [46, 56, 57]. In conclusion, LAR must be considered in children with typical AR symptoms and negative SPT/sIgE, but more studies with larger populations are required.

Pathophysiology

The immunopathology of LAR is not well understood. In 20–40% of patients with positive NAPT but absent systemic sensitization, sIgE has been found in the nasal secretions [26–28]. Nevertheless the source of this sIgE is not clear. The synthesis of all mature antibodies is induced in germinal center B cells in a process involving class switch recombination of their heavy chains, a phenomenon affecting the functional specialization of the antibody [58]. This step is followed by the somatic hypermutation (SH) of the variable regions of the antibody in order to increase the affinity for its cognate antigen [58]. These two processes require different enzymes such as *activation-induced cytidine deaminase and recombination-activating gene 1* or *2* [58]. During class switch recombination, DNA in the heavy-chain locus is rearranged to juxtapose distant DNA regions and to generate isotype-specific switch circles that are ultimately eliminated. Mature B cells exit the secondary lymphoid organs and differentiate into antibody-producing plasma cells or

Table 5.1 Clinical symptoms and signs of allergic rhinitis in children

Clinical symptoms and signs of allergic rhinitis	Cause
Adenoid face	Nasal obstruction
Oral breathing	
Gingival mucosa hypertrophy	
Chapped lips	
Dental malocclusion	
Transverse nasal crease	Nasal pruritus
Elevated nose tip	
"Allergic salute"	
Snoring	Sleep apnea
Fatigue	
Eye bags	
Infraorbital fold	

Table 5.2 Prevalence of local allergic rhinitis in children

Author	Year	Country	Study group	Age	Allergen	Positive response NPT (*n*, %)
Fuiano et al.	2012	Italy	36 NAR (perennial)	Children 4–18	Alternaria	23/36 (64%)
Buntarickporpan et al.	2015	Thailand	25 NAR (perennial)	Children 8–18	DP	0/25 (0%)
Blanca-López et al.	2016	Spain	61 NAR (seasonal)	Adults/ Children	Phleum	37/61 (61%)
Duman et al.	2016	Turkey	28 NAR (seasonal/ perennial)	Children 5–16	DP, DF, grass mix	7/28 (25%)
Zicari et al.	2016	Italy	18 NAR (perennial)	Children 6–12	DP, DF, Lolium	12/18 (66.6%)

DP Dermatophagoides pteronyssinus, DF Dermatophagoides farinae

memory B cells. The synthesis of IgE requires IL-4 and presents several differences compared to other immunoglobulin isotypes [59]. These features include increased apoptosis of germinal center-derived IgE+ B cells or impaired formation of IgE+ memory B cells that can result in a low frequency or insufficient affinity maturation of germinal center-derived IgE antibodies [59, 60]. Nevertheless, high-affinity IgE can be produced by IgG+ memory B cells in the mucosa following class switch recombination to IgE (εCSR) [59]. This sequential εCSR generates a switch circle different from that of direct εCSR [60] (Fig. 5.1). In the nasal mucosa of individuals with AR or CRSwNP markers of εCSR have been demonstrated [61, 62], and in AR patients, sIgE is usually detected in the nasal secretions [63]. In this regard, it is believed that high-affinity IgE in the bloodstream of allergic individuals is mainly derived from the mucosa rather than from the lymphoid organs [59, 64]. Although sIgE has been found in the nasal secretions of some LAR subjects [27], definitive evidence

for IgE synthesis in the nasal mucosa of these patients is lacking. Moreover the proportion of LAR patients with detectable nasal sIgE is consistently under 50% [26, 27], a fact partially explained by the dilutional effect of the methods necessary to collect nasal secretions. However, mechanisms such as immunoglobulin free light chains (FLC) have also been implicated in the development of chronic rhinitis in the absence of systemic atopy [65]. In patients with eosinophil dominated nasal diseases but without systemic IgE sensitization, higher levels of FLC were found both at the tissue level and serum as compared with healthy or atopic controls [66, 67]. Moreover anti-IL-5 treatment reduced local FLC concentrations in patients with CRSwNP [66], further relating FLC to type 2 responses. FLC are secreted by plasma cells together with whole antibodies, and similarly to IgE can sensitize mast cells for activation upon cross-linking by their cognate antigens [68]. The nature of FLC receptor on mast cells remains elusive but it differs from the ones binding IgE or IgG [65].

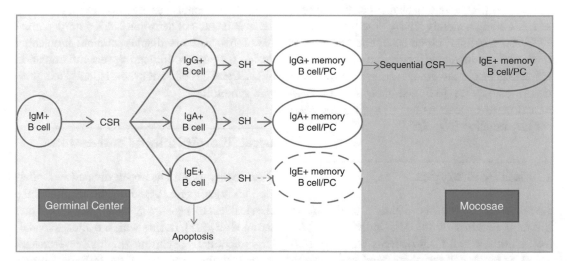

Fig. 5.1 Differential synthesis of high-affinity IgE with respect to other immunoglobulin isotypes. The interaction of IgM+ naïve B cells with activated T cells in the germinal centers of the secondary lymphoid organs induces the class switch recombination of IgM to generate activated IgG+, IgA+, or IgE+ B cells. IgG+ and IgA+ B cells undergo subsequent somatic hypermutation (SH) to generate circulating high-affinity IgG-producing and IgA producing memory B cells and plasma cells. IgE+ B cells in the germinal centers experience a high rate of apoptosis and deficient SH. These phenomena determine the low frequency and insufficient affinity maturation of circulating IgE derived from the secondary lymphoid organs. Nevertheless, high-affinity IgE can be generated in the mucosae upon IL-4 signaling and class switch recombination of IgG+ memory B cells to generate IgE+ plasma cells. Mucosal high-affinity IgE exerts its functions in the neighboring resident immune cells, but can also traffic through the lymphoid vessels and be detected in the bloodstream

Nevertheless, there is no evidence relating FLC to positive NAPT responses. Whether patients with FLC-driven rhinitis (if they exist at all) should be termed "atopic" or "allergic" is also a matter of debate [69]. Basophil activation test (BAT) uses flow cytometry to measure allergen triggered activation of peripheral basophils and is increasingly used in allergy diagnosis [70]. Because sIgE can enter the bloodstream from the nasal mucosa via the lymphatic vessels, circulating basophils can bind IgE and thus become sensitized [71]. In this regard, basophils could be the only carriers of circulating high-affinity IgE in LAR, whereas in AR IgE would be found at both free and basophil-bound states. Interestingly, basophil depletion in blood samples from AR subjects has significantly reduced sIgE in culture supernatants [64]. Studies from our group found that 66–50% of SPT-/serum sIgE-negative NAPT-positive individuals display positive BAT responses [72, 73]. Moreover, in a small group of those patients the IgE/FceRI-mediated activation of basophils was confirmed by inhibition experiments with wortmannin, a PI3Kinase blocker [73]. This finding challenges the concept of LAR being a merely "local" disease. Whether FLC can also bind blood basophils and trigger their antigen-mediated activation is unknown. Of note, FLC-specific antagonists have been described (F991) [68] and their use in BAT experiments appears as an interesting approach for investigation (Fig. 5.2).

Clinical Phenotypes

Local allergic rhinitis patients share many clinical features with AR individuals [31, 74]. Both AR and LAR patients can have seasonal or perennial symptoms, and reactivity to multiple allergens upon NAPT [28]. Studies from our group have demonstrated that in the Mediterranean areas grass and olive tree pollens are the most frequent allergens involved in seasonal LAR, whereas HDM, and to a lesser extent *Parietaria* pollen, and the mold *Alternaria* trigger most cases of perennial LAR [31, 46]. Epidemiological studies suggest that both LAR and AR tend to worsen over time [30, 31]. Allergic rhinitis, LAR, and NARES display very similar inflammatory patterns with markers of eosinophil infiltration and activation [2]. Both AR and LAR subjects have increased release of mast cell and eosinophil mediators after NAPT [26, 43]. As mentioned, individuals with perennial LAR fulfill the criteria for NARES diagnosis [2], and are often misclassified in this group if a NAPT is not performed. However, LAR and other NAR phenotypes share fewer clinical features and laboratory findings [8], and it has not been sufficiently studied whether LAR, similar to AR, can coexist with CRSwNP. On the other hand the coexistence of AR and LAR in the same individual is a frequent situation in our own experience (unpublished data), and we propose the term dual-allergic rhinitis (DAR) for this disease phenotype. Preliminary data from our group have identified DAR patient with perennial persistent moderate-to-severe LAR (often due to HDM reactivity) aggravated during the spring due to systemic IgE sensitization to pollens (olive tree and/or grass). Nevertheless other DAR phenotypes may also exist, including the coexistence of seasonal LAR with perennial AR. DAR patients display clinical worsening during the season, indicating that inflammation in LAR and AR can act synergistically to aggravate symptoms.

Local Allergic Rhinitis and Asthma

Historically, asthma has been divided into allergic and nonallergic, based on the results of the classical test to measure systemic atopy (SPT and serum sIgE) [75], in line with the allergic/nonallergic dichotomy of chronic rhinitis. Nevertheless, several studies performed by different groups have revealed that this asthma classification is not mirrored by a differential inflammatory pattern between the two asthma phenotypes. In fact, there are multiple similarities in the pathophysiological features of allergic and nonallergic asthma [76, 77].

Studies performed in bronchial tissue have demonstrated that the cellular infiltrate of the

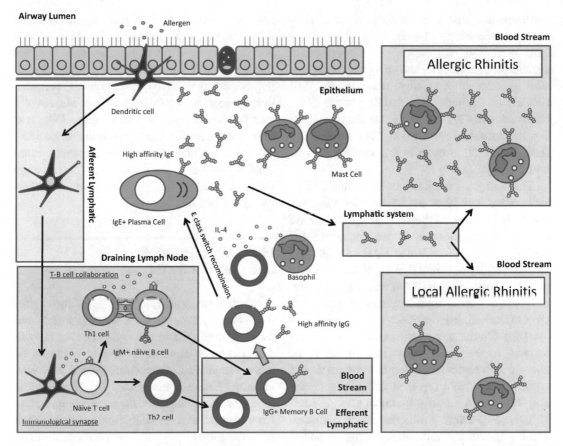

Fig. 5.2 Proposed pathophysiology of local allergic rhinitis (IgE mediated). Environmental allergens are caught up from the airway lumen by resident dendritic cells that also carry them to the lymph nodes through the afferent lymphatic vessels. Allergen-loaded dendritic cells activate allergen-specific naïve T cells in the lymph nodes and polarize them towards a Th1 or Th2 phenotype. In the germinal centers, activated Th1 and Th2 cells interact with IgM+ naïve B cells to generate IgG+ and IgE+ B cells, respectively. IgE+ B cells do not efficiently mature to memory B cells or plasma cells in the secondary lymphoid organs. Conversely, IgG+ B cells undergo somatic hypermutation and differentiate into memory B cells and antibody-producing plasma cells which traffic through the lymphatic and blood vessels and extravasate at the airway mucosa. Mucosal IgG+ memory B cells release high-affinity IgG to the lamina propria. Upon the influence of IL-4 provided by basophils or Th2 lymphocytes among other cells, IgG+ memory B cells can also undergo class switch recombination to IgE in the lamina propria to generate high amounts of high-affinity allergen-specific IgE. Mucosal IgE can bind to the surface receptors of resident mast cells and basophils, and sensitize them for activation upon allergen reexposure. Importantly, mucosal IgE can traffic through the lymphatic system to the bloodstream, where it can also sensitize circulating basophils. In allergic rhinitis patients, high-affinity IgE saturates the receptors of circulating basophils, and free IgE can be also found in the bloodstream and detected by commercial assays. Free IgE can also sensitize skin mast cells and give positive skin prick test responses in patients with allergic rhinitis. In local allergic rhinitis individuals, high-affinity IgE does not saturate the receptors on circulating basophils and free IgE is not detected in the bloodstream. Therefore, high-affinity IgE does not sensitize skin mast cells in local allergic rhinitis patients, but can give positive basophil activation test responses

bronchial mucosa in nonallergic asthma largely resembles that of allergic asthma [78]. In addition, the expression of cytokines such as IL-4, IL-5, and IL-13 is similarly increased in both asthma phenotypes [76, 78], together with other inflammatory mediators and chemokines such as eotaxin-1, eotaxin-2, monocyte chemotactic proteins (MCP)-3 and -4, and CCR3 [79].

Similar to rhinitis, IgE is suspected to play a pivotal role in asthma, and several studies have demonstrated that asthmatic individuals without systemic atopy display local synthesis of IgE, increased expression of ε heavy-chain germ line, local εCSR, and upregulated expression of the high-affinity receptor for IgE (FcεRI) on immune cells residing in the bronchial mucosa [77, 80]. These findings suggest that the bronchial mucosa might be a major site for IgE induction even in the absence of systemic atopy.

The antigen specificity of bronchial IgE in asthma has not been sufficiently investigated, and it is unknown whether this IgE can bind environmental allergens as was demonstrated for the nasal IgE in AR and LAR patients [81] and in CRSwNP individuals [82]. A study reported functional HDM-specific IgE in sputum samples from nonallergic asthma patients after bronchial provocation with *D. pteronyssinus* [83]. On the other hand, another study performed in bronchial mucosa specimens of allergic asthmatics, nonallergic asthmatics, and nonatopic controls reported that allergen-specific IgE could be only found in allergic individuals [84]. These conflicting results indicate that the specificity and affinity of the bronchial IgE in both allergic and nonallergic asthma warrant further research.

Similar to AR, available data suggests that bronchial symptoms are also common in LAR patients [27, 31, 44]. In these studies, typical symptoms of asthma are self-reported by 20–47% of LAR individuals. Nevertheless, asthma diagnosis was not the primary outcome of those studies, and an objective evaluation for bronchial hyperreactivity in LAR individuals was not performed. Moreover, the long-term follow-up studies published to date on large populations of LAR patients report an increase of self-reported bronchial symptoms after 5 years of LAR diagnosis, with a significantly higher proportion of patients requiring a visit to the emergency room due to wheezing and dyspnea [30].

The role of allergens as triggers of bronchial symptoms in LAR patients is not sufficiently investigated. A study performed in nonallergic asthmatics demonstrated the presence of functional sIgE in sputum, despite a negative clinical

response to the bronchial challenge with HDM [83]. Another study including patients with LAR and asthma confirmed by methacholine test found that 40% of the individuals displayed positive responses to HDM upon bronchial provocation (a decrease in $FEV_1 \geq 20\%$). Moreover a significant increase in methacholine PC_{20} was observed 24 h after the allergen challenge [85]. These observations strongly suggest that a bronchial equivalent to LAR may exist, even though studies with larger cohorts are required for definitive conclusions.

Local Allergic Rhinitis and Conjunctivitis

Many patients with LAR complain about conjunctivitis symptoms such as ocular itch and burning, tearing, and red eye [31]. Similarly to AR, ocular symptoms are more common in pollen-sensitive LAR patients than in individuals with HDM sensitivity [31, 74]. Nevertheless it is not clear whether these symptoms arise from true ocular sensitization or they result from the activation of nasal-ocular reflexes upon nasal allergen exposure [86]. In AR individuals the nasal allergen provocation can elicit ocular symptoms that can be dampened with intranasal administration of corticosteroids [87]. In our experience, LAR individuals can also experience ocular symptoms during NAPT [31, 48, 74]. On the other hand, the conjunctival epithelium naturally hosts a robust population of immune cells, including mast cells and T and B lymphocytes [88]. In allergic conjunctivitis, resident B cells produce sIgE to sensitize conjunctival mast cells for activation [89]. Additionally, sIgE and other inflammatory mediators may also traffic from the nasal mucosa to the conjunctiva via the lacrimal duct [89]. Whether conjunctival sensitization in addition to nasal-ocular reflexes works synergistically in LAR patients to induce ocular symptoms is not sufficiently investigated. Moreover, whether local allergic conjunctivitis can occur in the absence of nasal reactivity remains unstudied.

Natural Evolution

Several clinically relevant questions have been posed after LAR was first described: What is the natural history of LAR? Should LAR be considered the initial step in the development of AR and systemic atopy? Is LAR a risk factor for the development of asthma?

Currently only data from two studies is available to address these questions: (1) a long-term 10-year follow-up study with a cohort of 194 LAR patients and 130 age- and sex-matched healthy controls designed by our group in 2005 [30], and (2) a retrospective study undertaken in 19 LAR individuals by Sennekamp et al., in 2015 [53].

In 2005 our group designed the first 10-year follow-up study to investigate the natural history of LAR, its possible evolution to systemic atopy and AR, and its association with asthma over time [30]. In this study, LAR patients and healthy controls were yearly evaluated by self-administered questionnaires, skin tests, serum sIgE, lung function, and NAPT. The results of the first 5 years of follow-up revealed that LAR is a well-differentiated condition with a similar rate of conversion to AR than healthy controls (6.25% vs. 5.2%). LAR patients worsened over time, with increased impairment in quality of life, higher severity and longer duration of nasal symptoms, more frequent visits to the emergency room, and higher onset of conjunctivitis and asthma compared to healthy controls [30]. The survival bias is avoided in this study by the sole inclusion of LAR individuals whose diagnoses were established less than 2 years before recruitment. Thus, this study excludes LAR subjects who had already developed systemic atopy during the natural course of their disease.

The retrospective study by Sennekamp et al. of 19 LAR patients reported a 21% rate of long-term conversion to AR after more than 7 years of evolution [53]. This proportion is comparable to the 17% conversion rate detected in 7930 healthy subjects evaluated in the region where the study was conducted [90]. However, the retrospective design, lack of healthy control arm, surveillance bias, small number of patients included, high variability in patient age, and time interval between evaluations are all limitations of this study that dampen the significance of these data [91]. The results of the 10-year longitudinal follow-up study finalized in 2016 has confirmed that LAR is an independent phenotype with a similar rate of conversion to AR than healthy controls [92] which should shed more light into the natural history of LAR.

These findings together with the very positive results of allergen immunotherapy (AIT) trials for LAR (discussed in a separate section in this chapter) strongly indicate the need for an early diagnosis and identification of LAR individuals among rhinitis patients without systemic atopy.

Diagnostic Approach

Local allergic rhinitis should be considered in the differential diagnosis in patients with rhinitis symptoms suggestive of AR in the absence of systemic atopy [29, 93]. The initial approach should always include a detailed clinical history where the occurrence of bronchial and conjunctival symptoms, the pattern and severity of nasal complaints, and the evolution of the disease since the onset should be specifically questioned (Fig. 5.3). The former aspects are largely indistinguishable between AR and LAR subjects. On the other hand, several characteristics of LAR patients help differentiate them from other NAR individuals [31]. As previously discussed, LAR patients are more frequently young females, non-smokers, and urban dwellers and report a family history of atopy (Table 5.3). It is also very important to perform a thorough nasal examination including endoscopy and nasal anterior rhinoscopy and/or CT scan to rule out CRS and/or nasal polyps if needed.

The next step in the evaluation of LAR involves evaluating the response of the target organ to the allergen challenge. In LAR patients, the classical approach consisting of SPT and/or measurement of serum sIgE is clearly insufficient and leads to a significant rate of misdiagnosis [29]. Therefore, the NAPT is the gold standard for LAR diagnosis, along with the detection of

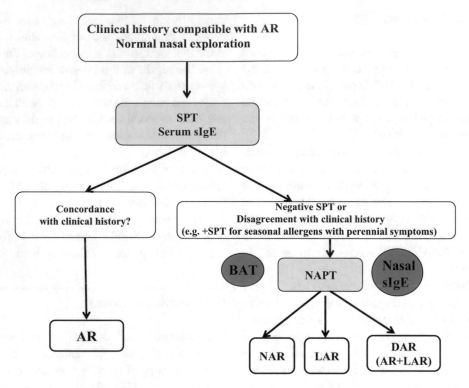

Fig. 5.3 Diagnostic approach in allergic rhinitis

Table 5.3 Clinical features for LAR identification

Local allergic rhinitis vs. nonallergic rhinitis	Local allergic rhinitis vs. allergic rhinitis
• Significantly younger and female predominance in LAR	In both phenotypes it is common:
• Symptoms in LAR are sneezing and pruritus, compared to blockage and rhinorrhea in NAR	• Frequent association with conjunctivitis and asthma
• Nonsmokers and with family history of atopy are more common in LAR	• Moderate-to-severe symptoms
• LAR have more severe symptoms	• Frequent onset during childhood
• Irritants are a common trigger in NAR	• Nasal pruritus, watery rhinorrhea, and sneezing
	• Evolution to worsening over time

sIgE in the nasal secretions [27, 29, 31, 44, 48, 85]. Nasal allergen provocation testing is a sensitive, specific, and reproducible technique, although it is time consuming and requires technical resources and trained staff. One option to increase the implementation of NAPT in the daily practice is to perform a nasal challenge with multiple allergens in order to rapidly identify patients without nasal reactivity. This procedure shortens the diagnostic workup by reducing the number of visits [28].

In a proportion of LAR individuals, sIgE in the nasal secretions is found, but the sensitivity of this measurement largely relies on the technique utilized to collect nasal secretions. With the classical nasal lavage, the quantification of sIgE has a very high specificity (>90%) but low sensitivity (22–40%) [27, 43, 44]. New methods to collect nasal secretions need to be explored to improve the sensitivity in this setting.

The basophil activation test (BAT) is a useful tool for LAR diagnosis as illustrated by the findings of several studies including patients with *D. pteronyssinus* and olive tree pollen nasal reactivity [72, 73]. In LAR patients reactive to *D. pteronyssinus,* BAT has a 50% sensitivity and it is even higher (66%) in subjects reacting to *Olea euro-*

paea upon nasal provocation. In both cases the specificity was >90%.

Therapeutics Options in Local Allergic Rhinitis

The treatment of airway allergy is complex and should involve patient's education, allergen avoidance, pharmacotherapy, and allergen immunotherapy (AIT).

Given the clinical and immunological similarities between LAR and AR patients it is reasonable to speculate that LAR patients will benefit from the same medications prescribed for AR individuals. The first-line therapy for LAR individuals should include antihistamines and inhaled corticosteroids, for nasal and bronchial symptoms, respectively [8, 74].

In daily clinical practice, the majority of LAR individuals are treated with health education, allergen avoidance measures, and pharmacological treatment including oral antihistamines and intranasal corticosteroids, all according to the Allergic Rhinitis and its Impact on Asthma (ARIA) guidelines and criteria. With this approach, LAR patients usually show a similar response to that of AR individuals in terms of symptom improvement and disease control [27, 30, 44]. However allergen avoidance is not always feasible, and the pharmacotherapy with either intranasal corticosteroids, oral antihistamines, or both does not prevent the progression of worsening disease. Of note, one-third of children and two-thirds of adults with AR do not achieve adequate disease control with pharmacotherapy alone [94, 95].

Long-term strategies such as immunomodulatory treatments affecting the natural course of the disease play an important role besides pharmacotherapy-based symptomatic treatment. Allergen immunotherapy (AIT) consists of the repeated administration of pure or modified allergen extracts to allergic individuals in order to boost immunomodulatory mechanisms and provide sustained clinical relief and a decrease in medication intake for disease control. This results in an improved quality of life during subsequent natural exposures to the allergen [96]. Allergen immunotherapy uniquely modifies the immune response towards the allergens and affects the long-term course of allergic rhinitis and asthma by activating several sequential immune mechanisms, such as increasing IgG4 blocking antibodies and increased production of cytokines that confer immune tolerance [97, 98]. The better understanding of AIT mechanisms should help identify early and late diagnostic biomarkers in order to select the patients who would obtain the maximum benefit from this treatment. Cellular and molecular events taking place during the course of AIT can be classified into three groups [97] (Fig. 5.4). The first group of events can start as soon as several hours after the administration of natural allergen extracts, and include a decrease in mast cell and basophil activation and granule exocytosis with a trend towards a lower rate of systemic anaphylaxis. The second group of events induce the generation of allergen-specific regulatory T cells (Treg) and B cells (Breg) which are able to suppress allergen-specific effector T cell subsets. The third group of events involves the regulation of the immunoglobulin isotypes synthetized against the specific allergens. It is demonstrated that AIT induces an early increase of allergen-specific IgE followed by a subsequent decrease, and an early and sustained production of blocking allergen-specific IgG_4 [97]. Initial administration of AIT results in an early decrease in mast cell and basophil granule exocytosis followed by increased generation of allergen-specific Tregs and suppression of allergen-specific Th2 cells among other effector cells [97].

Role of Allergen Immunotherapy in Allergic Rhinitis

Allergen immunotherapy is the only treatment for allergic rhinoconjunctivitis and asthma that has the potential to modify the natural course of disease [98–103].

The term "allergen immunotherapy" (AIT) has been proposed to universally refer to therapeutic strategies aimed at inducing a state of

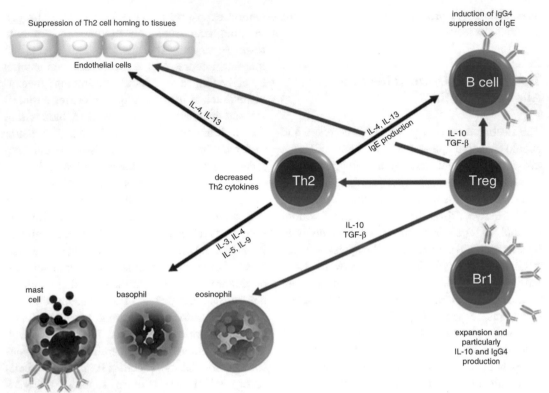

Direct and indirect suppressive effects on mast cells, basophils and eosinophils

Fig. 5.4 Mechanisms of allergen immunotherapy. Role of Treg and Breg cells in the suppression of allergic inflammation. The balance between Th2 and Treg cells is crucial for the development or suppression of allergic inflammation. Treg cells and their cytokines suppress Th2 immune responses and contribute to the control of allergic inflammation in several ways. *Red arrows* indicate the regulatory and suppressive effects of Treg cells, which can exert their functions by direct mechanisms or indirectly through the induction of IgG₄ and IgA synthesis and the suppression of IgE synthesis on B cells; Treg cells also act on vascular endothelium by suppressing Th2 cell homing to tissues, on mast cells, basophils, and eosinophils through direct and indirect suppressive effects. Moreover, they also antagonize by direct and indirect mechanisms the activation of epithelial cell and the release of proinflammatory mediators. In addition, Breg cells also suppress effector T cells and synthetize IgG₄. Reprinted from Journal of Allergy and Clinical Immunology, 133(3), Mübeccel Akdis, Cezmi A. Akdis, Mechanisms of allergenspecific immunotherapy: Multiple suppressor factors at work in immune tolerance to allergens, 621–631, Copyright 2014, with permission from Elsevier

immune tolerance towards one or more specific allergens [104]. Currently two types of AIT are available, defined by the route of allergen administration: subcutaneous immunotherapy (SCIT) and sublingual immunotherapy (SLIT). Both SCIT and SLIT have been shown to be effective and safe for the treatment of AR in adults and children [105]. The SCIT approach has been used worldwide for more than one century and has been demonstrated to be effective in controlling symptoms of AR, in preventing the development of more IgE sensitizations to environmental allergens and progression to allergic asthma, and in reducing some AR comorbidities such as recurrent sinusitis. Over the past two decades, the prescription of SLIT has increased considerably and is now the preferred route in several European countries [106]. Additional routes under active investigation include epicutaneous or intralymphatic AIT [107, 108].

According to the ARIA [109, 110], moderate-to-severe intermittent or persistent AR are indications for AIT, especially in those patients who do not respond well to pharmaco-therapy. Recent systematic reviews confirm that patients on AIT can achieve substantial clinical improvement manifested as reduction in nasal and ocular symptoms or medication requirements [105, 111]. It also improves quality of life, prevents progression of AR to asthma, and reduces the appearance of new sensitizations [112–115]. Moreover, several large studies have demonstrated that the clinical efficacy of AIT persists after therapy discontinuation [116, 117]. Contraindications for AIT include patients suffering from medical conditions increasing the risk of AIT-related severe anaphylactic reactions, such as those with poorly controlled asthma or significant cardiovascular diseases (e.g., unstable angina, recent myocardial infarction, significant arrhythmia, and uncontrolled hypertension). Furthermore, AIT should be administered with caution in patients receiving β-blockers or angiotensin-converting enzyme inhibitors. Chronic rhinosinusitis with or without nasal polyps is not a contraindication for AIT, as long as the IgE sensitizations are considered clinically relevant. Severe or uncontrolled asthma is the major independent risk factor for both nonfatal and fatal adverse reactions to AIT, and thus it is considered a major contraindication, especially for SCIT [118–120]. All patients undergoing AIT should be observed for at least 30 min after every injection to ensure the proper management of systemic reactions if they occur [98, 118].

Role of Allergen Immunotherapy in Local Allergic Rhinitis

As mentioned above, LAR is not a mild or trivial disease, and patients often complain of persistent moderate-severe rhinitis, with impairment of their quality of life, and frequently associated conjunctivitis and asthma [31]. The conversion rate to systemic atopy is low in LAR [53, 91], and there is a trend towards a clinical worsening of the disease over time, with development of more persistent and severe nasal symptoms, more fre-

quent visits to the emergency room, and onset of conjunctivitis and asthma [30]. Consequently a significant proportion of LAR patients needs continuous pharmacological treatment with nasal corticosteroids and/or oral antihistamines [27, 30, 44], and even with these therapeutic measures their disease is not always adequately controlled. Although the a priori evidence of a localized allergic response in LAR patients suggests that specific AIT would be beneficial, the efficacy of AIT in LAR needs to be corroborated by double-blind placebo-controlled clinical trials (DBPCCT).

A First Step: Observational Study

The first approach of our group to evaluate the potential role of AIT in LAR was an observational study performed in 20 adult patients (aged 19–45 years) with moderate or severe LAR due to grass pollen [121]. In this study ten patients were treated with pre-seasonal grass-SCIT and rescue medication was allowed during the spring; the ten remaining patients only received rescue medication at their own discretion [121]. The results showed that 6 months of grass-SCIT significantly improved the nasal tolerance to the allergen compared to rescue medication only, with higher threshold doses of grass pollen necessary for eliciting a positive NAPT. Of note, one-third of the SCIT-treated patients tolerated the maximum concentration of allergen, and were thus negative in the post-SCIT NAPT. Significant increases in the levels of sIgG to grass pollen in the serum of SCIT-treated patients were also detected. The SCIT-treated individuals reported a clinical improvement the following spring, with an important reduction in rhinoconjunctivitis symptom and rescue medication scores (Fig. 5.5) [121]. Although a placebo effect cannot be excluded, the changes of objective parameters such as an increase in nasal tolerance to the allergen and an increase in the serum levels of grass-specific IgG indicate that SCIT might also be beneficial in LAR individuals.

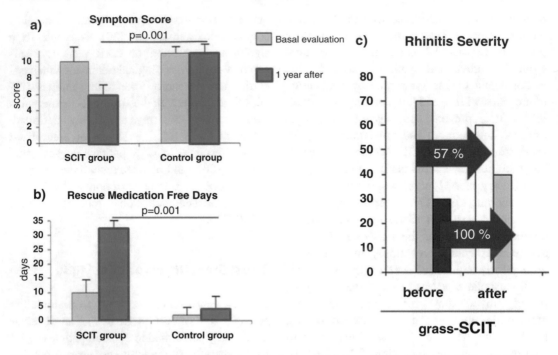

Fig. 5.5 Clinical effect of subcutaneous allergen immunotherapy with grass pollen in LAR individuals. (**a**) Symptom score; (**b**) rescue medication-free days; and (**c**) severity of rhinitis

Double-Blind Placebo-Controlled Clinical Trials

The interesting results of the above-mentioned observational study led us to conduct a phase II, randomized DBPCCT to investigate the safety and efficacy of 2-year SCIT treatment with *D. pteronyssinus* (SCIT-DP) compared to placebo in LAR patients reacting to HDM [122]. This study provided evidence for the sustained efficacy of AIT in LAR patients, with reduction in symptoms and need of rescue medication and increases in the number of medication-free days. The immunological effects of AIT included the production of allergen-specific IgG_4 and the decrease of serum sIgE with a strong increase in nasal tolerance to the allergen (Fig. 5.6). At the end of the study, two-thirds of the patients treated with AIT tolerated a nasal concentration of Der p 1 > 10 times higher than the concentration eliciting a positive NAPT at baseline. The NAPT was negative in 50% of the treated patients at the end of the study [122]. These results strongly indicate that LAR should be considered an indication for

AIT, and reinforce the need for early diagnosis and treatment of patients with rhinitis in the absence of systemic atopy.

Conclusion

The research undertaken on LAR and its comorbidities in the last decades is helping to understand this complex disease phenotype defined by the presence of allergic inflammation in the target organs in the absence of classical markers of systemic atopy. Nevertheless, the fact that a proportion of LAR patients display positive BAT results challenges the concept of LAR being merely a local disease, and reinforces the view of basophils as carriers of high-affinity IgE in the bloodstream. The allergic evaluation of the target organ is crucial for the proper diagnosis of this new entity in patients with a clinical history suggestive of airway allergy in the context of negative SPT and serum sIgE. However, many questions regarding disease pathophysiology remain to be elucidated, especially in relation to

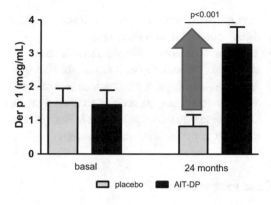
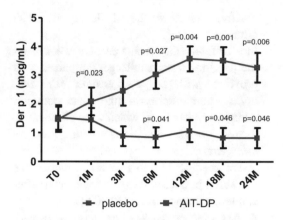

Fig. 5.6 Allergen tolerance to *Dermatophagoides pteronyssinus* induced by allergen immunotherapy in LAR individuals. (Left) Comparison between active and placebo groups at baseline and after 24 months of treatment. (Right) Increases in allergen tolerance throughout the study compared to baseline

the lower airways where the evidence of functional sIgE is still scarce. Additional research should investigate the presence of LAR in patients with occupational rhinitis with or without asthma.

Multicenter epidemiological studies will provide a more detailed patient phenotyping and the opportunity to explore the effect of environmental factors on the disease onset. The development of in vitro tests for an easy diagnosis in the clinical setting and the improvement of detection methods for nasal (or bronchial) sIgE would help the recognition of this disease by clinicians. In relation to AIT, it would be interesting to compare the clinical effect and the immunological response of different AIT routes, schedules, and allergen extract or components used.

Clinical Cases in Local Allergic Rhinitis

Case Presentation 1

A 34-year-old female, working as a secretary, nonsmoker, and with a family history of allergy, complains of a 10-year history of nasal pruritus, sneezing, watery rhinorrhea, and ocular symptoms during the spring. Symptoms worsen during outdoor activities and windy days. She also presents with symptoms of coughing, dyspnea, and wheezing unrelated to infectious episodes. She has been taking oral antihistamines for a while prescribed by her general practitioner, with clear improvement of her symptoms. She is referred to the allergist for diagnosis and management.

Allergy Workup

The allergist underwent a thorough examination of the patient, with the following studies:

- First, a *nasal exploration* by anterior rhinoscopy revealed septal deviation and turbinate hypertrophy. In order to rule out sinus disease, a CT scan was performed and was normal.
- *Skin prick testing* with a battery of common aeroallergens was performed (pollens, house dust mites, Alternaria, latex, cat and dog dander) and all were negative.
- *Total serum IgE*: 43 UI/mL.
- *Serum-specific IgE* for all the allergens tested by skin prick testing were all negative (<0.35 kU/L).
- *Spirometry* was normal.
- In this patient, having symptoms clearly compatible with allergic disease and negative skin testing/serum-specific IgE, the allergist suspected a case of local allergic rhinitis and performed the following studies:
- A *nasal provocation test* with grass extract (*Phleum pratense*) was performed, using sequential dilutions of 1/100, 1/10 y 1/1, with

positive result to the challenge at 1/100 dilution.

- In a different day separated by a week from the previous nasal challenge, the patient was provoked with *D. pteronyssinus, olive tree pollen*, and *Alternaria* (the most common allergens in her area) which were all negative (*nasal provocation test with multiple allergens*).
- *Nasal specific IgE* to *Phleum pratense* was measured in a nasal lavage sample taken after challenge, being positive (0.80 kU/L).
- A *basophil activation test* was performed, being positive to *Phleum pratense* and negative to *D. pteronyssinus, olive tree pollen*, and *Alternaria*.

Management/Outcome

In this case, after the confirmation of local allergic rhinitis, the following treatments and instructions were given to the patient:

- Avoidance of pollen exposure during the season.
- Pharmacological treatment: oral antihistamines, nasal corticosteroids, short-acting bronchodilators.
- Based on the published evidence, the patient was prescribed allergen immunotherapy with *Phleum pratense* for a minimum of 3 years and a maximum of 5 years.

After 1 year of treatment with immunotherapy with *Phleum pratense*, the patient reports an important improvement of the nasal-ocular and bronchial symptoms during the spring, with a decrease in the use of relief medication.

Clinical Pearls and Pitfalls

- If a patient reports typical symptoms of allergic rhinitis and displays negative skin prick test/serum-specific IgE, the possibility of local allergic rhinitis has to be explored.
- Also, chronic rhinosinusitis and/or nasal polyposis should be ruled out.
- The diagnosis of local allergic rhinitis has to be confirmed by means of nasal allergen prov-

ocation test, measurement of nasal specific IgE, or basophil activation test.

- Patients with local allergic rhinitis must be diagnosed correctly in order to establish a specific treatment (allergen avoidance and specific immunotherapy). A delay in the diagnosis can worsen the symptoms and lead to the onset of comorbidities such as asthma.

Case Presentation 2

A 28-year-old male who is a nonsmoker and works as an electrician was referred due to a 15-year history of nasal pruritus, sneezing, watery rhinorrhea, and ocular symptoms all year round. Symptoms started by being seasonal with clinical worsening during outdoor activities, but in the past 2 years symptoms were present all year round. Symptoms worsen in rainy days, and he refers to having moisture stains in his bedroom ceiling due to roof leakage. He has taken oral antihistamines for a while with clinical improvement. He was referred to the allergist for diagnosis.

Diagnosis

The allergist underwent a thorough examination of the patient, with the following studies:

- First, a *nasal exploration* by anterior rhinoscopy revealed a normal anatomy and no signs of chronic rhinosinusitis and/or polyposis.
- *Skin prick testing* was performed with a battery of common aeroallergens (pollens, house dust mites, *Alternaria*, latex, cat and dog dander), positive to olive tree pollen.
- *Total serum IgE*: 147 UI/mL.
- *Serum-specific IgE* for all the allergens tested by skin prick testing; only positive to olive tree pollen (20 kU/L).
- *Spirometry* was normal.

This patient has perennial AR symptoms with seasonal worsening with SPT/sIgE positive to olive tree pollen only, so two diagnostic possibilities exist:

1. Classical AR due to sensitization to seasonal allergens coexisting with mixed rhinitis (MR) or
2. Classical AR due to sensitization to seasonal allergens coexisting with LAR due to perennial allergens (dual-allergic rhinitis or DAR). Diagnosis was reached as follows:
   - A *nasal provocation test* with olive tree pollen was performed, using sequential dilutions of 1/100, 1/10 y 1/1, and found a positive result to the challenge at 1/100 dilution.
   - In different sessions separated by 1 week, the patient was challenged with perennial allergens (*D. pteronyssinus, Alternaria,* and *Parietaria*) being positive to *Alternaria* at 1/10 dilution.

Management/Outcome

In this case, after dual-allergic rhinitis was confirmed, the following treatments and recommendations were given to the patient:

- Avoidance of pollen exposure during the season
- Repairing of moisture damage in the house
- Pharmacological treatment: oral antihistamines, nasal corticosteroids, short-acting bronchodilators

After the house was repaired and a dehumidifier was placed in the bedroom, perennial symptoms decreased, with improvement of the nasal-ocular symptoms and no onset of bronchial symptoms.

Clinical Pearls and Pitfalls

- If there is a disagreement between clinical history and skin testing/sIgE, we should keep on studying the case since the patient could be a DAR (coexistence of LAR and AR) or a mixed rhinitis (coexistence of AR and NAR).
- Also, chronic rhinosinusitis and/or nasal polyposis should be ruled out.
- It is necessary to confirm the diagnosis by means of a nasal provocation test.
- Patients must be diagnosed correctly in order to establish a specific treatment plan.

References

1. Greiner AN, Hellings PW, Rotiroti G, Scadding GK. Allergic rhinitis. Lancet. 2011;378(9809): 2112–22.
2. Papadopoulos NG, Guibas GV. Rhinitis subtypes, endotypes, and definitions. Immunol Allergy Clin N Am. 2016;36(2):215–33.
3. Canonica GW, Bousquet J, Mullol J, Scadding GK, Virchow JC. A survey of the burden of allergic rhinitis in Europe. Allergy. 2007;62(Suppl 85):17–25.
4. Muraro A, Clark A, Beyer K, Borrego LM, Borres M, Lodrup Carlsen KC, et al. The management of the allergic child at school: EAACI/GA2LEN task force on the allergic child at school. Allergy. 2010;65(6):681–9.
5. de la Hoz Caballer B, Rodriguez M, Fraj J, Cerecedo I, Antolin-Amerigo D, Colas C. Allergic rhinitis and its impact on work productivity in primary care practice and a comparison with other common diseases: the Cross-sectional study to evAluate work Productivity in allergic Rhinitis compared with other common dIseases (CAPRI) study. Am J Rhinol Allergy. 2012;26(5):390–4.
6. Bousquet J, Van Cauwenberge P, Khaltaev N, Aria Workshop G, World Health O. Allergic rhinitis and its impact on asthma. J Allergy Clin Immunol. 2001;108(5 Suppl):S147–334.
7. Dykewicz MS, Hamilos DL. Rhinitis and sinusitis. J Allergy Clin Immunol. 2010;125(2 Suppl 2):S103–15.
8. Rondon C, Bogas G, Barrionuevo E, Blanca M, Torres MJ, Campo P. Nonallergic rhinitis and lower airway disease. Allergy. 2017;72(1):24–34.
9. Ellis AK, Keith PK. Nonallergic rhinitis with eosinophilia syndrome and related disorders. Clin Allergy Immunol. 2007;19:87–100.
10. Lacroix JS, Landis BN. Neurogenic inflammation of the upper airway mucosa. Rhinology. 2008;46(3):163–5.
11. Van Gerven L, Alpizar YA, Wouters MM, Hox V, Hauben E, Jorissen M, et al. Capsaicin treatment reduces nasal hyperreactivity and transient receptor potential cation channel subfamily V, receptor 1 (TRPV1) overexpression in patients with idiopathic rhinitis. J Allergy Clin Immunol. 2014;133(5):1332–9. 9 e1–3
12. Ellegard E, Karlsson G. Nasal congestion during pregnancy. Clin Otolaryngol Allied Sci. 1999;24(4):307–11.
13. Chhabra N, Houser SM. The diagnosis and management of empty nose syndrome. Otolaryngol Clin N Am. 2009;42(2):311–30. ix
14. Campo P, Aranda A, Rondon C, Donia I, Diaz-Perales A, Canto G, et al. Work-related sensitization and respiratory symptoms in carpentry apprentices exposed to wood dust and diisocyanates. Ann Allergy Asthma Immunol. 2010;105(1):24–30.

15. Grammer LC 3rd. Occupational rhinitis. Immunol Allergy Clin N Am. 2016;36(2):333–41.
16. Perez-Alzate D, Blanca-Lopez N, Dona I, Agundez JA, Garcia-Martin E, Cornejo-Garcia JA, et al. Asthma and rhinitis induced by selective immediate reactions to paracetamol and non-steroidal anti-inflammatory drugs in aspirin tolerant subjects. Front Pharmacol. 2016;7:215.
17. Graf P. Rhinitis medicamentosa: a review of causes and treatment. Treat Respir Med. 2005;4(1):21–9.
18. Cho SH, Bachert C, Lockey RF. Chronic rhinosinusitis phenotypes: an approach to better medical care for chronic rhinosinusitis. J Allergy Clin Immunol Pract. 2016;4(4):639–42.
19. Hamilos DL. Drivers of chronic rhinosinusitis: inflammation versus infection. J Allergy Clin Immunol. 2015;136(6):1454–9.
20. Zhang N, Van Zele T, Perez-Novo C, Van Bruaene N, Holtappels G, DeRuyck N, et al. Different types of T-effector cells orchestrate mucosal inflammation in chronic sinus disease. J Allergy Clin Immunol. 2008;122(5):961–8.
21. Davila I, Rondon C, Navarro A, Anton E, Colas C, Dordal MT, et al. Aeroallergen sensitization influences quality of life and comorbidities in patients with nasal polyposis. Am J Rhinol Allergy. 2012;26(5):e126–31. Epub 2012/11/22
22. Roberts G, Ollert M, Aalberse R, Austin M, Custovic A, DunnGalvin A, et al. A new framework for the interpretation of IgE sensitization tests. Allergy. 2016;71(11):1540–51.
23. Dordal MT, Lluch-Bernal M, Sanchez MC, Rondon C, Navarro A, Montoro J, et al. Allergen-specific nasal provocation testing: review by the rhinoconjunctivitis committee of the Spanish Society of Allergy and Clinical Immunology. J Invest Allergol Clin Immunol. 2011;21(1):1–12. quiz follow Epub 2011/03/05
24. Krajewska-Wojtys A, Jarzab J, Gawlik R, Bozek A. Local allergic rhinitis to pollens is underdiagnosed in young patients. Am J Rhinol Allergy. 2016;30(6):198–201.
25. Rondon C, Canto G, Blanca M. Local allergic rhinitis: a new entity, characterization and further studies. Curr Opin Allergy Clin Immunol. 2010;10(1):1–7. Epub 2009/12/17
26. Rondon C, Fernandez J, Lopez S, Campo P, Dona I, Torres MJ, et al. Nasal inflammatory mediators and specific IgE production after nasal challenge with grass pollen in local allergic rhinitis. J Allergy Clin Immunol. 2009;124(5):1005–11. e1. Epub 2009/10/03
27. Rondon C, Romero JJ, Lopez S, Antunez C, Martin-Casanez E, Torres MJ, et al. Local IgE production and positive nasal provocation test in patients with persistent nonallergic rhinitis. J Allergy Clin Immunol. 2007;119(4):899–905. Epub 2007/03/06
28. Rondon C, Campo P, Herrera R, Blanca-Lopez N, Melendez L, Canto G, et al. Nasal allergen provocation test with multiple aeroallergens detects polysensitization in local allergic rhinitis. J Allergy Clin Immunol. 2011;128(6):1192–7. Epub 2011/07/26
29. Campo P, Rondon C, Gould HJ, Barrionuevo E, Gevaert P, Blanca M. Local IgE in non-allergic rhinitis. Clin Exp Allergy. 2015;45(5):872–81.
30. Rondon C, Campo P, Zambonino MA, Blanca-Lopez N, Torres MJ, Melendez L, et al. Follow-up study in local allergic rhinitis shows a consistent entity not evolving to systemic allergic rhinitis. J Allergy Clin Immunol. 2014;133(4):1026–31.
31. Rondon C, Campo P, Galindo L, Blanca-Lopez N, Cassinello MS, Rodriguez-Bada JL, et al. Prevalence and clinical relevance of local allergic rhinitis. Allergy. 2012;67(10):1282–8. Epub 2012/08/24
32. Carney AS, Powe DG, Huskisson RS, Jones NS. Atypical nasal challenges in patients with idiopathic rhinitis: more evidence for the existence of allergy in the absence of atopy? Clin Exp Allergy. 2002;32(10):1436–40.
33. Bozek A, Ignasiak B, Kasperska-Zajac A, Scierski W, Grzanka A, Jarzab J. Local allergic rhinitis in elderly patients. Ann Allergy Asthma Immunol. 2015;114(3):199–202.
34. Fuiano N, Fusilli S, Passalacqua G, Incorvaia C. Allergen-specific immunoglobulin E in the skin and nasal mucosa of symptomatic and asymptomatic children sensitized to aeroallergens. J Investig Allergol Clin Immunol. 2010;20(5):425–30.
35. Huggins KG, Brostoff J. Letter: local IgE antibodies in allergic rhinitis. Lancet. 1975;2(7935):618.
36. Klimek L, Bardenhewer C, Spielhaupter M, Harai C, Becker K, Pfaar O. Local allergic rhinitis to Alternaria Alternata: evidence for local IgE production exclusively in the nasal mucosa. HNO. 2015;63(5):364–72. Lokale allergische Rhinitis auf Alternaria alternata: Nachweis bei Patienten mit persistierender nasaler Symptomatik
37. Powe DG, Jagger C, Kleinjan A, Carney AS, Jenkins D, Jones NS. 'Entopy': localized mucosal allergic disease in the absence of systemic responses for atopy. Clin Exp Allergy. 2003;33(10):1374–9.
38. Cheng KJ, Xu YY, Liu HY, Wang SQ. Serum eosinophil cationic protein level in Chinese subjects with nonallergic and local allergic rhinitis and its relation to the severity of disease. Am J Rhinol Allergy. 2013;27(1):8–12.
39. Powe DG, Bonnin AJ, Jones NS. 'Entopy': local allergy paradigm. Clin Exp Allergy. 2010;40(7):987–97.
40. van Rijswijk JB, Blom HM, KleinJan A, Mulder PG, Rijntjes E, Fokkens WJ. Inflammatory cells seem not to be involved in idiopathic rhinitis. Rhinology. 2003;41(1):25–30.
41. Blom HM, Godthelp T, Fokkens WJ, Klein Jan A, Holm AF, Vroom TM, et al. Mast cells, eosinophils and IgE-positive cells in the nasal mucosa of patients with vasomotor rhinitis. An immunohistochemical study. Eur Arch Otorhinolaryngol. 1995;252(Suppl 1):S33–9.

42. Huggins KG, Brostoff J. Local production of specific IgE antibodies in allergic-rhinitis patients with negative skin tests. Lancet. 1975;2(7926):148–50.
43. Lopez S, Rondon C, Torres MJ, Campo P, Canto G, Fernandez R, et al. Immediate and dual response to nasal challenge with Dermatophagoides pteronyssinus in local allergic rhinitis. Clin Exp Allergy. 2010;40(7):1007–14. Epub 2010/03/27
44. Rondon C, Dona I, Lopez S, Campo P, Romero JJ, Torres MJ, et al. Seasonal idiopathic rhinitis with local inflammatory response and specific IgE in absence of systemic response. Allergy. 2008;63(10):1352–8. Epub 2008/09/11
45. Wedback A, Enbom H, Eriksson NE, Moverare R, Malcus I. Seasonal non-allergic rhinitis (SNAR)--a new disease entity? A clinical and immunological comparison between SNAR, seasonal allergic rhinitis and persistent non-allergic rhinitis. Rhinology. 2005;43(2):86–92.
46. Blanca-Lopez N, Campo P, Salas M, Garcia Rodriguez C, Palomares F, Blanca M, et al. Seasonal local allergic rhinitis in areas with high concentrations of grass pollen. J Investig Allergol Clin Immunol. 2016;26(2):83–91.
47. Lee KS, Yu J, Shim D, Choi H, Jang MY, Kim KR, et al. Local immune responses in children and adults with allergic and nonallergic rhinitis. PLoS One. 2016;11(6):e0156979.
48. Rondon C, Campo P, Togias A, Fokkens WJ, Durham SR, Powe DG, et al. Local allergic rhinitis: concept, pathophysiology, and management. J Allergy Clin Immunol. 2012;129(6):1460–7. Epub 2012/04/21
49. Cruz Niesvaara D, Rondon C, Almeida Quintana L, Correa A, Castillo Sainz R, Melendez L, et al. Evidence of local allergic rhinitis in areas with high and permanent aeroallergens exposure. J Allergy Clin Immunol. 2012;129(2):AB111.
50. Roberts G, Xatzipsalti M, Borrego LM, Custovic A, Halken S, Hellings PW, et al. Paediatric rhinitis: position paper of the European academy of allergy and clinical immunology. Allergy. 2013;68(9):1102–16.
51. Kurukulaaratchy RJ, Karmaus W, Raza A, Matthews S, Roberts G, Arshad SH. The influence of gender and atopy on the natural history of rhinitis in the first 18 years of life. Clin Exp Allergy. 2011;41(6):851–9.
52. Arasi S, Pajno GB, Lau S, Matricardi PM. Local allergic rhinitis: a critical reappraisal from a paediatric perspective. Pediatr Allergy Immunol. 2016;27(6):569–73.
53. Sennekamp J, Joest I, Filipiak-Pittroff B, von Berg A, Berdel D. Local allergic nasal reactions convert to classic systemic allergic reactions: a long-term follow-up. Int Arch Allergy Immunol. 2015;166(2):154–60.
54. Fuiano N, Fusilli S, Incorvaia C. A role for measurement of nasal IgE antibodies in diagnosis of Alternaria-induced rhinitis in children. Allergol Immunopathol. 2012;40(2):71–4.
55. Buntarickpornpan P, Veskitkul J, Pacharn P, Visitsunthorn N, Vichyanond P, Tantilipikorn P, et al. The prevalence and clinical characteristics of local allergic rhinitis in Thai children. J Allergy Clin Immunol. 2015;135(2):AB282.
56. Zicari AM, Occasi F, Di Fraia M, Mainiero F, Porzia A, Galandrini R, et al. Local allergic rhinitis in children: novel diagnostic features and potential biomarkers. Am J Rhinol Allergy. 2016;30(5):329–34.
57. Duman H, Bostanci I, Ozmen S, Dogru M. The relevance of nasal provocation testing in children with nonallergic rhinitis. Int Arch Allergy Immunol. 2016;170(2):115–21.
58. Muramatsu M, Kinoshita K, Fagarasan S, Yamada S, Shinkai Y, Honjo T. Class switch recombination and hypermutation require activation-induced cytidine deaminase (AID), a potential RNA editing enzyme. Cell. 2000;102(5):553–63.
59. He JS, Narayanan S, Subramaniam S, Ho WQ, Lafaille JJ, Curotto de Lafaille MA. Biology of IgE production: IgE cell differentiation and the memory of IgE responses. Curr Topic Microbiol Immunol. 2015;388:1–19.
60. Tong P, Wesemann DR. Molecular mechanisms of IgE class switch recombination. Curr Topic Microbiol Immunol. 2015;388:21–37.
61. Cameron L, Hamid Q, Wright E, Nakamura Y, Christodoulopoulos P, Muro S, et al. Local synthesis of epsilon germline gene transcripts, IL-4, and IL-13 in allergic nasal mucosa after ex vivo allergen exposure. J Allergy Clin Immunol. 2000;106(1 Pt 1):46–52.
62. Gevaert P, Nouri-Aria KT, Wu H, Harper CE, Takhar P, Fear DJ, et al. Local receptor revision and class switching to IgE in chronic rhinosinusitis with nasal polyps. Allergy. 2013;68(1):55–63.
63. KleinJan A, Vinke JG, Severijnen LW, Fokkens WJ. Local production and detection of (specific) IgE in nasal B-cells and plasma cells of allergic rhinitis patients. Eur Respir J. 2000;15(3):491–7.
64. Eckl-Dorna J, Pree I, Reisinger J, Marth K, Chen KW, Vrtala S, et al. The majority of allergen-specific IgE in the blood of allergic patients does not originate from blood-derived B cells or plasma cells. Clin Exp Allergy. 2012;42(9):1347–55.
65. Groot Kormelink T, Thio M, Blokhuis BR, Nijkamp FP, Redegeld FA. Atopic and non-atopic allergic disorders: current insights into the possible involvement of free immunoglobulin light chains. Clin Exp Allergy. 2009;39(1):33–42.
66. Groot Kormelink T, Calus L, De Ruyck N, Holtappels G, Bachert C, Redegeld FA, et al. Local free light chain expression is increased in chronic rhinosinusitis with nasal polyps. Allergy. 2012;67(9):1165–72.
67. Powe DG, Groot Kormelink T, Sisson M, Blokhuis BJ, Kramer MF, Jones NS, et al. Evidence for the involvement of free light chain immunoglobulins in allergic and nonallergic rhinitis. J Allergy Clin Immunol. 2010;125(1):139–45. e1–3
68. Redegeld FA, van der Heijden MW, Kool M, Heijdra BM, Garssen J, Kraneveld AD, et al. Immunoglobulin-free light chains elicit imme-

diate hypersensitivity-like responses. Nat Med. 2002;8(7):694–701.

69. Rondon C, Canto G, Fernandez J, Blanca M. Are free light chain immunoglobulins related to nasal local allergic rhinitis? J Allergy Clin Immunol. 2010;126(3):677. Author reply -8. Epub 2010/08/10

70. Hoffmann HJ, Santos AF, Mayorga C, Nopp A, Eberlein B, Ferrer M, et al. The clinical utility of basophil activation testing in diagnosis and monitoring of allergic disease. Allergy. 2015;70(11):1393–405.

71. Min B, Paul WE. Basophils: in the spotlight at last. Nat Immunol. 2008;9(3):223–5.

72. Campo P, Villalba M, Barrionuevo E, Rondon C, Salas M, Galindo L, et al. Immunologic responses to the major allergen of Olea Europaea in local and systemic allergic rhinitis subjects. Clin Exp Allergy. 2015;45(11):1703–12.

73. Gomez E, Campo P, Rondon C, Barrionuevo E, Blanca-Lopez N, Torres MJ, et al. Role of the basophil activation test in the diagnosis of local allergic rhinitis. J Allergy Clin Immunol. 2013;132(4):975–6. e1–5

74. Campo P, Salas M, Blanca-Lopez N, Rondon C. Local allergic rhinitis. Immunol Allergy Clin N Am. 2016;36(2):321–32.

75. Jayaratnam A, Corrigan CJ, Lee TH. The continuing enigma of non-atopic asthma. Clin Exp Allergy. 2005;35(7):835–7.

76. Humbert M, Durham SR, Ying S, Kimmitt P, Barkans J, Assoufi B, et al. IL-4 and IL-5 mRNA and protein in bronchial biopsies from patients with atopic and nonatopic asthma: evidence against "intrinsic" asthma being a distinct immunopathologic entity. Am J Respir Crit Care Med. 1996;154(5):1497–504.

77. Humbert M, Grant JA, Taborda-Barata L, Durham SR, Pfister R, Menz G, et al. High-affinity IgE receptor (FcepsilonRI)-bearing cells in bronchial biopsies from atopic and nonatopic asthma. Am J Respir Crit Care Med. 1996;153(6 Pt 1):1931–7.

78. Bentley AM, Durham SR, Kay AB. Comparison of the immunopathology of extrinsic, intrinsic and occupational asthma. J Invest Allergol Clin Immunol. 1994;4(5):222–32.

79. Humbert M, Ying S, Corrigan C, Menz G, Barkans J, Pfister R, et al. Bronchial mucosal expression of the genes encoding chemokines RANTES and MCP-3 in symptomatic atopic and nonatopic asthmatics: relationship to the eosinophil-active cytokines interleukin (IL)-5, granulocyte macrophage-colony-stimulating factor, and IL-3. Am J Respir Cell Mol Biol. 1997;16(1):1–8.

80. Takhar P, Corrigan CJ, Smurthwaite L, O'Connor BJ, Durham SR, Lee TH, et al. Class switch recombination to IgE in the bronchial mucosa of atopic and nonatopic patients with asthma. J Allergy Clin Immunol. 2007;119(1):213–8.

81. Platts-Mills TA. Local production of IgG, IgA and IgE antibodies in grass pollen hay fever. J Immunol. 1979;122(6):2218–25.

82. Zhang N, Holtappels G, Gevaert P, Patou J, Dhaliwal B, Gould H, et al. Mucosal tissue polyclonal IgE is functional in response to allergen and SEB. Allergy. 2011;66(1):141–8.

83. Mouthuy J, Detry B, Sohy C, Pirson F, Pilette C. Presence in sputum of functional dust mite-specific IgE antibodies in intrinsic asthma. Am J Respir Crit Care Med. 2011;184(2):206–14.

84. Pillai P, Fang C, Chan YC, Shamji MH, Harper C, Wu SY, et al. Allergen-specific IgE is not detectable in the bronchial mucosa of nonatopic asthmatic patients. J Allergy Clin Immunol. 2014;133(6):1770–2. e11

85. Campo P, Antunez C, Rondon C, Mayorga C, Garcia R, Ruiz M, et al. Positive bronchial challenges to D. Pteronyssinus in asthmatic subjects in absence of systemic atopy. J Allergy Clin Immunol. 2011;127(2):AB6.

86. Baroody FM, Naclerio RM. Nasal-ocular reflexes and their role in the management of allergic rhinoconjunctivitis with intranasal steroids. World Allergy Org J. 2011;4(1 Suppl):S1–5.

87. Baroody FM, Shenaq D, DeTineo M, Wang J, Naclerio RM. Fluticasone furoate nasal spray reduces the nasal-ocular reflex: a mechanism for the efficacy of topical steroids in controlling allergic eye symptoms. J Allergy Clin Immunol. 2009;123(6):1342–8.

88. Galletti JG, Guzman M, Giordano MN. Mucosal immune tolerance at the ocular surface in health and disease. Immunology. 2017;150(4):397–407.

89. Leonardi A. Allergy and allergic mediators in tears. Exp Eye Res. 2013;117:106–17.

90. Nicolai T, Bellach B, Mutius EV, Thefeld W, Hoffmeister H. Increased prevalence of sensitization against aeroallergens in adults in West compared with East Germany. Clin Exp Allergy. 1997;27(8):886–92.

91. Rondon C, Campo P, Blanca-Lopez N, Torres MJ, Blanca M. More research is needed for local allergic rhinitis. Int Arch Allergy Immunol. 2015;167(2):99–100.

92. Rondon C, Campo P, Eguiluz-Gracia I, Plaza C, Bogas G, Galindo P, et al. Local allergic rhinitis is an independent rhinitis phenotype: the results of a 10-year follow-up study. Allergy. 2018;73(2):470–78.

93. Papadopoulos NG, Bernstein JA, Demoly P, Dykewicz M, Fokkens W, Hellings PW, et al. Phenotypes and endotypes of rhinitis and their impact on management: a PRACTALL report. Allergy. 2015;70(5):474–94.

94. Wheatley LM, Togias A. Clinical practice. Allergic rhinitis. N Engl J Med. 2015;372(5):456–63.

95. Meltzer EO, Blaiss MS, Derebery MJ, Mahr TA, Gordon BR, Sheth KK, et al. Burden of allergic rhinitis: results from the Pediatric Allergies in America survey. J Allergy Clin Immunol. 2009;124(3 Suppl):S43–70.

96. Committee for Medicinal Products for Human Use. European Medicines Agency Pre-Authorisation. Evaluation of Medicines for Human Use Guideline of the clinical development of products for specific

immunotherapy for the treatment of allergic diseases; 2008.

97. Akdis CA, Akdis M. Mechanisms of allergen-specific immunotherapy and immune tolerance to allergens. World Allergy Org J. 2015;8(1):17.

98. Jutel M, Agache I, Bonini S, Burks AW, Calderon M, Canonica W, et al. International consensus on allergy immunotherapy. J Allergy Clin Immunol. 2015;136(3):556–68.

99. Bousquet J, Khaltaev N, Cruz AA, Denburg J, Fokkens WJ, Togias A, et al. Allergic Rhinitis and its Impact on Asthma (ARIA) 2008 update (in collaboration with the World Health Organization, GA(2)LEN and AllerGen). Allergy. 2008;63(Suppl 86):8–160.

100. Walker SM, Pajno GB, Lima MT, Wilson DR, Durham SR. Grass pollen immunotherapy for seasonal rhinitis and asthma: a randomized, controlled trial. J Allergy Clin Immunol. 2001;107(1):87–93.

101. Frew AJ, Powell RJ, Corrigan CJ, Durham SR, Group UKIS. Efficacy and safety of specific immunotherapy with SQ allergen extract in treatment-resistant seasonal allergic rhinoconjunctivitis. J Allergy Clin Immunol. 2006;117(2):319–25.

102. Wallace DV, Dykewicz MS, Bernstein DI, Blessing-Moore J, Cox L, Khan DA, et al. The diagnosis and management of rhinitis: an updated practice parameter. J Allergy Clin Immunol. 2008;122(2 Suppl):S1–84.

103. Pfaar O, Bachert C, Bufe A, Buhl R, Ebner C, Eng P, et al. Guideline on allergen-specific immunotherapy in IgE-mediated allergic diseases: S2k Guideline of the German Society for Allergology and Clinical Immunology (DGAKI), the Society for Pediatric Allergy and Environmental Medicine (GPA), the Medical Association of German Allergologists (AeDA), the Austrian Society for Allergy and Immunology (OGAI), the Swiss Society for Allergy and Immunology (SGAI), the German Society of Dermatology (DDG), the German Society of Oto- Rhino-Laryngology, Head and Neck Surgery (DGHNO-KHC), the German Society of Pediatrics and Adolescent Medicine (DGKJ), the Society for Pediatric Pneumology (GPP), the German Respiratory Society (DGP), the German Association of ENT Surgeons (BV-HNO), the Professional Federation of Paediatricians and Youth Doctors (BVKJ), the Federal Association of Pulmonologists (BDP) and the German Dermatologists Association (BVDD). Allergo J Int. 2014;23(8):282–319.

104. Calderon MA, Casale T, Cox L, Akdis CA, Burks AW, Nelson HS, et al. Allergen immunotherapy: a new semantic framework from the European Academy of Allergy and Clinical Immunology/American Academy of Allergy, Asthma and Immunology/PRACTALL consensus report. Allergy. 2013;68(7):825–8.

105. Burks AW, Calderon MA, Casale T, Cox L, Demoly P, Jutel M, et al. Update on allergy immunotherapy: American Academy of Allergy, Asthma & Immunology/European Academy of Allergy and Clinical Immunology/PRACTALL consensus report. J Allergy Clin Immunol. 2013;131(5):1288–96. e3

106. Bernstein DI, Schwartz G, Bernstein JA. Allergic rhinitis: mechanisms and treatment. Immunol Allergy Clin N Am. 2016;36(2):261–78.

107. Casale TB, Stokes JR. Immunotherapy: what lies beyond. J Allergy Clin Immunol. 2014;133(3):612–9. quiz 20

108. von Moos S, Johansen P, Tay F, Graf N, Kundig TM, Senti G. Comparing safety of abrasion and tape-stripping as skin preparation in allergen-specific epicutaneous immunotherapy. J Allergy Clin Immunol. 2014;134(4):965–7. e4

109. Brozek JL, Bousquet J, Baena-Cagnani CE, Bonini S, Canonica GW, Casale TB, et al. Allergic Rhinitis and its Impact on Asthma (ARIA) guidelines: 2010 revision. J Allergy Clin Immunol. 2010;126(3):466–76.

110. Bousquet J, Schunemann HJ, Samolinski B, Demoly P, Baena-Cagnani CE, Bachert C, et al. Allergic Rhinitis and its Impact on Asthma (ARIA): achievements in 10 years and future needs. J Allergy Clin Immunol. 2012;130(5):1049–62.

111. Canonica GW, Cox L, Pawankar R, Baena-Cagnani CE, Blaiss M, Bonini S, et al. Sublingual immunotherapy: world allergy organization position paper 2013 update. World Allergy Org J. 2014;7(1):6.

112. Purello-D'Ambrosio F, Gangemi S, Merendino RA, Isola S, Puccinelli P, Parmiani S, et al. Prevention of new sensitizations in monosensitized subjects submitted to specific immunotherapy or not. A retrospective study. Clin Exp Allergy. 2001;31(8): 1295–302.

113. Des Roches A, Paradis L, Menardo JL, Bouges S, Daures JP, Bousquet J. Immunotherapy with a standardized Dermatophagoides pteronyssinus extract. VI. Specific immunotherapy prevents the onset of new sensitizations in children. J Allergy Clin Immunol. 1997;99(4):450–3.

114. Jacobsen L, Niggemann B, Dreborg S, Ferdousi HA, Halken S, Host A, et al. Specific immunotherapy has long-term preventive effect of seasonal and perennial asthma: 10-year follow-up on the PAT study. Allergy. 2007;62(8):943–8.

115. Horn A, Zeuner H, Wolf H, Schnitker J, Wustenberg E, GRAZAX LQ-study group. Health-related quality of life during routine treatment with the SQ-standardised grass allergy immunotherapy tablet: a non-interventional observational study. Clin Drug Invest. 2016;36(6):453–62.

116. Tahamiler R, Saritzali G, Canakcioglu S. Long-term efficacy of sublingual immunotherapy in patients with perennial rhinitis. Laryngoscope. 2007;117(6):965–9.

117. Marogna M, Spadolini I, Massolo A, Canonica GW, Passalacqua G. Long-lasting effects of sublingual immunotherapy according to its duration: a 15-year prospective study. J Allergy Clin Immunol. 2010;126(5):969–75.

118. Cox L, Nelson H, Lockey R, Calabria C, Chacko T, Finegold I, et al. Allergen immunotherapy: a prac-

tice parameter third update. J Allergy Clin Immunol. 2011;127(1 Suppl):S1–55.

119. Calderon MA, Simons FE, Malling HJ, Lockey RF, Moingeon P, Demoly P. Sublingual allergen immunotherapy: mode of action and its relationship with the safety profile. Allergy. 2012;67(3):302–11.

120. Calderon MA, Cox L, Casale TB, Moingeon P, Demoly P. Multiple-allergen and single-allergen immunotherapy strategies in polysensitized patients: looking at the published evidence. J Allergy Clin Immunol. 2012;129(4):929–34.

121. Rondon C, Blanca-Lopez N, Aranda A, Herrera R, Rodriguez-Bada JL, Canto G, et al. Local allergic rhinitis: allergen tolerance and immunologic changes after preseasonal immunotherapy with grass pollen. J Allergy Clin Immunol. 2011;127(4):1069–71. Epub 2011/02/01

122. Rondon C, Campo P, Salas M, Aranda A, Molina A, Gonzalez M, et al. Efficacy and safety of D. Pteronyssinus immunotherapy in local allergic rhinitis: a double-blind placebo-controlled clinical trial. Allergy. 2016;71(7):1057–61.

Occupational Rhinitis

6

Kristin Claire Sokol and Daniel L. Hamilos

Case Presentation 1

A 50-year-old male woodworker presents to the allergy clinic with complaints of nasal stinging and burning, watery nose, nasal congestion, and frequent sinus headaches. These symptoms have been ongoing for years. He has noticed that when he took a few months off from work due to a back injury, his nasal symptoms improved somewhat. He denies a history of seasonal allergies, asthma, or eczema. Other past medical history includes hypertension and hyperlipidemia. He reports a history of about one sinus infection requiring antibiotics every 2 or 3 years. He denies any other recurrent infections. He is taking a thiazide diuretic for his high blood pressure and a statin for his high cholesterol. He does not take any medications on a regular basis for his nasal complaints. He does take ibuprofen or a decongestant spray as needed for acute symptoms. He is a former smoker; he quit 15 years ago. He does not drink alcohol. On physical examination, his

inferior nasal turbinates are erythematous and boggy. His oropharynx is somewhat erythematous, but has no exudate or visible drainage. He has no facial tenderness on palpation. The rest of his HEENT examination is normal. CBC does not reveal eosinophilia or any other abnormalities. Nasal smear shows a predominance of neutrophils. CT sinus reveals small mucus retention cysts in his bilateral maxillary sinuses, but is otherwise normal. He is instructed to start daily saline nasal lavage, in addition to an intranasal corticosteroid once a day prior to going to work. He comes in for a follow-up visit 3 months later with moderate improvement in his symptoms.

Case Presentation 2

A 28-year-old female with a history of intermittent asthma, allergic rhinitis, and eczema presents to the allergy clinic with a 6-month history of worsening symptoms of watery nose, sneezing, watery/itchy eyes, and cough. She recently graduated from a school of pharmacy and started a new job about 1.5 years ago working in a hospital pharmacy with the main task of compounding antibiotics and other drugs. She is currently taking an oral antihistamine intermittently, and uses an intranasal corticosteroid daily without much relief. She does not smoke cigarettes or drink alcohol. She is not taking any additional medications. She does note that her symptoms improve

K. C. Sokol (✉)
National Institute of Allergy and Infectious Diseases, National Institutes of Health, Bethesda, MD
e-mail: kristin.sokol@nih.gov

D. L. Hamilos
Department of Rheumatology, Allergy & Immunology, Harvard Medical School, Massachusetts General Hospital, Boston, MA, USA
e-mail: dhamilos@partners.org

© Springer International Publishing AG, part of Springer Nature 2018
J. A. Bernstein (ed.), *Rhinitis and Related Upper Respiratory Conditions*,
https://doi.org/10.1007/978-3-319-75370-6_6

somewhat on weekends and they improved significantly when she took a vacation to the Caribbean 4 months ago. Physical examination reveals pale boggy inferior nasal turbinates, an absence of nasal polyps, cobblestoning in the oropharynx, and mild conjunctival erythema and watery eye drainage. Her lung exam reveals no wheezes, rhonchi, or rales. Specific IgE via skin prick testing reveals sensitization to several environmental allergens including dust mite, trees, and grasses. Spirometry reveals an FEV1 of 75% predicted with significant reversibility after an inhaled short-acting beta-agonist. After a detailed work history, it is determined that she is exposed to many different antibiotics, but also highly exposed to lactase, a disaccharide enzyme produced by *Aspergillus oryzae* and *A. niger*, which is used extensively in the food and drug industries [1]. Specifically, skin prick testing of several antibiotics and lactase only reveals sensitization to lactase. Nasal smear identifies a predominance of eosinophils. Her workplace is provided with this information and asked to reduce her exposure to lactase. She is also instructed to wear personal protective equipment when compounding any drug. She starts an oral antihistamine on a daily basis, and increases her nasal corticosteroid dose to two sprays in each nostril twice a day with proper technique. She comes in for follow-up 6 months later with markedly improved symptoms.

Introduction

Occupational rhinitis is defined as inflammation of the nasal mucosa that causes symptoms of rhinitis, such as nasal congestion, rhinorrhea, sneezing, and itching, due to causes associated with a particular work environment. This must be distinguished from work-exacerbated rhinitis where there is a preexisting history of rhinitis and symptoms worsen at work [2–4]. In 2009, the European Academy of Allergy and Clinical Immunology (EAACI) published a consensus paper that classified occupational rhinitis into two general types, allergic and nonallergic [5]. Allergic occupational rhinitis is characterized by a latency period

of months to years. It is attributed to an immune-mediated hypersensitivity reaction to a particular workplace exposure. The term "allergic occupational rhinitis" has traditionally been used to encompass occupational agents that can be either IgE mediated or non-IgE mediated. Nonallergic occupational rhinitis does not have a known underlying immunologic basis for disease.

Allergic Occupational Rhinitis

There are now over 200 agents that have been associated with occupational rhinitis; thus a review of each substance would be beyond the scope of this chapter. Occupational agents capable of causing allergic occupational rhinitis can be classified as either high-molecular-weight (HMW) (>5 kDa) or low-molecular-weight (LMW) (<5 kDa) agents [2]. The agents include the same high- and low-molecular-weight sensitizers that are known to cause occupational asthma.

High-Molecular-Weight Agents

HMW agents are organic biological substances derived from plants or animals, such as flour, grain dust, latex, mites, mold spores, laboratory animals, enzymes, and other sources. It is noteworthy that the prevalence of latex sensitization in healthcare workers (HCW) was found to be strongly related to the level of airborne latex allergen exposure [6]. Furthermore, an intervention designed to reduce airborne latex allergen exposure (use of powder-free latex gloves) was associated with a 16-fold reduction in the latex sensitization rate [6]. The profound reduction of latex sensitization among healthcare workers and susceptible patients is a testimony to how effective environmental control to prevent exposure and subsequent sensitization can be.

Common occupations associated with HMW agents include bakers, laboratory workers, veterinarians, seafood packagers and processors, farm workers, healthcare workers, and detergent industry workers [7]. High-molecular-weight agents can cause upper airway inflammation via an IgE-mediated immune response leading to Th2-driven inflammation. In healthcare workers, recently implicated causes of occupational rhinitis include ethylenediamine tetraacetic acid (EDTA)-containing detergent enzymes used for cleaning medical instruments and aliphatic or alicyclic amines used in cleaning products [8, 9]. In these reports, tetrasodium EDTA and certain of the amines were found to elicit positive nasal provocation testing in some of the affected healthcare workers.

Low-Molecular-Weight Agents

In contrast to HMW agents, low-molecular-weight (LMW) agents are mostly inorganic compounds and include synthetic chemicals, such as diisocyanates, persulfate salts, acid anhydrides, aldehydes, and drugs, as well as metallic agents and chemicals derived from wood dust. Common occupations associated with these agents include chemical workers, epoxy resin production workers, carpenters, furniture makers, painters, hairdressers, and textile workers [7]. Only a small number of LMW compounds have elicited an IgE-dependent mechanism [10], with many eliciting allergic disease through other immune mechanisms that remain to be fully characterized [11].

Nonallergic (Irritant-Induced) Occupational Rhinitis

Nonallergic occupational rhinitis, also known as irritant-induced occupational rhinitis, is caused by agents capable of producing mucosal inflammation without evidence of a latency phase or immunologic sensitization (Table 6.1). The mechanisms by which irritants can induce airway inflammation are far less known [2], but mechanisms involving epithelial damage and neurokinin release from nociceptive nerve fibers are thought to play a significant role [12]. It is known that sensory nerve fibers exist underneath the airway epithelium that express chemoreceptors

Table 6.1 Examples of agents implicated in occupational rhinitis

Allergic		Nonallergic
High-molecular-weight agents	Low-molecular-weight agents	Irritants
Natural rubber latex	Anhydrides	Ammonia
Psyllium	Diisocyanates	Cigarette smoke
Grain dust, flour dust, alpha-amylase	Abeitic acid/ colophony	Formaldehyde
Mold spores	Plicatic acid	Chlorine
Seafood proteins	Persulfates	Diesel exhaust
Pollens	Quaternary ammonium disinfectants	Wood dust
Animal proteins (urine, saliva, dander)	Cyanoacrylates	Solvent vapors
Insect antigens and mites	Wood dust	Sulfur dioxide
Proteolytic enzymes		Asphalt vapors
Lactase		

(i.e., transient response potential receptors or TRPs). When these chemoreceptors are activated by irritants and osmotic and mechanical stimuli, there is a local release of neuropeptides resulting in activation of their selective receptors located on mucosal blood vessels, submucosal glands, and inflammatory cells. The release of neuropeptides and signal transduction via nociceptive fibers through the central nervous system can cause increased parasympathetic activation and/or dampening of sympathetic responses resulting in increased blood vessel dilatation and oversecretion of mucus manifesting as upper respiratory symptoms such as rhinorrhea, nasal congestion, and sneezing [2].

Certain particulates, such as cigarette smoke, and certain water-soluble irritants, such as ammonia or sulfur dioxide vapors, organic acids, aldehydes, and chlorine, that readily dissolve in mucous membrane water, provoke these immediate irritant ocular and nasal responses [12]. Nonallergic occupational rhinitis, or irritant rhinitis, can be seen in a number of industries and professions including woodworkers, pulp mill workers, spice grinders, animal laboratory workers, antibiotic manufacturers, firefighters, health professionals, and cleaning workers [13, 14]. Occupational rhinitis is associated with strong irritants including ammonia, chlorine gas, solvent vapors, bleach, hydrochloric acid, nitrogen dioxide, hydrogen sulfide, and certain drugs [4, 14]. Reactive upper airway dysfunction syndrome (RUDS) is a type of nonallergic occupational rhinitis that can develop following a single exposure to a very high concentration of an irritant gas, vapor, or smoke. Biopsies of the nasal mucosa among these individuals have shown epithelial desquamation, defective epithelial junctions, and increased number of nerve fibers [13, 14]. Unlike reactive airway dysfunction syndrome (RADS) which is now an established clinical entity, RUDS is still a rather vague condition with unknown incidence and prevalence [2]. However, just like work-related rhinitis can be a precursor to and often coexist with work-related asthma, RUDS and RADS can occur in the same patient.

The risk factors associated with occupational rhinitis include exposure level, length of exposure, atopy status, and smoking history [7]. The risk of IgE-mediated sensitization to HMW agents is directly related to the level and duration of exposure in certain workers, especially detergent workers, bakers, and those that work with lab animals. These workers are at greater risk not only for sensitization but also for the development of rhinitis symptoms. Underlying atopy is also a risk factor for sensitization to HMW agents such as flour, lab animals, and latex [7]. The association between smoking and risk of occupational rhinitis remains unclear, as some studies revealed an enhanced risk of sensitization in smokers, whereas others failed to demonstrate this relationship [3, 7, 15].

It is also worth noting that work-related rhinitis may precede the development of work-related asthma [16], and, therefore, work-related rhinitis should be considered a potential risk factor of work-related asthma [11]. The prevalence of occupational rhinitis in patients with occupational asthma has been estimated to be between 76 and 92% of workers [10].

Scope of the Problem

It is difficult to assess the overall incidence and prevalence of occupational rhinitis, as the epidemiology is not well investigated mainly because it is not considered a serious disease. Occupational rhinitis does tend to be about 2–4 times more prevalent than occupational asthma [3, 10]. It has been estimated to affect anywhere from 2 to 87% of workers exposed to occupational allergic or irritant agents, depending on the industrial setting [10]. Studies have shown that the prevalence of occupational rhinitis ranged from 3 to 87% in various industries (Table 6.2) [10]. Two recent studies have revealed a prevalence of rhinitis ranging from 42 to 62% in hairdressers exposed to persulfates and ammonia [19, 20]. In one study, it was shown that pharmaceutical workers are exposed to lactase during the manufacturing of digestive aid products for individuals with lactose intolerance and this can lead to symptoms of rhinitis [1]. However, the true prevalence is difficult to determine as the diagnosis of occupational rhinitis is challenging. In one study, patients underwent specific inhalational challenge (SIC) tests for confirmation of both occupational asthma and occupational rhinitis. A positive nasal challenge was observed in 25 SIC tests and a positive bronchial challenge was observed in 17 SIC tests. In 13 cases, both the nasal and bronchial challenges were positive, and these concordant responses were more commonly seen when HMW agents were tested [21].

Diagnosis/Assessment

Occupational upper airway disorders, including occupational rhinitis, are diagnosed based on history and exposure at work, physical examination, and for some, specialized diagnostic tests. A careful exposure history is essential for recognition and diagnosis. A history of prior allergic disorders must be asked. The timing of the onset, worsening, and improvement of symptoms is important, especially noting if there is improvement away from the work environment. Also, a history of a high prevalence rate of symptoms

Table 6.2 Estimated prevalence of occupational rhinitis in various industries [2, 10, 13, 15, 17, 18]

Occupation	Agent	How exposure occurs	Prevalence	Exposure evaluation	Duration of exposure	Confirmation of allergy?
Laboratory animal workers	Rat, mouse, guinea pig, rabbit	Animal handling; urinary aeroallergens	9–42%	Total dust; rat urinary aeroallergens; hours per week	NA	Specific skin test and specific serum IgE
Swine confinement workers	Pig	Animal handling	8–23%	NA	NA	Not done
Farm workers/cattle farmers	Storage mite	Grain bins, animal feed	2–60%	NA	NA	Specific skin test and specific serum IgE
Grain elevator workers	Grain dust	Grain growing, handling, processing	9–64%	NA	NA	Specific skin test
Bakers	Flour, alpha amylase	Bakers and packers exposed to flour proteins	18–29%	Total dust; flour aeroallergens	NA	Specific skin test
Detergent manufacturing	Proteolytic enzymes, lactase, papain	Cleaning medical instruments	3–87%	NA	3–6 years	Specific serum IgE
Seafood industry	Trout, crustacea, fish food	Filleting of fish; clam, crab, and shrimp processing; aquarists	5–24%	Amount of *Chironomus thumn.* larvae used per month	NA	Specific skin test and specific serum IgE
Chemical workers	Reactive dyes, anhydrides	Reactive dye products; textile dyeing	10–48%	Dust concentration, duration of employment	NA	Specific skin test and specific serum IgE
Carpentry/furniture making	Wood dust, plicatic acid	Mansonia, western red cedar	10–36%	Total dust concentration	NA	Not done
Hairdressers	Persulfates, ammonia, paraphenylene-diamine (PPD)	Persulfate products	27%	NA	5 years	Specific skin test, specific inhalational challenge
Pharmaceutical workers	Spiramycin, lactase, psyllium	Drug compounding, packaging	9–40%	NA	NA	Specific skin test and specific serum IgE
Nondomestic cleaners, healthcare workers	Ethylenediamene tetraacetic acid (EDTA)	Aerosols	35%	NA	NA	Not done
Healthcare and glove manufacturing workers	Latex	Inhalation, latex thread contact	0.12–20%	NA	10 years	Specific skin test and specific serum IgE
Auto body workers/boat builders	Diisocyanates	NA	NA	Concentration of selected isocyanaces	NA	Specific serum IgE negative
Pepper mill workers	Capsaicin	Inhalation	100% (n = 1)	NA	4 years	Skin prick tests negative
Domestic waste collectors	Organic dust (bioaerosols)	Loading, driving	29–39%	NA	10 years	NA

NA information not available

among coworkers can support a diagnosis of irritant-induced occupational rhinitis. Another method to aid with history is the "work removal-work resumption" test where the patient is assessed after a period of a few weeks away from the suspected exposure and is reassessed again a few weeks after resumption of work [2]. There are specialized questionnaires including the Rhinoconjunctivitis Quality of Life Questionnaire (RQLQ) and the Sinonasal Outcome Test (SNOT) which can be used to assess symptoms and quality-of-life impairment [12], although questionnaires have a low specificity for diagnosing occupational rhinitis.

Physical examination, including anterior rhinoscopy and percussion of the maxillary and frontal sinuses, can help in diagnosis of rhinitis, but often does not delineate between allergic or irritant occupational rhinitis and other forms of rhinitis. Rhinolaryngoscopy and flexible rhinolaryngoscopy enable the physician to evaluate for nasal polyposis and vocal cord dysfunction, respectively. These tools can also be used to exclude other common causes of rhinitis such as structural factors like septal deviations and nasal valve dysfunction [2].

Beyond a detailed history and physical examination, specialized diagnostic tests can help with the diagnosis of occupational rhinitis. Allergy skin or serologic testing with documented reactivity to indigenous aeroallergens is important for determining the patient's allergic (atopic) status. It is also useful for testing a suspected occupational allergen which can confirm sensitization. However, a major limitation is the lack of standardized occupational allergens that can be used for testing. The immunological evaluation is more significant in high-molecular-weight (HMW) agents (i.e., animal or plant proteins, enzymes) and a few low-molecular-weight (LMW) agents (i.e., trimellitic anhydride, hexamethylene diisocyanate, platinum salts) in which IgE can be detected by skin prick testing and/or measurement of serum-specific IgE [22]. Often, symptoms of irritant-induced occupational rhinitis will mimic those of allergic rhinitis; however, it is usually difficult to determine responsible etiologic agents. In these situations, material data

safety sheets (MSDS) may be helpful for providing clues to which agent(s) might be responsible for triggering rhinitis symptoms. A laboratory workup reveals a lack of systemic eosinophilia and a predominance of neutrophils on nasal smear in irritant rhinitis. Nasal cytology has been used as a tool for diagnosing occupational rhinitis in certain workers. In a recent study, woodworkers were found to have more neutrophils in nasal smears than controls. It was also found that woodworkers exposed to wood dust for a longer period of time had more lymphocytes in their nasal smears [23]. Sinus computed tomography scans can rule out the presence of acute or chronic sinusitis, fungal sinusitis, and other structural or infectious abnormalities, but is not recommended in the initial evaluation.

Nasal peak flow measurements, although not used in clinical practice with much frequency, can be used to document the response to allergen or irritant exposures that the patient may be exposed to in the workplace. A causal relationship between exposure to a specific occupational agent and rhinitis can be established by specific nasal provocation testing (NPT) with the suspected agent. The European Academy of Allergy, Asthma, and Immunology Task Force on Occupational Rhinitis states that "in the presence of work-related rhinitis symptoms, objective assessment using nasal provocation challenges in the laboratory or at the work-place should be strongly recommended" [5]. This diagnostic test has been studied much more with high-molecular-weight agents than low-molecular-weight agents [5]. In addition, NPT is only utilized by a limited number of clinical centers, especially in the United States, and remains poorly standardized [2].

Management/Outcome

The management of occupational rhinitis is threefold. Since occupational rhinitis is a preventable condition, avoidance is the first step in management. Prevention of exposure to hazardous materials can, in many cases, prevent incident cases of occupational rhinitis [6]. Secondary prevention includes early detection of the symptoms and interruption of disease progression. Reduced exposure can be accomplished by improving ventilation systems, wearing appropriate protective clothing and masks, and, if possible, relocation of the patient to another job location [2]. For established occupational rhinitis, tertiary prevention usually implicates treatment which involves reducing exposure to the known or suspected allergen or irritant, supportive measures such as nasal saline lavage, and medications either used alone or in combination such as topical corticosteroids, topical antihistamines, and topical cholinergic blockers. There is very little evidence for any beneficial effects of specific allergic immunotherapy in occupational upper airway disease [2]. Although there are no published studies supporting the use of immuno therapy as a treatment option for IgE-mediated occupational rhinitis [24], immunotherapy may be beneficial in certain clinical settings, such as in laboratory animal workers and veterinarians who are sensitized to animal dander.

In addition to preventing or reducing nasal symptoms, the management of occupational rhinitis should also be aimed at decreasing the risk of occupational asthma onset [5]. The relationship between occupational rhinitis and occupational asthma has been examined and the frequency of association was higher for HMW compared with LMW agents [22]. Close follow-up with awareness for the progression of lower airway symptoms, including lung function testing, is required [2].

If persistence of exposure to an agent causing occupational rhinitis occurs, as stated above, occupational asthma can develop. Because of this, the European Academy of Allergy, Asthma, and Immunology (EAACI) Task Force on occupational rhinitis has proposed that patients with occupational rhinitis be considered impaired on a permanent basis for the job that caused the condition as well as for jobs with similar exposures. Although some countries offer compensation of occupational rhinitis, available data has shown that financial compensation does not adequately offset the socioeconomic consequences of the disease. Compensation systems should be directed at offering the worker an alternative job within the same company without the possibility of exposure to the offending agent [3].

If avoidance of the causative agent can be achieved, the prognosis of the patients with occupational rhinitis is generally good [15]. In a prospective study of 20 individuals with allergic or nonallergic occupational rhinitis, when suspected exposures were eliminated, the individuals noted both decreased nasal symptoms and improved quality of life [21]. Studies have not addressed the prevention of onset of development of asthma [21].

Clinical Pearls and Pitfalls

- There are two forms of work-related rhinitis: occupational rhinitis, which is defined as rhinitis symptoms due to causes associated with a particular work environment, and work-exacerbated rhinitis, in which the individual had preexisting rhinitis made worse by exposures in the workplace.
- Occupational rhinitis is often underestimated and underdiagnosed.
- More than 300 substances have been identified as possible agents producing occupational rhinitis [22].
- Allergic occupational rhinitis can be caused by high- or low-molecular-weight agents.
- Nonallergic occupational rhinitis can occur with one high-level exposure to an irritant, and this disorder is termed RUDS, or reactive upper airway dysfunction syndrome.
- The distinction between irritant occupational rhinitis from allergic occupational rhinitis in clinical practice is often difficult but might be distinguished by the predominance of irritant symptoms (rather than itching and sneezing), a high prevalence of symptoms among co-workers, a negative laboratory workup, the predominance of neutrophils on nasal smear, and when applicable a lack of in vivo or in vitro reactivity to identifiable workplace allergens.
- A detailed history is essential when evaluating a patient suspected of having occupational

rhinitis, including documented improvement away from the workplace.

- There are three forms of prevention of occupational rhinitis: primary, secondary, and tertiary prevention.
- Exposure prevention is the most practical and effective method for the primary prevention of occupational rhinitis. Early symptom identification and exposure reduction are the most practical and effective methods for the secondary prevention of occupational rhinitis. Tertiary prevention involves treatment of symptoms in the form of supportive care and/or medications.
- Early diagnosis is critical in the prevention of progression into occupational asthma or possibly rhinosinusitis.
- The prognosis of occupational rhinitis seems to be good with significant reduction or avoidance of the offending exposure.

References

1. Bernstein JA, Bernstein DI, Stauder T, Lummus Z, Bernstein IL. A cross-sectional survey of sensitization to Aspergillus oryzae-derived lactase in pharmaceutical workers. J Allergy Clin Immunol. 1999;103(6):1153–7.
2. Hox V, Steelant B, Fokkens W, Nemery B, Hellings PW. Occupational upper airway disease: how work affects the nose. Allergy. 2014;69:282–91.
3. Moscato G, Vandenplos O, Van Wijk RG, Malo JL, Quirce S, Walusiak J, et al. EAACI task force on occupational rhinitis. Allergy. 2008;63:969–80.
4. Stevens WW, Grammer LC. Occupational rhinitis: an update. Curr Allergy Asthma Rep. 2015;15:487.
5. Moscato G, Vandenplas O, Van Wijk RG, Malo JL, Perfetti L, Quirce S, et al. EAACI position paper on occupational rhinitis. Respir Res. 2009;10:16.
6. Kelly KJ, Wang ML, Klancnik M, Petsonk EL. Prevention of IgE sensitization to latex in health care workers after reduction of antigen exposures. J Occup Environ Med. 2011;53(8):934–40.
7. Sublett JW, Bernstein DI. Occupational rhinitis. Immunol Allergy Clin N Am. 2011;31:787–96.
8. Laborde-Castérot H, Rosenberg N, Dupont P, Garnier R. Is the incidence of aliphatic amine-induced occupational rhinitis and asthma underestimated? Am J Ind Med. 2014;57(12):1303–10.
9. Laborde-Castérot H, Villa AF, Rosenberg N, Dupont P, Lee HM, Garnier R. Occupational rhinitis and asthma due to EDTA-containing detergents or disinfectants. Am J Ind Med. 2012;55(8):677–82.
10. Siracusa A, Desrosiers M, Marabini A. Epidemiology of occupational rhinitis: prevalence, aetiology, and determinants. Clin Exp Allergy. 2000;30:1519–34.
11. Mazurek JM, Wiessman DN. Occupational respiratory allergic diseases in healthcare workers. Curr Allergy Asthma Rep. 2016;16:77.
12. Zhao YA, Shusterman D. Occupational rhinitis and other work-related upper respiratory tract conditions. Clin Chest Med. 2012;33:637–47.
13. Shusterman D. Occupational irritant and allergic rhinitis. Curr Allergy Asthma Rep. 2014;14:425.
14. Siracusa A, Folletti I, Moscato G. Non-IgE-mediated and irritant-induced work-related rhinitis. Curr Opin Allergy Clin Immunol. 2013;13:159–66.
15. Grammer LC. Occupational rhinitis. Immunol Allergy Clin N Am. 2016;36:333–41.
16. Karjalainen A, Martikainen R, Klaukka T, Saarinen K, Uitti J. Risk of asthma among Finnish patients with occupational rhinitis. Chest. 2003;123(1):283–8.
17. Nam YH, Jin HJ, Hwang EK, Shin YS, Ye YM, Park HS. Occupational rhinitis induced by capsaicin. Allergy Asthma Immunol Res. 2012;4(2):104–6.
18. Schantora AL, Casjens S, Deckert A, van Kampen V, Neumann HD, Bruning T, et al. Prevalence of work-related rhinmo-conjuncitivits and respiratory symptoms among domestic waste collectors. Adv Exp Med Biol. 2015;834:53–61.
19. Foss-Skiftesvik MH, Winther L, Johnsen CR, Sosted H, Mosbech HF, Zachariae C, et al. High occurrence of rhinitis symptoms in hairdressing apprentices. Int Forum Allergy Rhinol. 2017;7(1):43–9.
20. Neilsen J, Milsson P, Dahlman-Hoglund A, Kronholm Diab K, Albin M, Karedal M, et al. Dust-free bleaching powder may not prevent symptoms in hairdressers with bleaching-associated rhinitis. J Occup Health. 2016;58(5):470–6.
21. Castano R, Trudeau C, Castellanos L, Malo JL. Prospective outcome assessment of occupational rhinitis after removal from exposure. J Occup Environ Med. 2013;55(5):579–85.
22. Gomez F, Rondon C, Salas M, Campo P. Local allergic rhinitis: mechanisms, diagnosis, and relevance for occupational rhinitis. Curr Opin Allergy Clin Immunol. 2015;15:111–6.
23. Staffieri C, Lovato A, Aielli F, Bortoletto M, Giacomelli L, Carrieri M, et al. Investigating nasal cytology as a potential tool for diagnosing occupational rhinitis in woodworkers. Int Forum Allergy Rhinol. 2015;5(9):814–9.
24. Moscato G, Pala G, Boillat MA, Folletti I, Gerth van Wijk R, Olgiati-Des Gouttes D, et al. EAACI position paper: prevention of work-related respiratory allergies among pre-apprentices or apprentices and young workers. Allergy. 2011;66(9):1164–73.

Rhinosinusitis Without Polyposis

Abdullah Al-Bader, Roy R. Casiano, and Lauren Fine

Case Presentation 1

A 43-year-old male presents to the clinic complaining of nasal obstruction and bilateral maxillary facial pain. He also reports decreased sense of smell, discolored nasal discharge, and feeling subjectively febrile. His symptoms began 10 days ago and have worsened over the last 3 days without seeking any medical attention.

He has had similar symptoms at least four to five times a year for the past 3 years, usually requiring antibiotics for resolution. He denies a history of chronic rhinitis symptoms or allergic rhinitis. There is no seasonal pattern to his symptoms other than that they tend to occur in the fall and winter, especially following viral upper respiratory syndromes. His medical history is significant only for hypertension diagnosed 1 year ago, controlled on losartan. He denies a history of recurrent local or systemic infections other than sinusitis. He has a family history of hypertension. He denies any allergies.

He is a high school teacher, never used tobacco nor used any recreational drugs, and is sexually active with his wife only and never had any unprotected intercourse.

His vitals were as follows: BP of 123/78, heart rate of 82, temperature of 100.1 F, and respiratory rate of 18. He was alert and oriented, and head exam normocephalic and atraumatic with normal neurologic evaluation. The chest exam revealed good air movement bilaterally with no wheezes or rhonchi and his abdominal and musculoskeletal examinations were unremarkable. He had normal tympanic membranes bilaterally and his oral pharyngeal examination was normal other than hyponasal speech. Nasal examination revealed erythematous and edematous nasal mucosa and turbinates bilaterally. Nasolaryngoscopy was performed and revealed moderate mucosal edema and mucopurulent secretions in the osteomeatal complexes bilaterally. The laryngeal mucosa appeared normal. A sample of his purulent secretions was collected and sent for microbiology evaluation.

Evaluation

A basic metabolic panel and complete blood count were obtained. The complete blood count revealed the following: hemoglobin of 16 g/dL, white blood cell count of 12.1×10^9/L, neutrophil count of 10×10^9/L, and lymphocyte count of

A. Al-Bader · R. R. Casiano
Department of Otolaryngology-Head and Neck Surgery, University of Miami, Miami, FL, USA
e-mail: Rcasiano@med.miami.edu

L. Fine (✉)
Division of Pulmonology, Department of Allergy, Critical Care and Sleep Medicine,
University of Miami, Miami, FL, USA
e-mail: LFine1@nova.edu

© Springer International Publishing AG, part of Springer Nature 2018
J. A. Bernstein (ed.), *Rhinitis and Related Upper Respiratory Conditions*,
https://doi.org/10.1007/978-3-319-75370-6_7

1.6×10^9/L with normal other cell counts and blood parameters.

Given the recurrent episodes of similar symptomatology, the patient was diagnosed with recurrent acute bacterial rhinosinusitis and was referred for an allergy and immunology evaluation. The patient had normal immunoglobulin M, G, E, and A levels with normal complement, albumin, and total protein levels. He had previously received the pneumococcal vaccine and demonstrated protective titers for 17 of 23 serotypes. All testing was performed while not on any immunosuppressants such as systemic corticosteroids, and he was felt to be immunocompetent. Skin prick testing to aeroallergens was negative.

Penicillin-sensitive *Streptococcus pneumoniae* was grown from his sampled secretions. A diagnosis of acute bacterial rhinosinusitis was established and the patient was treated with oral amoxicillin for 10 days accordingly. He was also prescribed a short course of oxymetazoline spray, nasal saline irrigations, and intranasal corticosteroids (INCS). His symptoms began to improve within 48 h of treatment.

Discussion

There are more than 30 million cases of sinusitis annually in the United States [1]. Acute rhinosinusitis causes a healthcare expenditure of more than $3.0 billion per year in the United States [2], with the direct cost of managing acute and chronic sinusitis exceeding $11 billion per year apart from the additional expenses from lost productivity, reduced job effectiveness, and impaired quality of life [1].

Based on recent adult sinusitis guidelines, rhinosinusitis is classified by duration into acute rhinosinusitis (ARS) if less than 4 weeks or as chronic rhinosinusitis (CRS) if lasting more than 12 weeks [1, 3]. ARS can be further classified based on etiology into acute bacterial (ABRS) or viral rhinosinusitis [1, 3]. Determining the etiology of rhinosinusitis is essential in order to evaluate the appropriateness of antibiotic therapy.

ABRS is a clinical diagnosis reached when patients have symptoms or signs of ARS (purulent nasal drainage accompanied by nasal obstruction,

facial pain/pressure, or both) that persist for more than 7 days without improvement or if symptoms and signs worsen within 10 days after initial improvement [1, 4].

Patients may also experience repeated ARS episodes. When patients develop three [5], four [1, 3, 4], or more annual episodes of ARS, with symptom-free periods in between, the condition is termed recurrent ARS (RARS) [1, 3, 4]. RARS is estimated to affect 1 in every 3000 Western adults, but despite its prevalence RARS remains poorly studied [6]. The underlying risk factors for developing RARS are poorly understood, although host defense mechanisms and genetics and infectious and environmental factors are potentially implicated [7].

Microbiology for ABRS is well established, with the major causative pathogens being the aerobic and facultative bacteria *Streptococcus pneumoniae*, *Haemophilus influenza*, and *Moraxella catarrhalis*. However, the microbiology of RARS is poorly studied. One small study using repeated sinus aspirates revealed the bacterial etiology of RARS to be similar to ABRS, with the addition of *Staphylococcus aureus* in RARS. The study has also shown an increase in antibiotic resistance and persistent colonization, which may also contribute to the pathophysiology of RARS [8].

Management

To date, there is paucity of data relating to the optimal management of RARS [6]. As mentioned earlier, ABRS is a clinical diagnosis. Investigations are not routinely required unless other diagnoses are suspected. However, for RARS, some investigations can be considered. Based on recent guidelines, radiographic imaging should not be obtained for ARS unless complications or alternative diagnoses are suspected [1, 4]. Patients with RARS can also be evaluated for other factors that may contribute to the development of and modify the management of RARS such as allergic or nonallergic rhinitis, asthma, cystic fibrosis, ciliary dyskinesia, and immunodeficiency [1, 4].

In the absence of factors that may predispose to recurrent infections, radiographic imaging may be considered to rule out structural obstruction of the sinuses or signs of ongoing sinonasal inflammation indicating chronic rhinosinusitis.

Similar to ABRS, the treatment of RARS can generally be divided into medical and surgical management.

Medical

Antibiotics

Observation and watchful waiting is an option prior to the use of antibiotics in ABRS, provided that close follow-up is ensured to avoid complications. Antibiotics can generally be considered for the treatment of ABRS symptoms mainly when symptoms fail to improve within 7 days, or there are worsening or severe symptoms [1, 4]. Severity of symptoms can be determined based on duration, intensity, and impact on patient's quality of life. Antibiotics can also be considered for ABRS episodes in patients experiencing RARS. Amoxicillin with or without clavulanate can be considered for ABRS as a first-line treatment option [1, 3, 4]. Amoxicillin-clavulanate can also be considered for potentially complicated infections or when resistant organisms are suspected [3]. Trimethoprim-sulfamethoxazole or macrolides can be considered as first-line antibiotic treatment for patients with proven penicillin allergy after proper allergy evaluation by allergy specialists. As there is no evidence to support specific antibiotic therapy in RARS, antimicrobial treatment in RARS should be based upon guidelines used for individual ABRS episodes [9].

Intranasal Corticosteroids (INCS)

INCS may be recommended for symptomatic relief of ABRS [1, 4]. For ABRS with mild-to-moderate severity, treatment can be initiated with INCS alone with reassessment of effect of treatment within 72 h [4]. When combined with antibiotic therapy, INCS improve the resolution of signs and symptoms of rhinosinusitis [2, 4]. INCS may also accelerate the relief of symptoms in patients with RARS, although the evidence for the benefit of INCS in RARS is rather limited [2].

Surgical

Surgical management has been shown to improve the quality of life in those with RARS [10]. In a retrospective study, Costa et al. compared RARS patients who underwent medical, surgical, or combined treatment (medical treatment followed by surgical) groups. Costa reported statistically significant improvement in sinonasal outcome test scores (SNOT-22) across all groups. RARS patients who underwent surgery demonstrated greater improvement in their SNOT-22 scores than the medically treated groups alone. In the combined treatment group, patients who elected to undergo surgery after suboptimal results with medical management have shown evident statistical improvements after crossing over from medical treatment to surgical treatment [6].

There is scarcity of evidence regarding the optimal management of RARS with poorly studied medical and surgical therapies. The main goal is to treat acute episodes of RARS similar to ABRS, rule out other causes contributing to recurrent infections (immunodeficiency, cystic fibrosis, ciliary dyskinesia), and rule out other conditions that may resemble rhinosinusitis such as chronic rhinitis (whether allergic or nonallergic).

Clinical Pearls and Pitfalls

- ABRS is mainly a clinical diagnosis.
- RARS is defined as three to four or more episodes of ARS in a year with symptom-free periods in between episodes.
- RARS patients may be evaluated for factors that may affect management such as allergy, immunodeficiency, asthma, cystic fibrosis, and ciliary dysfunction.
- Radiological imaging is preserved for complicated rhinosinusitis and when other diagnoses are suspected.
- Treatment for RARS is divided into medical and surgical. Antibiotics and adjunctive

treatments can be considered prior to referring for surgery.

- Medical and surgical management offers potential improvements for RARS with possibly superior results in surgical treatments for select patients.

Case Presentation 2

A 31-year-old female presents to clinic with a 3-year history of profuse anterior and posterior rhinorrhea associated with bilateral nasal congestion, nasal airway obstruction, intermittent diffuse headaches, intermittent aural fullness, and cough that are worse at night. She describes her rhinorrhea to be clear, mucoid, persistent, and produced bilaterally. Her symptoms are not affected by seasonal changes but can be aggravated by exposure to strong odors and fragrances such as perfumes. She is treated with antibiotics three to four times a year for a presumed diagnosis of acute sinusitis but has never had any imaging or a nasal endoscopy to confirm this diagnosis.

When asked about allergic symptoms, she mentioned mild sneezing attacks but denied any symptoms consistent with ocular conjunctivitis such as itching or watering. Review of systems was otherwise unremarkable. She is otherwise healthy and her past medical history is not significant for any chronic illnesses. Family history is significant for a sibling who was diagnosed with asthma. There is no other atopic history in the family.

She has seen her primary care physician who ordered an in vitro IgE-specific antibody test to local aeroallergens, which were negative. She also reports very minimal improvement of her symptoms in response to loratadine 10 mg daily, fluticasone nasal spray (two sprays each side daily), and nasal saline irrigations prescribed 4 weeks ago by her primary care physician. She still uses the prescribed treatment and takes no other medications. She works as an office manager, denies smoking tobacco or drug abuse, is not sexually active, and has no known allergies to any medications. She also denied a personal history of smoking, second-hand smoke exposure, or exposure to irritants at work such as industrial fumes.

Physical Examination

Her vital signs were as follows: BP 118/77, HR 65, temperature 98 F, and RR 18. The patient had hyponasal speech. She was alert and oriented and in no distress. Cranial nerves II–XII were intact. Her head was normocephalic and atraumatic. Head and neck exam was notable for normal canals and normal tympanic membranes bilaterally. Ocular exam including conjunctiva was normal bilaterally. Nasal examination revealed boggy and pale nasal mucosa with bilateral clear mucoid secretions and hypertrophied inferior turbinates. Skin examination was normal; she did not show signs of atopic dermatitis, dermatographia, or allergic shiners. On chest auscultation, she had normal air entry bilaterally with no wheezes or rhonchi. Her cardiovascular, abdominal, and musculoskeletal examinations were also unremarkable.

Investigations

Complete blood count revealed hemoglobin of 12 g/dL, white blood cell count of 9×10^9/L, platelet count of 310×10^9/L, neutrophils of 7×10^9/L, lymphocytes of 3.1×10^9/L, and eosinophils of 0.2×10^9/L. Electrolytes were within normal limits. Serum immunoglobulin E (IgE) level was 78 IU/mL. A nasal smear was obtained and showed >20% eosinophils. Skin prick testing was negative to a panel of seasonal and perennial environmental allergens in the presence of normal saline and histamine controls.

Management

A diagnosis of nonallergic rhinitis with eosinophilia syndrome (NARES) was established. The diagnosis was supported by the patient's symptoms worsening with exposure to certain nonallergic irritants, a negative atopic history, negative skin prick and specific IgE testing, and predominant eosinophils on nasal smears.

She was counseled about her diagnosis with proper education to stress the importance of avoiding any irritants that may trigger her symptoms. Intranasal corticosteroids (INCS) were continued and she was instructed on the proper technique of administering the medication to maximize the benefit. Azelastine nasal spray was also prescribed in conjunction with the nasal corticosteroid for the relief of local symptoms based on its clinical effect in nonallergic rhinitis and studies showing a synergistic benefit with INCS [11, 12]. Loratadine 10 mg was replaced with chlorpheniramine 4 mg daily to decrease drainage.

Discussion

Chronic rhinitis affects upward of 70 million individuals in the United States making it one of the most prevalent medical disorders in the country [13]. An estimated 44–87% of people with rhinitis have mixed rhinitis, a combination of allergic and nonallergic rhinitis [14]. Rhinitis can generally be divided into allergic rhinitis (AR) and nonallergic rhinitis (NAR). Allergic rhinitis can follow a perennial or seasonal pattern induced by well-defined indoor and outdoor aeroallergens. Nonallergic rhinitis may be infectious, such as that caused by viruses, bacteria, or other microbial organisms, or it may be nonallergic/noninfectious induced by weather changes such as temperature or barometric pressure and a spectrum of odorants and irritants [15]. Patients that manifest symptoms in response to allergic and nonallergic triggers are referred to as having mixed rhinitis [13].

Chronic nonallergic rhinitis is defined by nasal symptoms such as obstruction, sneezing, and anterior or posterior rhinorrhea that occur in relation to nonallergic, noninfectious triggers such as weather or temperature changes, exposure to caustic odors or cigarette smoke, barometric pressure differences, and others [14]. It tends to be adult onset, with the typical age of

presentation between 30 and 60 years; however, children can also have NAR [16]. Historically, NAR variants have been divided into two groups based on nasal cytology: NAR with eosinophilia syndrome (NARES) and non-NARES. However, nasal cytology is rarely performed in clinical practice today due to issues with reproducible sample collection methodologies [16]. Nonallergic rhinitis can also be classified into two broad categories—inflammatory and noninflammatory—that can be differentiated by nasal swab or biopsy [17]. Based on anatomy, a third category has also been reported as structurally related rhinitis. This includes patients with nasal septal deviation, turbinate deformity, nasal valve dysfunction, neoplasms, foreign body, choanal atresia or stenosis, adenoid hypertrophy among other conditions [18].

It is postulated that NAR results from abnormalities in the autonomic nervous system of the nose including adrenergic, cholinergic, and/or nonadrenergic, noncholinergic innervation. These abnormalities have been reported in both inflammatory and noninflammatory forms of rhinitis. However, they are most predominant in the noninflammatory form [17]. The dysautonomia results in diminished sympathetic activity with or without parasympathetic overactivity and altered expression or activity of transient receptor potential (TRP) channels which are calcium ion channel receptors that are present at peripheral nerve terminals [13, 17]. TRP vanilloid 1 (TRPV1) and TRP Ankyrin 1 (TRPA1) are of particular note as they play a major role in transmitting the neural stimuli that trigger symptoms. When autonomic nerves fibers are exposed to inflammatory mediators, the G-coupled receptors activate kinase and phospholipase systems that prime TRPV1. Priming of TRPA1 is currently less defined. Once primed, TRP receptors become more susceptible to activation by endogenous and exogenous compounds, leading to calcium influx, depolarization, and active release of neurotransmitter. This process comprises the major component of neurogenic inflammation [17]. The topical antihistamine azelastine was found to activate TRPV1 receptors in in vitro studies and with continuous exposure can desensitize receptors. The inflammatory form of NAR is further divided into eosinophilic and non-eosinophilic. Nasal biopsies commonly show increased eosinophils, mast cells, and mast cell degranulation. These histologic findings may be associated with different clinical manifestations. For example, predominant eosinophilia may indicate increased responsiveness to glucocorticoids, whereas mast cell predominance may be associated mainly with nasal pruritus [17].

Noninflammatory NAR can be further classified into nine subtypes: drug-induced rhinitis (including rhinitis medicamentosa), gustatory rhinitis (rhinorrhea associated with eating), hormonal induced rhinitis, infectious rhinitis, NARES, occupational rhinitis, senile rhinitis, atrophic rhinitis, and vasomotor rhinitis (VMR) [16].

The symptoms and physical exam of AR and NAR can overlap and therefor these two rhinitis subtypes may appear very similar clinically. Although the diagnosis of AR and NAR is mainly clinical, blood or skin allergy testing may be utilized to both support and differentiate between these two disorders. Distinguishing features of AR and NAR are summarized in Table 7.1.

The diagnosis of NAR is based on a history consistent with NAR such as the development of symptoms in response to odorant and irritant triggers in the absence of an allergic etiology. The most common diagnostic tests used to distinguish allergic from nonallergic rhinitis are percutaneous skin tests and allergen-specific IgE antibody testing, both of which are negative in NAR. Less commonly utilized tests are nasal provocation test, nasal cytology, nasolaryngoscopy, and intracutaneous skin testing [13, 19]. Skin testing involves introducing controlled amounts of allergen into the epidermis. It yields rapid results and is convenient, safe, and widely accepted. IgE-mediated diseases such as AR involve both an immediate response caused by the release of constitutive mast cell and basophil mediators such as histamine, and a late response due to the production of newly formed mediators such as leukotrienes and chemokines 4–8 h later [19].

Allergen-specific IgE antibody testing is highly specific and correlates well with skin prick

Table 7.1 Distinguishing features of allergic and nonallergic rhinitis[a]

Nonallergic rhinitis	Allergic rhinitis
More common after age 20	Presents in childhood
No familial pattern	Family history of atopy
More common in females	Affects males and females equally
Mostly perennial with little seasonal variation	Seasonal variation common
Negative skin and /or serum IgE testing	Positive skin and/or serum IgE testing
Broad range or irritants	Mainly aeroallergen triggers
Symptoms: • Nasal congestion, sneezing, rhinorrhea • Postnasal drainage with or without cough • Infrequent eye symptoms • Minimal itching • More headaches • Eustachian tube dysfunction	Symptoms: • Nasal: congestion, sneezing, rhinorrhea and nasal itch • Ocular: conjunctivitis, watering and itch
Physical examination: • Mucosa can be normal, erythematous, or atrophic, with increased watery secretions • Mucosa may also be boggy and edematous similar to that in allergic rhinitis	Physical examination: • Mucosa may be boggy, pale, and edematous • Allergic shiners

[a]Adapted from [13]

testing. Intracutaneous testing is used in situations where patients have a negative prick skin test but a compelling history of an allergy to the suspected allergen. Specific IgE testing is useful if percutaneous testing is not practical due to lack of expertise by the clinician or if the patient is taking a medication that interferes with skin testing (tricyclic antidepressants or antihistamines) [19]. It is also preferred over skin testing when the risk of severe allergic reaction is high, and in those patients with skin conditions or dermatographia which might interfere with skin testing [13, 17]. IgE might also be locally produced referred to as localized reAR, which can be detected by nasal response to allergen-specific nasal challenge [17]. For NAR, imaging is not generally required unless structural issues are suspected or in situations where treatment is not effective.

Several comorbidities and complications are associated with chronic rhinitis such as acute and chronic sinusitis, headaches, worsening asthma, chronic cough secondary to postnasal drip, acute and chronic otitis media, eustachian tube dysfunction, sleep apnea, and decreased quality of life [13]. Managing NAR consists of avoidance of triggers in combination with medical and surgical treatments. Avoidance is not as effective for NAR as it is for AR although avoiding respiratory irritants such as strong odors (soap, paint, and perfumes) and air pollutants (fumes and tobacco smoke) is recommended for patients who find that exposure to these irritants worsens their symptoms [14]. Figures 7.1 and 7.2 summarize the classification and treatment of allergic and nonallergic rhinitis, respectively.

Corticosteroids

Nonallergic rhinitis is generally less responsive to medical treatment conventionally used to treat AR. A combination of INCS and topical antihistamine (azelastine or olopatadine) is probably the

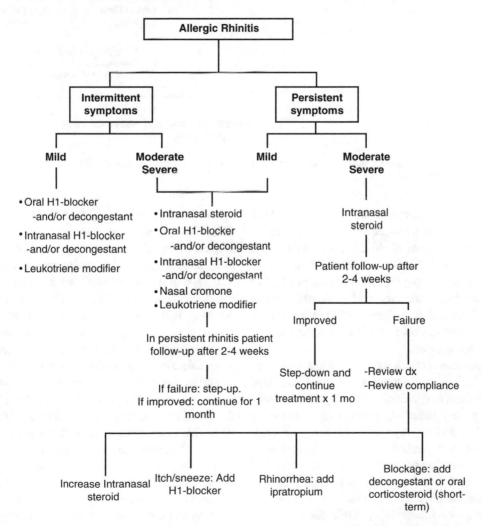

Fig. 7.1 Algorithmic considerations for pharmacologic treatment of allergic rhinitis. Reprinted from [20] with permission from Elsevier

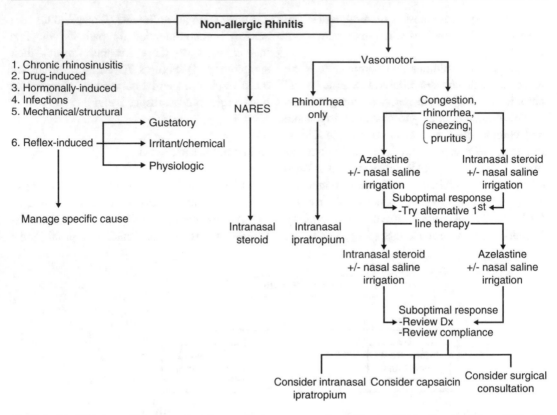

Fig. 7.2 Algorithmic considerations for pharmacologic treatment of nonallergic rhinitis. Reprinted from [20] with permission from Elsevier

most effective treatment for NAR to date [17]. Intranasal corticosteroids are most useful in the inflammatory form of NAR but have been found to be clinically effective in studies for NAR overall as a treatment [17, 20]. Patients need to be informed that it takes up to 48–72 h before INCSs take effect and symptoms start to improve [14]. For this reason, using INCSs as needed day to day is not advised.

Intranasal corticosteroids decrease inflammation mainly by decreasing arachidonic acid metabolism and reducing the degree of inflammatory cell infiltrate, particularly eosinophils [21]. The INCSs, especially the currently available second-generation agents (mometasone furoate, fluticasone propionate, ciclesonide, and fluticasone furoate), are considered generally safe and have favorable pharmacokinetic characteristics that minimize systemic bioavailability (<1%) compared to older INCS and oral CS

agents, thus minimizing systemic adverse effects [22]. The Food and Drug Administration has also labeled budesonide nasal spray as a Category B drug, indicating its safety during pregnancy [23]. The intranasal corticosteroids are associated with various topical side effects, affecting 5–10% of patients. These include nasal dryness, burning, hoarseness, sneezing, and aftertaste. Other less common side effects include headache, nausea, local infection (especially *Candida albicans*), epistaxis, and nasal septal perforation. Some of the topical adverse effects of INCSs are directly the result of poor technique of drug administration, which further emphasizes the importance of patient education on the proper use of these agents. Techniques for ensuring proper delivery of an INCS are to use the contralateral hand for each nostril, avoid applying pressure on the nasal septum, and direct the spray towards the ipsilateral ear for maximal effect.

Antihistamines

Nonsedating second-generation H1 antihistamines are not as effective in NAR compared with AR largely because the mechanistic pathways are neurogenic rather than histaminergic [17]. However, first-generation antihistamines may have some therapeutic benefit due to their anticholinergic activity which is helpful for drying up postnasal drainage. Due to the sedating side effects of first-generation antihistamines, they are not often used as first-line treatment for AR but for NAR may be necessary and if they are used should be dosed at bedtime. Topical antihistamines have also been found to be very effective in the treatment of NAR. Azelastine has shown to be more efficacious than olopatadine for treating NAR and is often combined with INCS such as fluticasone for further control of symptoms [11, 14].

Decongestants

There is lack of evidence for the benefit of decongestants [20]; thus, they should be considered as adjunctive therapy for NAR mainly to relieve nasal congestion [14, 17]. Oral decongestants can be considered for use of controlling nasal congestion not responsive to the use of INCS, topical antihistamines, or a combination of both [17]. However, these agents have many intolerable side effects such as tachycardia, insomnia, increased blood pressure, and in some cases thromboembolic events. Thus it is recommended to use these agents with caution and to review potential side effects with patients prior to starting. Intranasal decongestants may cause rebound congestion when used for extended periods of time. However, recent studies have found that when they are used in conjunction with an INCS agent they can be used for an extended period of time without development of rhinitis medicamentosa. Evidence has demonstrated that INCS prevent downregulation of alpha-adrenergic receptors, thereby preventing tolerance [20, 24, 25].

Anticholinergic

Intranasal ipratropium bromide spray is recommended when rhinorrhea is the main symptom. It is primarily indicated for gustatory rhinorrhea and rhinorrhea due to cold exposure [14, 17]. It can be used in conjunction with INCS and/or intranasal antihistamines for the treatment of anterior or posterior rhinorrhea [14].

Nasal Saline Lavage

Nasal saline lavage has been found to have modest effect in selected patients [14, 17]. It is best performed prior to INCS or azelastine use so that secretions are cleared prior to application of medications [14] Saline lavage significantly improves nasal symptoms including congestion [17]. It is hypothesized that this improvement might result from increasing mucociliary function, decreasing mucosal edema and inflammatory mediators, as well as clearance of inspissated mucus and exogenous inflammatory or irritant triggers [26].

Capsaicin

Capsaicin use for the treatment of NAR is still investigational; however, there is mounted evidence that intranasal application of this homeopathic agent is effective in NAR [25, 27]. It is believed to have a role in desensitization of TRPV1 ion channels and depletion of neuropeptide mediators such as substance P, thus decreasing nasal hyperreactivity [14, 17].

Surgery

Surgical management is reserved for select recalcitrant cases of NAR, mainly when patients fail 6–12 months of medical therapy. Surgery can be considered in the presence of surgically correctable comorbidities such as nasal obstruction due to nasal septal deviation, inferior turbinate or adenoid hypertrophy, or refractory sinusitis due to osteomeatal complex disease.

Clinical Pearls and Pitfalls

- Chronic rhinitis is one of the most prevalent medical disorders in the United States that can lead to recurrent sinusitis if not diagnosed and treated properly.
- Chronic rhinitis can be allergic or nonallergic.
- Diagnosis of NAR is mainly clinical and supported by negative skin prick or allergen-specific IgE testing.
- A combination of INCS and topical antihistamine is possibly the most effective treatment for NAR.
- First-generation oral antihistamines may be of benefit to some patients due to their anticholinergic effects. Second-generation antihistamines are not as effective for NAR compared with AR.

References

1. Rosenfeld RM, Piccirillo JF, Chandrasekhar SS, Brook I, Kumar KA, Kramper M, Orlandi RR, Palmer JN, Patel ZM, Peters A, Walsh SA, Corrigan MD. Clinical practice guideline (update): adult sinusitis executive summary. Otolaryngol Head Neck Surg. 2015;15:598–609.
2. Van Loon JW, van Harn RP, Venekamp RP, Kaper NM, Sachs AP, Van der Heijden GJ. Limited evidence for effects of intranasal corticosteroids on symptom relief for recurrent acute rhinosinusitis. Otolaryngol Head Neck Surg. 2013;149:668–73.
3. Orlandi RR, Kingdom TT, Hwang PH. International consensus statement on allergy and rhinology: rhinosinusitis executive summary. Int Forum Allergy Rhinol. 2016;6:S3–21.
4. Desrosiers M, Evans GA, Keith PK, Wright ED, Kaplan A, Bouchard J, Ciavarella A, Doyle PW, Javer AR, Leith ES, Mukherji A, Robert Schellenberg R, Small P, Witterick IJ. Canadian clinical practice guidelines for acute and chronic rhinosinusitis. J Otolaryngol Head Neck Surg. 2011;40:S99–193.
5. Peters AT, SS JH, Hamilos DL, Baroody F, Chandra RK, Grammar LC, Kennedy DW, Cohen NA, Kaliner MA, Wald ER, Karagianis A, Slavin RG. Diagnosis and management of rhinosinusitis: a practice parameter update. Ann Allergy Asthma Immunol. 2014;113:347–85.
6. Costa ML, Psaltis AJ, Nayak JV, Hwang PH. Medical therapy vs surgery for recurrent acute rhinosinusitis. Int Forum Allergy Rhinol. 2015;5:667–73.
7. Loftus PA, Lin J, Tabaee A. Anatomic variants of the paranasal sinuses in patients with recurrent acute rhinosinusitis. Int Forum Allergy Rhinol. 2016;6:328–33.
8. Brook I, Frazier EH. Microbiology of recurrent acute rhinosinusitis. Laryngoscope. 2004;114:129–31.
9. Kaper NM, Breukel L, Venekamp RP, Grolman W, Van der Heijden GJ. Absence of evidence for enhanced benefit of antibiotic therapy on recurrent acute rhinosinusitis episodes: a systematic review of the evidence base. Otolaryngol Head Neck Surg. 2013;149:664–7.
10. Bhattacharyya N. Surgical treatment of chronic recurrent rhinosinusitis: a preliminary report. Laryngoscope. 2006;116:1805–8.
11. Banov CH, Liberman P. Efficacy of azelastine nasal spray in the treatment of vasomotor (perennial nonallergic) rhinitis. Ann Allergy Asthma Immunol. 2001;86:28–35.
12. Hampel FCRP, Van Bavel J, Amar NJ, Daftary P, Wheeler W, Sacks H. Double-blind, placebo-controlled study of azelastine and fluticasone in a single nasal spray delivery device. Ann Allergy Asthma Immunol. 2010;105:168–73.
13. Greiwe JM, Jonathan A, Bernstein MD. Nonallergic rhinitis diagnosis. Immunol Allergy Clin N Am. 2016;36:289–303.
14. Tran NP, Vickery J, Blaiss MS. Management of rhinitis: allergic and non-allergic. Allergy, Asthma Immunol Res. 2011;3:148–56.
15. Becker S, Rasp J, Eder K, Berghaus A, Kramer MF, Groger M. Non-allergic rhinitis with eosinophilia syndrome is not associated with local production of specific IgE in nasal mucosa. Eur Arch Otorhinolaryngol. 2016;273:1469–75.
16. Scarupa MD, Kaliner MA. Nonallergic rhinitis, with a focus on vasomotor rhinitis clinical importance, differential diagnosis and effective treatment recommendations. World Allergy Organ J. 2009;2:20–5.
17. Lieberman PL, Smith P. Nonallergic rhinitis: treatment. Immunol Allergy Clin N Am. 2016;36:305–19.
18. Salib RJ, Harries PG, Nair SB, Howarth PH. Mechanisms and mediators of nasal symptoms in non-allergic rhinitis. Clin Exp Allergy. 2008;38:393–404.
19. Quillen DM, Feller DB. Diagnosing rhinitis: allergic vs nonallergic. Am Fam Physician. 2006;73:1583–90.
20. Greiner AN, Meltzer EO. Pharmacologic rationale for treating allergic and nonallergic rhinitis. J Allergy Clin Immunol. 2006;118:985–98.
21. Petty DA, Blaiss MS. Intranasal corticosteroids topical characteristics: side effects, formulation and volume. Am J Rhinol Allergy. 2013;27:510–3.
22. Sastre J, Mosqes R. Local and systemic safety of intranasal corticosteroids. J Investig Allergol Clin Immunol. 2012;22:1–12.
23. Namazy JA, Schatz M. The safety of intranasal steroids during pregnancy: a good start. J Allergy Clin Immunol. 2016;138:105–6.

24. Vaidyanathan S, Williamson P, Clearie K, Khan F, Lipworth B. Fluticasone reverses oxymetazoline-induced tachyphylaxis of response and rebound congestion. Am J Respir Crit Care Med. 2010;182:19–24.
25. Singh U, Bernstein J. Intranasal capsaicin in management of nonallergic (vasomotor) rhinitis. Prog Drug Res. 2014;68:147–70.
26. Nguyen SA, Psaltis AJ, Schlosser RJ. Isotonic saline nasal irrigation is an effective adjunctive therapy to intranasal corticosteroid spray in allergic rhinitis. Am J Rhinol Allergy. 2014;28:308–11.
27. Fokkens W, Hellings P, Segboer C. Capsaicin for rhinitis. Curr Allergy Asthma Rep. 2016;16(8):60.

Chronic Rhinosinusitis with Polyposis: Diagnosis and Treatment

8

Wytske Fokkens

Case Presentation 1

A 47-year-old man presents with a chronic cough and nasal congestion with postnasal drip. His nose is usually relatively open but when eating he has difficulty breathing through his nose. There is usually no rhinorrhea, except when walking outside and at the end of the day. He has associated facial pain that he describes as a pressure over the forehead and behind the eyes. This discomfort is decreased when he takes painkillers. He uses fluticasone propionate nasal spray two puffs BID but does not think this really improves his symptoms. He occasionally rinses his nose with saline but takes no other medication for his nose.

He also has a history of asthma, which requires daily use of salbutamol and formoterol as needed but is on no controller therapy. He has felt poorly the entire winter, like he has a continuous cold. His primary care physician has been treating his worsening asthma with antibiotics (clarithromycin for 3 weeks) and periodic bursts of prednisone (10 mg for 1 week). Occasionally, he takes aspirin or ibuprofen, which does not appear to affect his breathing. He has no other chronic medical problems and does not take other medications.

He does not smoke, and only uses alcohol on occasion, which does not appear to increase his symptoms.

In 2012 he had functional endoscopic sinus surgery (FESS) with suboptimal results.

He completed a *SNOT-22*, which showed a total score of 23 (Table 8.1).

The asthma control questionnaire (ACQ) revealed an average score of 2.3 (Table 8.2).

Nasal endoscopy showed chronic rhinosinusitis with polyposis (CRSwNP) gr 1-2 on the right side and gr 1 on the left side covered with yellow crusts. The ostia to the maxillary sinus were non-obstructed, but the mucosa was clearly thickened. The nasopharynx did not show any abnormalities and during the examination there was no evidence of a postnasal drip. The Eustachian tube openings did not show any abnormalities and the rest of the otolaryngeal examination was also normal.

Skin prick testing showed marginal sensitization to HDM (1+) and Aspergillus (1+).

PNIF: 100 mL/s (normal value >100 mL/s, mean for his length and age: 140 mL/s).

Smell (Sniffin' Sticks Screening 12 Test): 11/12 good (normosmia).

CT sinus: There was full opacification of the frontal sinus bilaterally, and partial opacification of the ethmoids bilaterally with an unobstructed olfactory fossa and infundibulum. The maxillary sinus mucosa was thickened bilaterally and the sphenoid sinus was opacified on the right side and clear on the left. There were no bony defects

W. Fokkens (✉)
Department of Otorhinolaryngology, Academic Medical Centre, Amsterdam, The Netherlands
e-mail: w.j.fokkens@amc.nl

© Springer International Publishing AG, part of Springer Nature 2018
J. A. Bernstein (ed.), *Rhinitis and Related Upper Respiratory Conditions*,
https://doi.org/10.1007/978-3-319-75370-6_8

Table 8.1 SNOT-22, case 1

Item	Score
Need to blow nose	1
Nasal blockage	2
Sneezing	0
Runny nose	0
Cough	4
Postnasal discharge	3
Thick nasal discharge	0
Ear fullness	1
Dizziness	0
Ear pain	0
Facial pain/pressure	2
Decreased sense of smell/taste	3
Difficulty falling asleep	0
Wake up at night	3
Lack of a good night's sleep	2
Wake up tired	1
Fatigue	0
Reduced productivity	0
Reduced concentration	0
Frustrated/restless/irritable	1
Sad	0
Embarrassed	0
Total score	23

or signs of significant ostitis, especially in the frontal sinuses (Fig. 8.1).

Consultation from a pulmonologist confirmed the diagnosis of asthma and prescribed a combination corticosteroid/long-acting bronchodilator inhaler.

Discussion

Diagnostic Approach

Questionnaire Evaluation: We always ask our patients to fill in the SNOT-22 and an asthma questionnaire with general questions on asthma, and the six-item ACQ [1, 2]. These questionnaires provide important information about the patient's QOL and ensure that all relevant questions are asked related to asthma, including assessment of asthma control.

Specifically, the SNOT-22 is a modification of the 31-item RSOM, containing 22 nose, sinus, and general items. The instrument is validated and has been demonstrated to be reliable and easy to use [3].

Table 8.2 ACQ, case 1

On average, during the past week:	
How often were you woken by your asthma during the night?	A few times (2)
How bad were your asthma symptoms when you woke up in the morning?	Moderate symptoms (3)
How limited were you in your activities because of your asthma?	Moderately limited (3)
How much shortness of breath did you experience because of your asthma?	A moderate amount (3)
How much of the time did you wheeze?	A moderate amount of the time (3)
How many puffs of short-acting bronchodilator (e.g., ventolin) have you used each day?	3 ± 4 puffs most days (2)
Average score	2.3

The six-item Asthma Control Questionnaire (ACQ) has been validated to measure the goals of asthma management as defined by international guidelines (minimization of day- and nighttime symptoms, activity limitation, beta(2)-agonist use, and bronchoconstriction). Responses are given on a 7-point scale and the overall score is the mean of the responses (0 = totally controlled, 6 = severely uncontrolled). Patients with a score of under 1.0 are considered controlled and patients with a score over 1.5 are inadequately controlled [4].

Nasal Airway Obstruction Assessment: We routinely obtain a PNIF to objectively check for nasal airway obstruction. PNIF is an inexpensive, fast, portable, and simple technique, which does not depend on computers to analyze the data [5]. PNIF is a modification of the Wright peak flow meter and consists of a face mask which the patient applies over the nose without touching the nose.

It has good reproducibility with a correlation coefficient up to 92%. The PNIF provides a measure of nasal airflow and a direct measure of nasal obstruction which can be used unilaterally with the mouth closed. Patients must be encouraged to inhale as hard and fast as they can through the mask keeping the mouth closed starting from the end of a full expiration. The best of three satisfactory maximal inspirations is usually taken as the PNIF [6]. In patients with chronic rhinosinusitis,

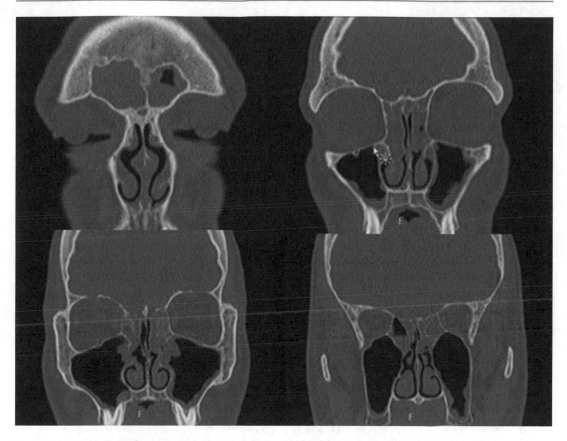

Fig. 8.1 CT scan of case 1

PNIF significantly improves after treatment and has been shown to correlate with the SNOT-22 total score. It also has a moderate-to-strong correlation with nasal obstruction VAS grading during the treatment period [7]. PNIF gives comparable data to acoustic rhinometry and rhinomanometry in healthy and obstructed noses [5, 6].

Allergic Assessment: Skin prick testing should be performed in all patients with CRS, with and without nasal polyps [8]. Although allergic rhinitis is not more prevalent in patients with CRSwNP than in the general population, the symptoms of allergic rhinitis when present do contribute to the patient's overall symptom load and therefore should be prevented as much as possible. Also, when there is a considerable allergic rhinitis component, treatment differs from CRSwNP treatment. For example, patients with allergic rhinitis can be given antihistamines or allergen immunotherapy to improve their symptoms and quality of life (QoL).

Olfactory Testing: For routine smell testing we use the Sniffin' Sticks Screening 12 Test [9]. This test is based on the identification of everyday odors in the scope of a "multiple-forced-choice" method. The time required for the execution and evaluation of the test is between 3 and 4 min. It is important to do objective smell testing as like this patient there is sometimes a discrepancy between subjective and objective smell evaluation. When no objective reduction in smell is observed it is usually difficult to improve the patient's smell with medications such as corticosteroids.

Laboratory Testing: Routine laboratory testing is generally not warranted. However, for patients where disease is not responding to initial treatment laboratory testing depends on unanswered relevant clinical issues. Peripheral eosinophils and total IgE are the most frequent tests obtained.

Radiologic Testing: A CT scan of the sinuses was performed in this patient. CT scanning of the paranasal sinuses is the modality of choice for optimal displaying of air, bone, and soft tissue. However, it should not be regarded as the primary step in diagnosis of the condition, except where there are unilateral signs and symptoms or other sinister clinical signs. Rather a CT scan of the sinuses is obtained to corroborate the patient's history and endoscopic examination after failure of medical therapy. Much attention has recently been given to the radiation exposure associated with CT scans, the use of which have increased 20-fold in the past 30 years. Thus, several protocols have been developed to decrease radiation exposure with comparable or improved resolution [10]. Cone beam technology is becoming increasingly available and is associated with lower radiation exposure than conventional imaging [11, 12].

Final Diagnosis

This is a patient with CRSwNP and asthma. He primarily complains about cough and postnasal drip. His total SNOT-22 score is 23. Nasal endoscopy shows grade 1–2 nasal polyps and purulent crusting. He is not performing saline rinsing adequately and not using optimal medical treatment. There are no signs of serious disease or complications by CT scanning other than confirmation of sinus opacification consistent with nasal polyps. There is no relevant sensitization to aeroallergens. The patient's medical treatment was optimized, which included adding an inhaled corticosteroid to improve his asthma control [13, 14].

Treatment

The patient was advised to start rinsing his nose twice daily with saline supplemented with corticosteroids in the rinsing solution. Treatment with systemic corticosteroids was not recommended because it was felt that the symptoms he was complaining of would not significantly improve with this treatment. It was also discussed with the patient that treatment with systemic antibiotics would not be of significant benefit as this time [15]. A nasal or sinus culture was not performed in our patient and is not routinely done in our patients, which may in part be due to the very low prevalence of antibiotic resistance in the Netherlands [16, 17]. We also did not advise to add other medications other than local corticosteroids to the rinsing solution. We discussed the option of adding xylitol, but this was deferred until response to rinsing with corticosteroid could first be determined. Surgical options involving the ethmoid and frontal recesses were also discussed but it was felt that the chances of significant clinical improvement of his symptoms, especially the PND and cough, were small. The patient felt that the impact of his facial pain/pressure did not sufficiently impact his QoL to warrant surgery prior to first optimizing his medical treatment.

Follow-Up

The patient was seen in follow-up 3 months later. The crusting had mostly resolved and he had grade one nasal polyps bilaterally. He still had occasional facial pain but his cough had significantly improved with the rinsing and inhaled corticosteroids. He was satisfied with his overall care, and it was recommended he continue his current medical treatment.

Discussion About Treatment Options

It has been suggested that patients with a preoperative SNOT-22 score higher than 30 points receive a greater than 75% chance of achieving a clinically relevant decrease of symptoms (MCID >9) and on average obtain a 45% relative improvement in their QoL after ESS but that patients with SNOT-22 score of less than 20 do not experience improved QoL from ESS [18, 19]. Recently an international, multidisciplinary panel of ten experts in CRS using the RAND/UCLA appropriateness methodology has developed a list of appropriateness criteria to offer ESS as a treatment option during management of uncomplicated adult CRS [20]. They recommended having a SNOT-22 score of ≥ 20 in conjunction with persistent relevant CT scan abnormalities after treatment which should include at least 8 weeks of topical corticosteroids and a short course of systemic corticosteroids. These are the minimal threshold criteria required to make ESS a treatment option but do not imply that all patients meeting these criteria require surgery. The decision to perform ESS should be made after an informed patient makes a preference-sensitive decision to proceed with surgery. It is important for the patient to understand which symptoms are likely to improve after surgery (e.g., facial pain) and which symptoms are more difficult to influence (smell, PND). Although there were abnormalities on the sinus CT scan involving primarily the frontal sinus, we did not feel that his limited symptoms of facial pain/pressure warranted a second FESS.

Nasal Irrigation

Nasal saline is used to cleanse the nose, getting rid of purulent mucus and crusts that support the vicious cycle of irritation leading to chronic inflammation leading to increased cellular and mucus debris. Patients with CRSwNP are often incapable of removing this debris out of the sinuses because the chronic inflammation results in impaired mucociliary clearance and obstruction of the sinus ostia.

Although evidence is limited, a Cochrane review on treatment of CRS (with or without polyps) symptoms has reported that high-volume isotonic or hypertonic solution is beneficial even when used as monotherapy [21]. However, there was no difference in benefit of a low-volume (5 mL) nebulized saline spray over intranasal corticosteroids [21].

Several modifications and additions to the nasal saline irrigation have been investigated.

Modern topical corticosteroid therapy does not have systemic side effects, although locally there might be some nasal irritation, dryness of the nasal passages, or epistaxis [22, 23]. Adequate delivery and therapeutic effect depend on several factors. For example, delivery is better after ESS as an ostial size of ≥ 4 mm is required for the irrigation fluid to penetrate into the maxillary sinuses [24].

Distribution of irrigation fluid to obstructed sinuses regardless of the delivery device used is limited (2–3%), with nasal sprays being the least effective of all [21]. Post-surgery rinsing distribution appears to be best with higher volume and positive pressure devices [21]. Sodium hypochlorite (NaOCl) is a well-known disinfecting agent effective against several organisms including *S. aureus* and *P. aeruginosa*. A 0.05% NaOCl-containing saline solution has been found to be significantly more effective than isotonic saline alone in CRS patients [25, 26].

Xylitol has been found to reduce nasal bacterial carriage, and rinsing with 12 mg of xylitol mixed with 240 mL of distilled water results in significant improvement of CRS symptoms compared to saline irrigation alone [27]. Xylitol 5% reduced biofilm biomass, inhibited biofilm formation, and reduced growth of planktonic bacteria (*S. epidermidis*, *S. aureus*, and *P. aeruginosa*) [28].

The idea that surfactants may dissolve biofilms by their potential to reduce water surface tension was tested in a non-randomized open-label trial using nasal irrigations containing baby shampoo and showed 46% subjective symptom improvement [29]. A commercialized version of this product however was later removed from the market because of possible side effects, most notably loss of smell.

In general, nasal rinsing is an important measure in the treatment of CRSwNP and should be incorporated as a supplement to other more disease-specific therapies [30]. At the same time additions to nasal irrigation fluid convert it into more active pharmacotherapy with promising results which has revived interest in the development of more optimal nasal drug delivery techniques [31].

Corticosteroids

Corticosteroids and especially topical nasal corticosteroid are the mainstay of pharmacotherapy for CRSwNP. They directly reduce eosinophil viability and activation as well as indirectly act to decrease the secretion of chemotactic cytokines of nasal and polyp epithelial cells [32].

Biologically, corticosteroids activate intracellular glucocorticoid receptors (GR), of which α and β isoforms exist [33]. The GRα receptor is anti-inflammatory by repressing pro-inflammatory and promoting anti-inflammatory gene transcription [34]. The nose has a rich supply of blood vessels and therefore in the presence of inflammation hyperemia resulting in increased blood flow and microvascular permeability resulting in edema formation can occur very quickly.

Corticosteroid therapy in CRS is used in two modalities, systemic and topical. Systemic therapy makes the drug available throughout the whole paranasal system and is by far the most effective approach but is associated with a much greater risk of systemic side effects like insomnia, weight gain, gastrointestinal disturbance, adrenal suppression, osteoporosis, mood changes, and corticosteroid-induced diabetes mellitus [35–37]. High-volume corticosteroid nasal irrigations are a good option in difficult-to-treat CRS control of disease, reaching 81.3% success control and significant improvement of SNOT-22 and Lund-Kennedy scores [38, 39]. Post-surgery distribution appears to be best with higher volume and positive pressure devices (21). Daily high-volume sinonasal budesonide irrigations fail to produce evidence of HPA axis suppression with prolonged use greater than 2 years [40].

The Cochrane meta-analyses for local corticosteroids in CRS (most studies with NP) show improvement for all symptoms, a moderate-sized benefit for nasal blockage, and a small benefit for rhinorrhea. The risk of epistaxis is increased, but these data included all levels of severity including small streaks of blood which may not be a major concern for patients and is often not clinically relevant. It is unclear from the evidence whether the risk of local irritation is larger when using intranasal corticosteroid compared to placebo. There is little information about the effect of topical corticosteroid therapy on QoL [22]. In another Cochrane review, insufficient evidence was found to suggest that one type of intranasal corticosteroid is more effective than another in patients with CRS (with or without nasal polyps), nor that the effectiveness of a spray differs from an aerosol. There was also insufficient evidence to suggest that the different types of corticosteroid molecules or spray versus aerosol delivery have different effects. In daily practice, the use of high-volume NaCl rinsing with local corticosteroid seems to be most effective and has been shown to be very safe [40].

Clinical Pearls and Pitfalls

- CRS (with or without nasal polyps) patients with a SNOT-22 score of less than 20 do not experience improved QoL from ESS.
- High-volume nasal saline irrigation has an important place in the treatment of CRS.
- Diagnosis and treatment of asthma is an important aspect in the care of CRSwNP patients.

Case Presentation 2

A 61-year-old man was seen in consultation for loss of smell, nasal blockage, rhinorrhea, and postnasal drainage. Approximately 7 years ago, he developed symptoms of obstructive sleep apnea syndrome (OSAS) requiring CPAP. Over the past few months he developed trouble using his CPAP because his nose was so congested. In addition, he has severe asthma with frequent requirement for bursts of systemic corticosteroids. He has aspirin intolerance and 2 years ago had a near-fatal asthma attack when he accidentally took an NSAID for joint pain. He is sensitized to HDM and pollen but not to fungi including Aspergillus species or Alternaria. During the tree season, he has symptoms of sneezing, worsening rhinorrhea, and itchy watery eyes.

His total SNOT-22 score was 40 (for details see Table 8.3).

The patient regularly performs nasal rinses with saline-containing corticosteroids. When he receives systemic corticosteroids for his asthma, he notices that his nasal symptoms become progressively better, as does his sense of smell, although the effect of the latest short course of corticosteroids did not last as long, nor did it yield the magnitude of response he had previously experienced with respect to decreased congestion and improved smell. He sees a pulmonologist for his asthma, and is on maintenance combination inhaled corticosteroid/long-acting beta-2-agonist controller therapy. Previously he had tried montelukast without noticeable improvement in his symptoms. He occasionally uses an oral second-generation antihistamine mainly during the spring pollen season.

Table 8.3 SNOT-22, case 2

Item	Score	Most important items
Need to blow nose	3	
Nasal blockage	4	×
Sneezing	2	
Runny nose	3	
Cough	4	×
Post-nasal discharge	4	
Thick nasal discharge	4	×
Ear fullness	0	
Dizziness	0	
Ear pain	0	
Facial pain/pressure	2	
Decreased sense of smell/taste	5	×
Difficulty falling asleep	2	
Wake up at night	3	×
Lack of a good night's sleep	1	
Wake up tired	0	
Fatigue	1	
Reduced productivity	1	
Reduced concentration	1	
Frustrated/restless/irritable	0	
Sad	0	
Embarrassed	0	
Total score	40	

He has no other medical problems and does not use other medications.

He does not smoke, and drinks two to three glasses of wine every night, which do not appear to impact his symptoms.

Previously he underwent a nasal septoplasty and 4 years ago he underwent FESS to remove nasal polyps. After the surgery, he could not smell but his nasal blockage was completely relieved. In the last 2 years, he has had frequent exacerbations of his CRS that in his opinion cause his asthma exacerbations.

Nasendoscopy confirmed CRSwNP grade 3–4 bilaterally (the polyps do not touch the floor of the nose) (Fig. 8.2). There is watery mucus but the nasopharynx examination was normal without evidence of postnasal drip. The remaining ENT examination including the ears was normal.

Skin prick test showed sensitization to HDM, grass, and tree pollen.

PNIF: 50 mL/s (normal value >100 mL/s).

Smell: (Sniffin' Sticks Screening 12 Test): 3/12 consistent with anosmia.

The *CT scan* of the sinuses (performed after 14 days of prednisone 30 mg daily) still demonstrates almost total opacification of the sinuses but there are no bony defects or signs of significant osteitis including in the frontal sinus (Fig. 8.3).

Diagnosis

This is a patient with aspirin triad which includes CRSwNP, severe asthma (FEV1 66%), and aspirin intolerance also known as NSAID exacerbated respiratory disease (NERD). His total SNOT-22 score was 40. Nasal endoscopy demonstrated grade 3–4 nasal polyps. He has significant symptoms despite using optimal medical treatment and his asthma is deteriorating. The patient requests revision surgery, and it is agreed that this is probably the best option. We performed a full-house FESS including full anterior and posterior ethmoidectomy, infundibulotomy, endoscopic opening of the frontal sinus (Draf IIa), and sphenoid.

Discussion

Nonsteroidal anti-inflammatory drug (NSAID)-exacerbated respiratory disease (NERD), also still referred to as aspirin triad or Samter's triad, is a syndrome of airway inflammation characterized by rhinosinusitis with polyposis, asthma, and nonsteroidal anti-inflammatory drug (NSAID) intolerance [41]. Approximately 9% of patients with CRSwNP will also have aspirin-exacerbated respiratory disease (AERD) making prompt identification, diagnosis, and management of this syndrome important for controlling disease progression [42, 43].

The pathophysiology of CRS is complex and includes local, systemic, microbial, environmental, genetic, and iatrogenic factors. Recognition of the heterogeneity of CRS has promoted the concept that CRS consists of multiple "endotypes," which are defined by distinct pathophysiologic mechanisms that might be identified by corresponding biomarkers.

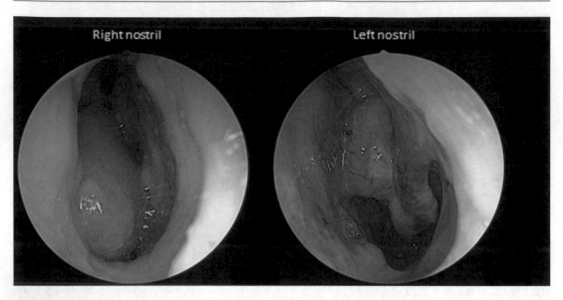

Fig. 8.2 Nasendoscopy view of both sides of the nose

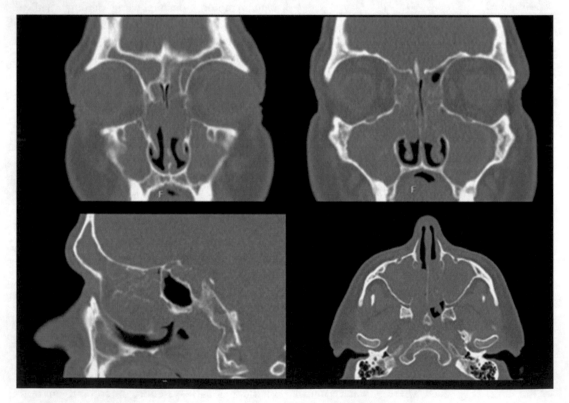

Fig. 8.3 CT scan of case 2

In the past several years, cluster analysis of CRS has shown that this condition like asthma is a complex disease consisting of several disease variants with different underlying pathomechanisms [44–46]. In Europe and the USA most patients with CRSwNP associated with NERD/AERD have a TH2 profile characterized by high eosinophilia and IL-5 levels [44].

Treatment

A full-house FESS including Draf IIa and sphenoidectomy was performed. Fortunately, the frontal sinus contained very thick glue that was able to be completely removed by meticulous rinsing, but there was no evidence of nasal polyps. Postoperatively the patients received 2 weeks of Augmentin and 2 weeks of prednisolone 30 mg per day. Very soon after surgery he again developed significant symptoms of nasal obstruction and loss of smell. Although endoscopy did not reveal any nasal polyps, the entire nasal mucosa was significantly swollen. One year postoperatively he again began to experience CRS exacerbations leading to worsening asthma. At that time the patient's pulmonologist recommended subcutaneous anti-IgE therapy for his asthma. In the months after starting the anti-IgE treatment, swelling of the nasal mucosa noticeably was reduced and the patient could breathe properly through his nose and better tolerate the CPAP even though his smell remained poor. After approximately 2 years his smell became optimal (smell test 8/12) and his CRS and asthma exacerbations subsided. The patient is still on anti-IgE treatment and his upper airway symptoms are minimal. Last year he only had one exacerbation where he needed systemic corticosteroids for his asthma.

Discussion

The evidence related to the effectiveness that different types of sinus surgery versus medical treatment for adults with CRSwNP is better than the other is primarily in the form of patient-reported symptom scores and QoL measurements [47]. Studies showing that more aggressive surgery is more effective are lacking, although there are some studies supporting this approach [48, 49]. Most experienced surgeons indicate that the extent of surgery should be tailored to the extent of the disease. For that reason, a full-house FESS was performed in this revision case.

In revision surgery, the regular anatomical landmarks as taught in basic FESS techniques are usually absent. Therefore, stable anatomical landmarks must be identified and used. A few of these landmarks can always be found even when extensive surgery has been performed earlier. Identifying these landmarks and going from one landmark to the other during revision surgery ensure safety. In revision surgery, it is mandatory to carefully study the CT scan and MRI, if available. Important landmarks to identify in revision surgery are the level of the skull base in relationship to the maxillary sinus roof, lamina papyracea (defects), sphenoid, onodi cells, optic nerve, carotid artery and attachments of septa to it, slope of the skull base and height of the lateral lamella (Keros classification), anterior ethmoid artery (nipple sign), and anatomy of the frontal recess.

It is important to discuss the objective of the surgery with the patient prior to operating. Goals of surgery can be to improve symptoms like nasal obstruction, smell, pain, or rhinorrhea. Often the goal of the surgeon can also be to decrease the amount of diseased mucosa or opening the sinus ostia for local treatment. It is important to discuss the goals of the surgery and expectations of the patient. Certain concepts are especially important that may require extra attention such as emphasizing that surgery is a step in the treatment sequence but that surgery itself seldom results in a CRS cure. When the main goal of the patient is to improve smell, we explain to the patient that traditionally nasal obstruction of the olfactory cleft with nasal polyps has been postulated to be a contributing cause of CRS-associated olfactory loss but the degree of anosmia does not always correlate with the degree of blockage, and therefore removal of polyps does not reliably improve olfaction [50]. If there is a question regarding the possible improvement in smell, initial treatment with a short course of systemic corticosteroids prior to surgery can determine the likelihood of smell improving after surgery [51]. In addition, histologic studies of olfactory mucosa in patients with CRS have demonstrated changes in the olfactory epithelium, and that markers of eosinophils are elevated in the superior turbinate of patients with CRSwNP that correlate with the degree of olfactory loss [52–54].

Another option in the treatment of patients with NERD is aspirin desensitization [55, 56]. Two small studies have shown efficacy of aspirin desensitization with 300–625 mg aspirin daily in patients with

CRSwNP and aspirin intolerance [57, 58]. However, daily intake of lower doses did not change symptomatology or need for surgery [59]. Optimal results of aspirin desensitization have been reported after sinus surgery and reduction of nasal polyposis. Contrary to the indication of cardiology patients requiring low-dose aspirin, we do not routinely offer patients aspirin desensitization mainly because of the risk of serious gastrointestinal (GI) events including GI bleeding, ulcers, and perforation. Furthermore, patients with severe uncontrolled asthma (FEV1 < 70%) are not optimal candidates for this therapy. Only for very aggressive CRSwNP cases that do not react favorably to other treatments and for those patients who do not qualify for biologicals do we discuss the option of aspirin desensitization. However, other centers around the world have different experiences and thresholds for recommending this treatment. Other risk factors for GI ulcer development like advanced age, history of ulcer or GI bleed, and concomitant use of systemic corticosteroids or anticoagulants are carefully taken into account before performing. Co-therapy with a PPI is advised [60].

Despite aggressive surgery, the symptoms and signs of disease recurred quickly in this patient.

Prior to the availability of monoclonal antibodies, we would likely have performed a drill-out procedure of the frontal sinus (Draf III procedure) to reduce inflammatory load [61].

Treatment with Monoclonal Antibodies

Patients with severe CRSwNP, certainly in Europe and the USA, have a TH2-type inflammation consisting of higher total IgE, increased eosinophils, and Th2 cytokines (e.g., IL-5 and IL4/IL-13). The development of monoclonal antibody treatments targeting IgE and TH2 cytokines has rapidly progressed over the last few years, and major advances using these therapies have been reported for the treatment of several allergic diseases including asthma [62].

A number of studies have been performed investigating the effects of the monoclonal antibodies, omalizumab (anti-IgE) [63], mepolizumab (anti-Il-5) [64], reslizumab (anti-Il-5) [65], and dupilumab (IL-4 receptor alpha and interfering with both IL-4 and IL-13 pathways), in CRSwNP patients [66]. All these studies have shown a positive effect on reducing polyp size, and also on improving CT scores [63, 64, 66], symptoms [63, 66], SNOT-22 QOL questionnaire [63, 66], and olfactory testing [63, 66]. These therapies are well tolerated with very limited side effects. Asthma patients in most of these studies also achieved significantly improved pulmonary function and asthma symptom reduction. In most countries omalizumab and mepolizumab are now approved for treating patients with severe asthma. In the future, biomarkers may allow us to personalize patient care by identifying which patient endotype would respond best to one monoclonal therapy over another resulting in substantially better clinical outcomes with far fewer side effects than present treatment options [67, 68].

Clinical Pearls and Pitfalls

- Phenotyping and endotyping of CRSwNP can result in precision management.
- It is important to discuss with the patient the goals of the surgery prior to operating.
- A trial with short-term systemic corticosteroids may predict whether surgery will have a potential favorable impact on improving smell postoperatively.
- Biologics targeting IgE and TH2 cytokines should be considered in the treatment of patients with severe CRSwNP and asthma.

References

1. Juniper EF, O'Byrne PM, Guyatt GH, Ferrie PJ, King DR. Development and validation of a questionnaire to measure asthma control. Eur Respir J. 1999;14(4):902–7.
2. Juniper EF, Svensson K, Mork AC, Stahl E. Measurement properties and interpretation of three shortened versions of the asthma control questionnaire. Respir Med. 2005;99(5):553–8.
3. Hopkins C, Gillett S, Slack R, Lund VJ, Browne JP. Psychometric validity of the 22-item Sinonasal Outcome Test. Clin Otolaryngol. 2009;34(5):447–54.
4. Juniper EF, Bousquet J, Abetz L, Bateman ED. Identifying 'well-controlled' and 'not well-controlled' asthma using the Asthma Control Questionnaire. Respir Med. 2006;100(4):616–21.

5. Ottaviano G, Fokkens WJ. Measurements of nasal airflow and patency: a critical review with emphasis on the use of peak nasal inspiratory flow in daily practice. Allergy. 2016;71(2):162–74.
6. Ottaviano G, Scadding GK, Coles S, Lund VJ. Peak nasal inspiratory flow; normal range in adult population. Rhinology. 2006;44(1):32–5.
7. Proimos EK, Kiagiadaki DE, Chimona TS, Seferlis FG, Maroudias NJ, Papadakis CE. Comparison of acoustic rhinometry and nasal inspiratory peak flow as objective tools for nasal obstruction assessment in patients with chronic rhinosinusitis. Rhinology. 2015;53(1):66–74.
8. Heinzerling L, Frew AJ, Bindslev-Jensen C, Bonini S, Bousquet J, Bresciani M, et al. Standard skin prick testing and sensitization to inhalant allergens across Europe—a survey from the GALEN network. Allergy. 2005;60(10):1287–300.
9. Hummel T, Sekinger B, Wolf SR, Pauli E, Kobal G. 'Sniffin' sticks': olfactory performance assessed by the combined testing of odor identification, odor discrimination and olfactory threshold. Chem Senses. 1997,22(1):39–52.
10. Hoxworth JM, Lal D, Fletcher GP, Patel AC, He M, Paden RG, et al. Radiation dose reduction in paranasal sinus CT using model-based iterative reconstruction. Am J Neuroradiol. 2014;35(4):644–9.
11. Fakhran S, Alhilali L, Sreedher G, Dohatcu AC, Lee S, Ferguson B, et al. Comparison of simulated cone beam computed tomography to conventional helical computed tomography for imaging of rhinosinusitis. Laryngoscope. 2014;124(9):2002–6.
12. Al Abduwani J, ZilinSkiene L, Colley S, Ahmed S. Cone beam CT paranasal sinuses versus standard multidetector and low dose multidetector CT studies. Am J Otolaryngol. 2016;37(1):59–64.
13. Reddel HK, Levy ML. The GINA asthma strategy report: what's new for primary care? NPJ Primary Care Respir Med. 2015;25:15050.
14. Reddel HK, Bateman ED, Becker A, Boulet LP, Cruz AA, Drazen JM, et al. A summary of the new GINA strategy: a roadmap to asthma control. Eur Respir J. 2015;46(3):622–39.
15. Head K, Chong LY, Piromchai P, Hopkins C, Philpott C, Schilder AG, et al. Systemic and topical antibiotics for chronic rhinosinusitis. Cochrane Database Syst Rev. 2016;(4):Cd011994.
16. Blommaert A, Marais C, Hens N, Coenen S, Muller A, Goossens H, et al. Determinants of between-country differences in ambulatory antibiotic use and antibiotic resistance in Europe: a longitudinal observational study. J Antimicrob Chemother. 2014;69(2):535–47.
17. Goossens H, Ferech M, Vander Stichele R, Elseviers M. Outpatient antibiotic use in Europe and association with resistance: a cross-national database study. Lancet. 2005;365(9459):579–87.
18. Rudmik L, Soler ZM, Mace JC, DeConde AS, Schlosser RJ, Smith TL. Using preoperative SNOT-22 score to inform patient decision for endoscopic sinus surgery. Laryngoscope. 2015;125(7):1517–22.
19. Dessouky O, Hopkins C. Surgical versus medical interventions in CRS and nasal polyps: comparative evidence between medical and surgical efficacy. Curr Allergy Asthma Rep. 2015;15(11):66.
20. Rudmik L, Soler ZM, Hopkins C, Schlosser RJ, Peters A, White AA, et al. Defining appropriateness criteria for endoscopic sinus surgery during management of uncomplicated adult chronic rhinosinusitis: a RAND/UCLA appropriateness study. Rhinology. 2016;54(2):117–28.
21. Chong LY, Head K, Hopkins C, Philpott C, Glew S, Scadding G, et al. Saline irrigation for chronic rhinosinusitis. Cochrane Database Syst Rev. 2016;(4):Cd011995.
22. Chong LY, Head K, Hopkins C, Philpott C, Schilder AG, Burton MJ. Intranasal steroids versus placebo or no intervention for chronic rhinosinusitis. Cochrane Database Syst Rev. 2016;(4):Cd011996.
23. Chong LY, Head K, Hopkins C, Philpott C, Burton MJ, Schilder AG. Different types of intranasal steroids for chronic rhinosinusitis. Cochrane Database Syst Rev. 2016;(4);Cd011993.
24. Harvey RJ, Goddard JC, Wise SK, Schlosser RJ. Effects of endoscopic sinus surgery and delivery device on cadaver sinus irrigation. Otolaryngol Head Neck Surg. 2008;139(1):137–42.
25. Yu MS, Kim BH, Kang SH, Lim DJ. Low-concentration hypochlorous acid nasal irrigation for chronic sinonasal symptoms: a prospective randomized placebo-controlled study. Eur Arch Otorhinolaryngol. 2017;274(3):1527–33.
26. Raza T, Elsherif HS, Zulianello L, Plouin-Gaudon I, Landis BN, Lacroix JS. Nasal lavage with sodium hypochlorite solution in Staphylococcus aureus persistent rhinosinusitis. Rhinology. 2008;46(1):15–22.
27. Weissman JD, Fernandez F, Hwang PH. Xylitol nasal irrigation in the management of chronic rhinosinusitis: a pilot study. Laryngoscope. 2011;121(11):2468–72.
28. Jain R, Lee T, Hardcastle T, Biswas K, Radcliff F, Douglas R. The in vitro effect of xylitol on chronic rhinosinusitis biofilms. Rhinology. 2016;54(4):323–8.
29. Chiu AG, Palmer JN, Woodworth BA, Doghramji L, Cohen MB, Prince A, et al. Baby shampoo nasal irrigations for the symptomatic post-functional endoscopic sinus surgery patient. Am J Rhinol. 2008;22(1):34–7.
30. Giotakis AI, Karow EM, Scheithauer MO, Weber R, Riechelmann H. Saline irrigations following sinus surgery—a controlled, single blinded, randomized trial. Rhinology. 2016;54(4):302–10.
31. Rudmik L, Hoy M, Schlosser RJ, Harvey RJ, Welch KC, Lund V, et al. Topical therapies in the management of chronic rhinosinusitis: an evidence-based review with recommendations. Int Forum Allergy Rhinol. 2013;3(4):281–98.
32. Benson M. Pathophysiological effects of glucocorticoids on nasal polyps: an update. Curr Opin Allergy Clin Immunol. 2005;5(1):31–5.
33. Oakley RH, Sar M, Cidlowski JA. The human glucocorticoid receptor beta isoform. Expression, biochemical properties, and putative function. J Biol Chem. 1996;271(16):9550–9.

34. Grzanka A, Misiolek M, Golusinski W, Jarzab J. Molecular mechanisms of glucocorticoids action: implications for treatment of rhinosinusitis and nasal polyposis. Eur Arch Otorhinolaryngol. 2011;268(2):247–53.

35. Pundir V, Pundir J, Lancaster G, Baer S, Kirkland P, Cornet M, et al. Role of corticosteroids in functional endoscopic sinus surgery—a systematic review and meta-analysis. Rhinology. 2016;54(1):3–19.

36. Head K, Chong LY, Hopkins C, Philpott C, Schilder AG, Burton MJ. Short-course oral steroids as an adjunct therapy for chronic rhinosinusitis. Cochrane Database Syst Rev. 2016;(4):Cd011992.

37. Head K, Chong LY, Hopkins C, Philpott C, Burton MJ, Schilder AG. Short-course oral steroids alone for chronic rhinosinusitis. Cochrane Database Syst Rev. 2016;(4):Cd011991.

38. Kosugi EM, Moussalem GF, Simoes JC, Souza Rde P, Chen VG, Saraceni Neto P, et al. Topical therapy with high-volume budesonide nasal irrigations in difficult-to-treat chronic rhinosinusitis. Brazilian J Otorhinolaryngol. 2016;82(2):191–7.

39. Rawal RB, Deal AM, Ebert CS Jr, Dhandha VH, Mitchell CA, Hang AX, et al. Post-operative budesonide irrigations for patients with polyposis: a blinded, randomized controlled trial. Rhinology. 2015;53(3):227–34.

40. Smith KA, French G, Mechor B, Rudmik L. Safety of long-term high-volume sinonasal budesonide irrigations for chronic rhinosinusitis. Int Forum Allergy Rhinol. 2016;6(3):228–32.

41. Makowska JS, Burney P, Jarvis D, Keil T, Tomassen P, Bislimovska J, et al. Respiratory hypersensitivity reactions to NSAIDs in Europe: the global allergy and asthma network (GA2 LEN) survey. Allergy. 2016;71(11):1603–11.

42. Morales DR, Guthrie B, Lipworth BJ, Jackson C, Donnan PT, Santiago VH. NSAID-exacerbated respiratory disease: a meta-analysis evaluating prevalence, mean provocative dose of aspirin and increased asthma morbidity. Allergy. 2015;70(7):828–35.

43. Rajan JP, Wineinger NE, Stevenson DD, White AA. Prevalence of aspirin-exacerbated respiratory disease among asthmatic patients: a meta-analysis of the literature. J Allergy Clin Immunol. 2015;135(3):676–81.e1.

44. Tomassen P, Vandeplas G, Van Zele T, Cardell LO, Arebro J, Olze H, et al. Inflammatory endotypes of chronic rhinosinusitis based on cluster analysis of biomarkers. J Allergy Clin Immunol. 2016;137(5):1449–56.e4.

45. Wang X, Zhang N, Bo M, Holtappels G, Zheng M, Lou H, et al. Diversity of TH cytokine profiles in patients with chronic rhinosinusitis: a multicenter study in Europe, Asia, and Oceania. J Allergy Clin Immunol. 2016;138(5):1344–53.

46. Lou H, Meng Y, Piao Y, Zhang N, Bachert C, Wang C, et al. Cellular phenotyping of chronic rhinosinusitis with nasal polyps. Rhinology. 2016;54(2):150–9.

47. Rimmer J, Fokkens W, Chong LY, Hopkins C. Surgical versus medical interventions for chronic rhinosinusitis with nasal polyps. Cochrane Database Syst Rev. 2014;(12):CD006991.

48. Shen PH, Weitzel EK, Lai JT, Wormald PJ, Lin CH. Retrospective study of full-house functional endoscopic sinus surgery for revision endoscopic sinus surgery. Int Forum Allergy Rhinol. 2011;1(6):498–503.

49. Jankowski R, Pigret D, Decroocq F, Blum A, Gillet P. Comparison of radical (nasalisation) and functional ethmoidectomy in patients with severe sinonasal polyposis. A retrospective study. Rev Laryngol Otol Rhinol (Bord). 2006;127(3):131–40.

50. Downey LL, Jacobs JB, Lebowitz RA. Anosmia and chronic sinus disease. Otolaryngol Head Neck Surg. 1996;115(1):24–8.

51. Schriever VA, Merkonidis C, Gupta N, Hummel C, Hummel T. Treatment of smell loss with systemic methylprednisolone. Rhinology. 2012;50(3):284–9.

52. Yee KK, Pribitkin EA, Cowart BJ, Vainius AA, Klock CT, Rosen D, et al. Neuropathology of the olfactory mucosa in chronic rhinosinusitis. Am J Rhinol Allergy. 2010;24(2):110–20.

53. Lavin J, Min JY, Lidder AK, Huang JH, Kato A, Lam K, et al. Superior turbinate eosinophilia correlates with olfactory deficit in chronic rhinosinusitis patients. Laryngoscope. 2017;127(10):2210–8.

54. Kern RC. Chronic sinusitis and anosmia: pathologic changes in the olfactory mucosa. Laryngoscope. 2000;110(7):1071–7.

55. Fokkens WJ, Lund VJ, Mullol J, Bachert C, Alobid I, Baroody F, et al. European position paper on rhinosinusitis and nasal polyps 2012. Rhinol Suppl. 2012;(23):3 p preceding table of contents, 1–298.

56. Fokkens WJ, Lund VJ, Mullol J, Bachert C, Alobid I, Baroody F, et al. EPOS 2012: European position paper on rhinosinusitis and nasal polyps 2012. A summary for otorhinolaryngologists. Rhinology. 2012;50(1):1–12.

57. Swierczynska-Krepa M, Sanak M, Bochenek G, Strek P, Cmiel A, Gielicz A, et al. Aspirin desensitization in patients with aspirin-induced and aspirin-tolerant asthma: a double-blind study. J Allergy Clin Immunol. 2014;134(4):883–90.

58. Esmaeilzadeh H, Nabavi M, Aryan Z, Arshi S, Bemanian MH, Fallahpour M, et al. Aspirin desensitization for patients with aspirin-exacerbated respiratory disease: a randomized double-blind placebo-controlled trial. Clin Immunol (Orlando, Fla). 2015;160(2):349–57.

59. Rozsasi A, Polzehl D, Deutschle T, Smith E, Wiesmiller K, Riechelmann H, et al. Long-term treatment with aspirin desensitization: a prospective clinical trial comparing 100 and 300 mg aspirin daily. Allergy. 2008;63(9):1228–34.

60. Baker TW, Quinn JM. Aspirin therapy in aspirin-exacerbated respiratory disease: a risk-benefit analysis for the practicing allergist. Allergy Asthma Proc. 2011;32(5):335–40.

61. Georgalas C, Hansen F, Videler WJ, Long FWJ. Terms results of Draf 3 procedure. Rhinology. 2011;49(2):195–201.

62. Tan HT, Sugita K, Akdis CA. Novel biologicals for the treatment of allergic diseases and asthma. Curr Allergy Asthma Rep. 2016;16(10):70.

63. Gevaert P, Calus L, Van Zele T, Blomme K, De Ruyck N, Bauters W, et al. Omalizumab is effective in allergic and nonallergic patients with nasal polyps and asthma. J Allergy Clin Immunol. 2013;131:110–6.e1.

64. Gevaert P, Van Bruaene N, Cattaert T, Van Steen K, Van Zele T, Acke F, et al. Mepolizumab, a humanized anti-IL-5 mAb, as a treatment option for severe nasal polyposis. J Allergy Clin Immunol. 2011;128:989–95.e1–8.

65. Gevaert P, Lang-Loidolt D, Lackner A, Stammberger H, Staudinger H, Van Zele T, et al. Nasal IL-5 levels determine the response to anti-IL-5 treatment in patients with nasal polyps. J Allergy Clin Immunol. 2006;118(5):1133–41.

66. Bachert C, Mannent L, Naclerio RM, Mullol J, Ferguson BJ, Gevaert P, et al. Effect of subcutaneous dupilumab on nasal polyp burden in patients with chronic sinusitis and nasal polyposis: a randomized clinical trial. JAMA. 2016;315(5):469–79.

67. Muraro A, Fokkens WJ, Pietikainen S, Borrelli D, Agache I, Bousquet J, et al. European symposium on precision medicine in allergy and airways diseases: report of the European Union parliament symposium (October 14, 2015). Rhinology. 2015;53(4):303–7.

68. Muraro A, Fokkens WJ, Pietikainen S, Borrelli D, Agache I, Bousquet J, et al. European symposium on precision medicine in allergy and airways diseases: report of the European Union parliament symposium (October 14, 2015). Allergy. 2016;71(5):583–7.

Rhinitis and Cough

Peter K. Smith

> Love and a cough cannot be hid.
>
> George Herbert (British Poet 1593–1633)

A cough is a complex neurogenic reflex that forms part of the innate protective mechanisms of the airways. The function of coughing is to clear the airways of noxious stimuli (microbes, chemicals, and physical); however, many medical conditions, including those of the upper airways, evoke cough, which in itself may be a major symptom of the particular disease state. This chapter is structured to overview the neural and molecular mechanisms involved in the detection and reaction to stimuli, causes of cough with a focus on upper airway etiologies, and two case studies to contextualize this information.

Case Presentation 1

A 47-year-old non-smoking male presents with a history of mild allergic rhinitis that was previously well controlled with the as-needed use of oral second-generation antihistamines and intranasal corticosteroids. Other medications include over-the-counter antacids. He complains of an 8-week history of cough and postnasal drip. He has some maxillary tenderness and has noticed yellow discolored thick nasal mucus. He has had one course of oral antibiotics (amoxicillin), which lightened the color of the nasal mucus, but

the thick discolored mucus returned. His cough also did not improve on oral antibiotics. He has noticed that cold air and the smell of smoke aggravate his cough. The cough also worsens upon lying down. His wife thinks that dairy products make the cough worse, but ceasing all sources of dairy for 2 weeks did not reduce his cough. Overall, he thinks the cough is worsening. He has experienced several prolonged bouts of severe coughing spasms lasting several minutes resulting in trouble breathing during which he felt like he was going to pass out and in a couple instances like he was going to die. On specific inquiry, his breathing difficulty is more pronounced with deep inspiration than expiration, and the tightness is felt in his throat rather than in his chest. He also notes dysphonia with these episodes. He has tried using his son's albuterol inhaler during these episodes; it appeared to yield partial improvement of his symptoms.

Physical Examination

The patient has allergic conjunctivitis with vascular injection and mucosal hypertrophy of the bulbar conjunctiva. Rhinoscopy revealed moderate edema of the inferior turbinates and of the head of the middle turbinates bilaterally, the latter finding suggestive of an inhalant allergy [1]. There is mucosal hypertrophy manifesting as a pale, edematous cobblestone speckled

P. K. Smith (✉)
Department of Clinical Medicine, Griffith University, Southport, QLD, Australia

© Springer International Publishing AG, part of Springer Nature 2018
J. A. Bernstein (ed.), *Rhinitis and Related Upper Respiratory Conditions*,
https://doi.org/10.1007/978-3-319-75370-6_9

appearance on the turbinates. There is thick mucopurulent discharge in the area of the middle meatus bilaterally. There was no evidence of nasal polyposis. There is no cervical lymphadenopathy. Pharyngeal and indirect laryngeal examination was normal. Chest cavity shape is normal with good air movement, and breath sounds on auscultation were normal.

Investigations

Skin prick testing revealed large reactions to dust mite, birch, ragweed, and timothy grass. Nasal swabs grew a heavy mixed growth of *Streptococcus pneumonia* and *Haemophilus influenzae*, which were sensitive to Augmentin and Cefaclor. CT scan of sinuses confirmed turbinate swelling and revealed thickening of the maxillary and frontal sinuses with the presence of fluid levels. The ethmoid sinuses were opaque. Spirometry showed normal lung function without change after bronchodilators. He did endorse difficulty taking a deep inspiration, which aggravated coughing. His inspiratory loop did not reveal the characteristic inspiratory "chink" observed with vocal cord dysfunction. This does not exclude vocal cord dysfunction but merely indicates the absence of symptoms at the time of evaluation.

Impression

Based on clinical history, this patient would appear to have several conditions that are contributing to his postnasal drip, acute respiratory distress, and cough. He has allergic rhinitis, acute rhinosinusitis (based on EPOS definition of sinusitis symptoms persisting less than 12 weeks) [2], and provisional diagnoses of vocal cord dysfunction (VCD), and gastroesophageal reflux disease. The diagnosis of VCD requires direct laryngeal assessment during an episode, where the vocal cords can be observed to be in a restricted adducted state. Gastroesophageal reflux disease should be further assessed via endoscopy and/or a pH probe if symptoms persist, as acid reflux may stimulate to laryngeal and pharyngeal cough reflexes.

Management

The patient was advised to use nasal saline lavages and a nasal decongestant (oxymetazoline) and nasal steroid spray (fluticasone furoate) but with strict instructions to cease the decongestant spray after 5 days. The patient was counselled that antibiotics and oral corticosteroids could be considered if there was fever or severe facial pain; however, most cases of ARS will resolve without the need for oral antibiotics. Reflux disease was treated with the use of a PPI for 4 weeks to see if the cough improves, and, if not, it was recommended to follow up with a gastroenterologist. The condition of vocal cord dysfunction was explained, and the patient was reassured that although the severe inability to breathe can cause a degree of anxiety, it is not a condition known to cause fatal attacks. Treatment of GERD, allergic rhinitis, and sinusitis improved symptoms and the patient was trained in VCD breathing exercises. The patient was advised to continue use of the intranasal corticosteroid if there were active allergic rhinitis symptoms, and allergen immunotherapy was discussed.

VCD Breathing Exercises

1. Remove yourself from the irritant if possible (such as cold air or smoke).
2. If possible, sit down, and drop the shoulders (to try to encourage the patient to relax).
3. Hold your hands to the diaphragm (making the patient focus on their breathing).
4. Purse your lips and take three short sharp breaths in within a second: "sip-sip-sip" (this focuses breathing to the lips rather than the patient having pharyngeal tension, and short breaths are easier to move air through the adducted vocal cords).
5. Exhale three times slowly through pursed lips: "blow-blow-blow."

6. Repeat five to ten times and the spasm should reduce. Practice this method several times a day so it is automatic when needed.
7. Other alternative methods include a panting form of breathing or simply trying to relax and breathe air in through the nasal airways.

Discussion

The complexity and interrelationship of the nose, sinuses, pharynx, larynx, and reflux disease were reviewed in this case. A summary diagram (Fig. 9.1) illustrates these interrelationships. The patient experienced acute rhinosinusitis, which most likely occurred after a viral infection; allergic upper airway disease possibly further contributed

to impaired sinus ventilation and drainage, resulting in bacterial colonization. Atopy appears to increase the risk of infection and the development of ARS [3, 4]. The use of decongestants and nasal lavages has been reported to be of benefit in reducing ARS symptoms, but not in all studies [2]. EPOS 2012 guidelines indicate that the use of intranasal corticosteroids is helpful in ARS and recommend reserving the use of antibiotics for patients with fever, pain, or invasive sinus disease. Vocal cord dysfunction can be difficult to differentiate from asthma, and up to 40% of cases of VCD will have coexistent asthma. A history and response to VCD breathing exercises help to define the condition; however, if there are persistent symptoms of dysphonia and laryngeal irritation, an otolaryngology examination is

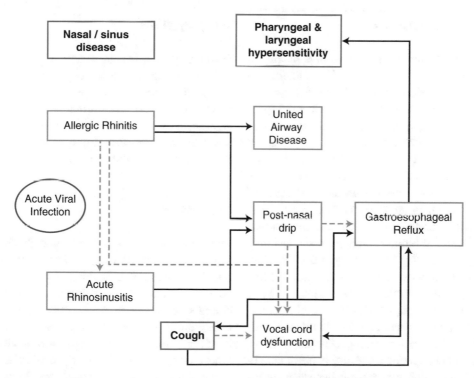

Fig. 9.1 In case 1, the patient develops acute rhinosinusitis on top of mild allergic rhinitis and gastroesophageal reflux disease. Because of allergic airway disease, the patient already has more reactive airways to allergic stimuli from the upper airways to the bronchi. Inflammatory mediators present in the postnasal drip fluid contribute to cough and chemoreceptors in the pharynx and larynx. Both coughing and swallowed mucus increase GER and the acidity of the reflux lowers

the activation threshold of the TRPV1 receptors to chemo-sensation in the larynx and pharynx. Coughing may activate mechanoreceptors in both the lower and upper airways. Obstruction of the upper airways from allergic rhinitis can reduce the warming, filtration, and humidifying functions of the nose, making the pharynx, larynx, and lower airways more vulnerable to exogenous irritants. Solid lines are well-defined entities and dotted lines are speculative in this case required to exclude laryngeal pathology. Acidity from reflux lowers the activation threshold of cough receptors, and reflux has also been reported to possibly contribute to sinusitis as gastric by-products have been found in sinus lavage fluid [5].

Although it is often suspected by patients, there is no evidence to support that cow's milk allergy is causing chronic rhinitis [6]. Caseins in cow's milk protein are quite insoluble and might attach to pharyngeal mucus, increasing the sensation of the mucus, rather than being a cause of mucus secretion. Harvey and colleagues have reported that rhinitis patients who complain of postnasal drip actually are less sensitive to changes in viscosity than healthy controls, so sensitivity is likely due to other factors other than mucus thickening [7].

Case Presentation 2

A 17-year-old female patient with a history of mild asthma and allergic rhinitis experienced a severe bout of viral bronchitis 5 weeks ago. She now has a persistent cough that is triggered spontaneously, but also by strong smells such as solvents and perfume, cold air, and change in temperature. At 2 weeks into the illness, because of ongoing rhinitis, and a dry nonproductive cough, cultures were performed that revealed adenovirus on nasal aspirate. Her chest X-ray was normal, and serology for mycoplasma was negative. A full blood examination showed only mild lymphopenia consistent with a viral infection. She has not experienced fever since the first 4 days of the illness. She was given a 5-day course of prednisolone in addition to the combination long-acting beta-agonist and inhaled corticosteroid spray she was taking. She does not have wheezing but experiences severe bouts of coughing spasms which are causing her sleep disturbance and missed school because the frequent cough was considered disruptive in class. She is an elite swimmer and has not been able to return to the pool, as this environment also appears to aggravate her cough. The cough remains nonproductive and is easily triggered. The only relief that she has obtained is use of cough lozenges. She is also taking non-sedating antihistamines,

cough syrups, acetaminophen, and nonsteroidal anti-inflammatory medications. She is a non-smoker and is not on any other medications. There is a cat in her home, which does appear to aggravate her cough.

Physical Examination

Physical exam reveals frequent staccato bursts of a dry cough with inspiration. Her nasal passages are pale, and the inferior and middle turbinates have pallor and edema. There is abundant nasal mucus. She has allergic-appearing conjunctiva and several small petechial hemorrhages on the bulbar conjunctiva. Her chest shape is normal, and there is good air movement without wheeze.

Investigations

Spirometry was obtained with some difficulty because of the frequent coughing, which prevented the patient from taking a deep breath. However, this test was normal and there was no significant change after a beta-agonist. Skin testing was positive for strong wheat and flare responses to dust mite and cat.

Impression

The patient has allergic rhinitis and also triggers suggestive of nonallergic, noninfectious rhinitis. She has post-viral bronchitis. She was culture positive for adenovirus, a known cause of bronchiolitis obliterans; however, there are noninfectious causes of this condition. She appears to have a low threshold to cough from inhaled irritants known as a "hair-trigger" cough. Her bouts of coughing appear to propagate coughing.

Management

Coughing is likely to be causing mechanosensory cough trigger receptors in the lower airways. Due to viral induced inflammation and allergy the chemical receptors TRPA1 and TRPV1 on sensory nerves are increased. Epithelial inflammation is also going to increase the release of epithelial acetylcholine, which then lowers the threshold of activation of sensory nerves and submucosal mast cells. With sustained and strong stimuli of vagal sensory afferents from the lower airways, a phenomenon of brainstem sensory activation occurs where upper airway afferents can stimulate cough (a "hair-trigger" cough). Management is to exclude active infection, reduce airway inflammation, and reduce sensory neural activation. Allergen avoidance measures for dust mite and cat were discussed, and the use of a dual-agent nasal corticosteroid/antihistamine spray was initiated (fluticasone/azelastine). Her asthma controller therapy was continued. Montelukast 10 mg was added, and she was permitted to continue cough medications. Her mother purchased a cough linctus that contained codeine, which the patient was advised not to take because of the associated risk of developing neuromuscular blocking drug anesthetic allergy [8]. A 5-day course of prednisolone 50 mg was given.

Cough Suppression Exercises

1. If the patient is able to catch their breath between coughs, breathe all the way out and bend forward to "squeeze" as much air as possible from the lungs.
2. Instruct the patient to hold their breath out as long as possible.
3. When ready to breathe in, instruct the patient to take a long slow breath ensuring that air is being inhaled through the nose.
4. Then breathe out—this can be done via the mouth or nose.
5. Continue to inspire through the nose.
6. This exercise should only be done once every few hours.

Reevaluation after 1 week revealed that the patient has some improvement but there was still disruptive coughing and a feeling of ticking in her throat, causing an ongoing cough. Low-dose amitriptyline 25 mg was initiated at bedtime,

which helped reduce her cough. Her sleep immediately and her "hair-trigger" cough abated over 2 weeks, allowing her to return to school and sporting activities. At 4 weeks both montelukast and amitriptyline were discontinued. She continued her asthma combination LABA/ICS and her nasal corticosteroid/antihistamine spray.

Discussion

This case demonstrates four important factors: (1) the united airway disease with upper and lower airways being involved in allergic and inflammatory responses; (2) the threshold for activation of sensory nerves is reduced in the presence of inflammation, and this is recognized to occur to both allergic and nonallergic triggers, heightening neurogenic reflex responses; (3) the nose is critical to warm, filter, and humidify inspired air, and without this function the pharynx, larynx, and lower airways are more reactive to chemical and physical irritants; and (4) neural hyper-receptivity occurs both peripherally and centrally, which may require specific medications to reduce nerve activation.

Montelukast has been reported to be useful in reducing post-viral cough in childhood [9]; however, a recent review in adults did not find an effect [10]. Montelukast does reduce eosinophil activation, and eosinophils are a potent source of nerve growth factor, which increase the expression of TRPV1. Corticosteroids reduce inflammatory responses, and induce apoptosis of inflammatory cells such as lymphocytes and eosinophils, but also have an effect in reducing epithelial acetylcholine production acting as a nerve stabilizer. A tricyclic antidepressant was utilized in this patient which appeared to be the final factor that helped resolve the cough. It can often take several weeks for these types of medications to resolve the central neural activation. This medication has peripheral and central nerve activation. The use of lozenges and cough sweets is interesting—menthol agonizes the TRPA1 receptor but also has effects on the mu opioid and TRPM8 receptors. This possibly "distracts" the TRPA1 receptor's response to more activating compounds, as there is a period of reduced activation after agonist stimulation. Note that TRPA1 activation has "U"-shaped kinetics, meaning there is not a linear response to agonists. Other common rhinitis and cough remedies have actions that are effected via sensory ion channels [11, 12]. Ginger and horseradish also agonize TRPA1. Allicin in garlic agonizes both the TRPA1 and TRPV1 receptors and citric acid (such as in lemon juice) has an agonist action on the TRPV1 receptor but it may also work on acid-sensing ion channels in the upper airways. There is little clinical trial evidence of these products in rhinitis-associated cough, but subjectively patients may feel better and they are low in cost with a very safe profile.

Physiology of Cough

Afferent stimuli for cough can be provoked by mechanical and chemical stimuli that are detected mainly via the vagus nerve and travel to the solitary nucleus of medulla oblongata in the brainstem. Projections radiate to the pre-Bötzinger complex and raphe nucleus, which are involved in the cough response. Cough pattern is also regulated by stimuli from the pontine respiratory group, lateral tegmental field, and deep cerebellar nuclei [13, 14]. The ability to consciously suppress cough indicates a degree of cortical control of the reflex; however, forced coughing does not seem to activate the aforementioned medullary centers [15].

The motor component of cough is a coordinated contraction of the diaphragm (phrenic nerve) and external intercostal muscles (segmental intercostal nerves) that is synchronized from the nucleus retroambiguus, and the glottis (recurrent laryngeal nerve), which is directed from the nucleus ambiguus. These efferent effectors combine to increase the pressure within the lower airways. The vocal cords and glottis then relax and air is expelled at up to 160 km (100 miles) an hour, helping to clear irritants.

Most information on cough receptors has been obtained from animal models rather than from humans [15]. There is significant heterogeneity of afferent receptors, but in a broad classification mechanical and chemical types of receptors are recognized [15]. Within the mechanosensors, there are two types of low-threshold receptors: the slow-adapting receptors and rapid-adapting receptors that are activated by light touch, inspiration, and bronchospasm. Slow-adapting receptor activation can reduce cholinergic activation of bronchial smooth muscle, decreasing airway tone [16]. Generally, low-threshold receptors do not become activated with chemical stimuli unless there is mechanical distortion of the nerve terminal (that might occur in processes that cause mucosal inflammation or injury), alteration in smooth muscle tone, or mucus production [17, 18]. Mechanosensors are distributed throughout the lower airways, but vagal afferents, which influence cough, are also present in the pharynx, larynx, external auditory canal (the basis of the Arnold reflex where light touch of the external auditory canal can induce cough), paranasal sinuses, and cardiac and esophageal branches from the diaphragm [18]. The majority of mechanoreceptors signal via alpha-delta fibers; however, chemical stimuli can also signal via these types of nerves [19]. The above sensory centers, their stimuli, and motor response elements are summarized in Fig. 9.2. This figure introduces the effect of multiple stimuli causing cough hypersensitivity [20].

The majority of cough receptors in the airways are chemoreceptors [21, 22]. The predominant chemosensitive receptor is the transient receptor potential vanilloid receptor (TRPV1), which is sensitive to acid, heat, capsaicin, and several other exogenous compounds [21]. TRPV1 ion channels are predominantly expressed on unmyelinated C-fibers but also are expressed in alpha-delta fibers, and co-localize with neuropeptides such as substance P, calcitonin gene-related peptide, and nerve growth factor receptor [22]. Many endogenous mediators such as histamine, bradykinin, and eicosanoids that are produced with allergic and inflammatory airway disease lower the threshold for activation of TRPV1 to agonists [12, 13, 23]. It is also worthwhile to note that agonist signals can be cumulative. Clinically we see this with acid reflux

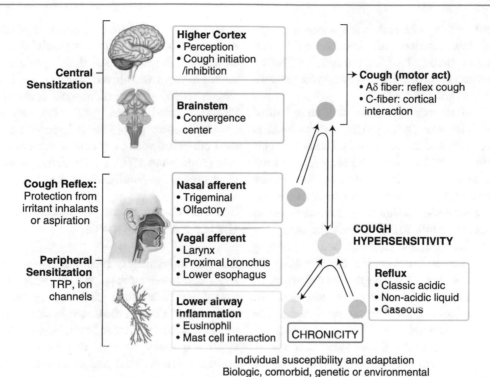

Fig. 9.2 Cough sensors, brainstem, and higher center involved in cough and motor response elements. Adapted from [20]

disease—where the activation threshold of the TRPV1 to stimulant such as capsaicin or temperature is reduced in the presence of gastric acid [24, 25].

There are several other types of sensory ion channels that populate airway sensory nerves including the transient receptor ankyrin one receptor (TRPA1) [24–28], the two pore domain potassium channels [29], acid-sensing ion channels [30, 31], and the ATP ligand-gated purinoreceptors [32, 33]. These receptors combine to provide an alert-and-response mechanism to exogenous and endogenous chemicals, and mechanical and thermal stimuli.

TRPV1 is increased in the airways of patients with chronic cough, which is reflected by increased sensitivity to capsaicin, and this sensitivity decreases with resolution of cough [34, 35]. TRPA1 is also reported to be important in cough responses as many of the ligands that bind to it such as cold air and components of smoke (such as acrolein) agonize it to cause cough [36]. Both TRPV1 and TRPA1 receptors have increased

expression on sensory nerves with inflammation, particularly as a result of nerve growth factor (NGF) [37–39]. The main source of NGF in humans is eosinophils, so allergic airway inflammation can increase receptors involved in cough afferent signalling [40]. The neurotrophins released locally as a response to TRPV1 or TRPA1 ion activation can cause chemotaxis and activation of eosinophils, so an amplification loop can occur at this level [41]. TRPV1 expression also increases in the presence of tumor necrosis factor (TNF) [42]. Both TRPA1 and TRPV1 ion channels induce activation of the MUC5 gene, a major gene involved in the production of mucus [43].

All epithelium, including that in the airways, engages innate and adaptive immune responses by damage- and pathogen-associated molecular pattern molecules (DAMPs, PAMPs) and alarmins [44]. Pro-allergic mediators including IL-33, IL-25, and TSLP can engage pro-allergic responses [45]. TSLP directly appears to activate the TRPA1 receptor on sensory nerves providing a rapid warning of threat in the presence of epithelial inflammation [46]. Inflamed epithelium can be a source of TNF that can increase TRPV1 expression and reduce the threshold for sensory nerve activation [42, 47].

It is often underappreciated that up to half of the acetylcholine (ACh) produced in the body is from non-epithelial sources [48]. The airway epithelium secretes pico-liter concentrations at the basal aspect which helps to stimulate sensory nerves and, at low levels, ACh stabilizes submucosal mast cells, making them more resistant to degranulation [49, 50]. With epithelial injury, the level of acetylcholine increases, both stimulating sensory nerves and lowering the threshold for activation and also lowering the activation threshold for mast cells to allergic stimuli [49, 50]. Glucocorticoids reduce the release of acetylcholine from epithelial cells [51]. Acetylcholine can induce cough via activation of nicotinic receptors [52] and lowers the activation threshold for TRPV1 and TRPA1 [53]. Note that bothTRPV1 and nicotinic ACh receptors are heavily co-expressed in vagal sensory neurons [53]. Acetylcholine is also produced by leukocytes and is involved in B and T lymphocyte, monocyte, and granulocyte function [54, 55].

A summary illustration of major sensory receptors involved in cough afferents is presented in Fig. 9.3.

Cough Convergence

In addition to the increase in numbers of sensory receptors, and lowered threshold of activation with airway inflammation discussed above, central sensitization has been described. With multiple cough afferents converging to the brainstem and higher centers, there is ongoing activation of the brainstem and higher centers and it has been proposed that this causes a reduced threshold for activation of cough by stimuli that would not normally cause a cough [15, 16, 56, 57]. Under these conditions, otherwise innocuous upper airway stimuli such as cold air, singing, or laughing can induce a cough [58], a so-called hair-trigger cough. Higher centers are involved in suppres-sion of cough, and there may be a lack of control of suppression of cough in some individuals with chronic cough [16, 20]. Another important study related to vagal stimuli and upper airway inflammation found that esophageal acid stimuli increased nasal mucus production and nasal symptom scores [59]. This is important as acid can both activate cough by acid-sensing ion channels (ASIC) and TRPV1 stimulation as well as via central neurogenic mechanisms [31].

United Airway Disease

A strong inflammatory relationship between the upper and lower airways was elegantly demonstrated by Braunstahl and colleagues, who showed that allergen challenge in the nasal airways increased cellular inflammation in both the upper and lower airways, and local bronchial challenge caused local and nasal inflammation, as well as increasing eosinophil activation in the peripheral blood [60–63]. The clinical importance of this association is that if there is upper airway inflammation, it is likely that the lower airways will also become inflamed and induce sensitization and activation of chemical and mechanical cough receptors via the above-described mechanisms.

Cough in Disease

A triad of asthma, rhinitis, and gastroesophageal reflux should be thought about in patients with chronic cough; however, not all patients with these conditions alone or in combination will have cough [20]. The American College of Chest Physicians has excellent guidelines on the causes, investigation, and management of cough [64]. Causes of cough involving the lower airways and non-respiratory causes of cough require consideration. Viral and bacterial infection of the airways will induce inflammation and mechanical receptor stimulation (more so in the lower airways), and epithelial and leucocyte mediators result in activation of chemical receptors throughout the airways to either cause cough or to reduce

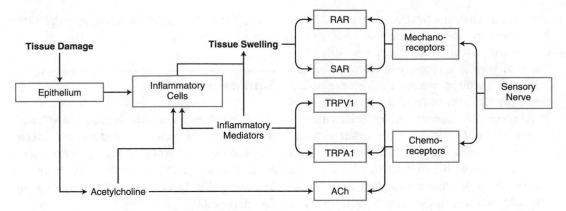

Fig. 9.3 Schematic diagram of key mechanisms in activation of sensory neural receptors and sensory nerves involved in cough. Epithelial injury (usually from infective or inflammatory sources) results in the recruitment of inflammatory cells. Alarmins including acetylcholine activate inflammatory cells, and acetylcholine also primes and/or activates sensory nerves. Inflammatory mediators either activate TRPA1 or TRPV1 directly or lower their threshold for activation. Tissue swelling and process of coughing can activate mechanoreceptors. Not shown because of complexity of image: Acid reflux also lowers TRPV1 activation threshold. Neuromediators such as substance P and calcitonin gene-related peptide are released by axon reflexes, which contribute to cellular inflammation and reduced neuronal activation threshold

the threshold for cough receptors in response to normal stimuli. Convergence of allergic airway disease requires consideration. The act of coughing increases reflux, and reflux induces coughing. Hyperinflation of the airways in asthma increases reflux, and beta-agonists used in the treatment of asthma and cough also reduce lower esophageal sphincter tone and further increase reflux [65].

Both allergic and nonallergic rhinitides are associated with cough. Both conditions can coexist as mixed rhinitis; therefore, not addressing a nonallergic rhinitis component can be a cause of "medical failure" in allergic rhinitis. Postnasal drip stimulates cough, but this is from laryngeal irritation rather than aspiration unless the patient is unconscious. Rhinosinusitis can be associated with cough, and in pediatric cases cough can be the major presenting symptom [2], along with rhinorrhea, nasal congestion, and postnasal drip [66]. In contrast, GERD can cause laryngeal reflux and an inflammatory bronchitis and laryngitis.

Other specific causes of rhinitis related to cough can include gustatory rhinitis, senile rhinitis, exercise, and medications. Cough and rhinitis can be a feature of systemic illness such as Wegener's granulomatosis (other nasal symptoms include nosebleeds, crusting, sinusitis, and congestion) and may precede lung symptoms. Ciliary dysmotility may also present with cough. More detailed causes of rhinitis, their investigation, and management are detailed in other chapters.

Management of Cough and Rhinitis

If the cough and rhinitis appear to worsen around irritants such as smoke or chemicals, reduce exposure where possible. Smokers should stop smoking and counselling for cessation should be provided. The upper airways have the physiological role to warm, filter, and humidify the air for respiration [67]. If the upper airway is obstructed, this normal physiology is compromised and cough threshold to irritants becomes lower. In acute cough where rhinitis is predominant, the clinician should investigate for infection including testing for respiratory viruses and pertussis. The American Academy of Chest Physicians indicates that subacute cough, in the absence of infection, should be managed like a chronic cough [64]. In patients with chronic cough, empiric first-line treatment of the common causes of cough such as asthma, gastroesophageal reflux disease (GERD) , and upper airway disease is appropriate, and these treatments can be additive. It is important to emphasize that treatment of GERD with antiacid treatments may still allow reflux of pepsin, a proteolytic enzyme that can irritate epithelium; therefore, a barrier reflux treatment may also be required. Progress should be reviewed and unsuccessful treatments discontinued. In the treatment of the upper airways, larger volume sinus lavages (>150 mL) may help chronic rhinosinusitis [68]. As opioids work via the mu and kappa opioid receptors, codeine can also help reduce cough thresholds [69]. There has been a link between use of pholcodine and risk of subsequent neuromuscular blocking agents causing anaphylaxis, which has led to the discontinuation of this medication for the treatment of cough [8]. Several compounds used in herbal and home remedies for rhinitis and cough influence neural sensitivity. Menthol is an agonist for the TRPA1 and can induce decreased signalling [70]. It also has effects on the kappa opioid receptor [71]. It is important to note that there is a bimodal effect on TRPA1 when stronger concentrations are used, which can cause irritation [72]. Capsaicin helps in the management of nonallergic rhinitis via desensitization of overexpressed TRPV1 ion channels but has not been as effective for allergic rhinitis [73]. Garlic and honey have antibacterial effects [74]; however, an ingredient in garlic called allicin has agonist effects on both TRPV1 and TRPA1 ion channels [11]. The TRPV1 ion channel is heat sensitive, so use of antipyretics may help increase the cough threshold in the febrile patient, but paradoxically nonsteroidal anti-inflammatory medications and aspirin can cause rhinitis and cough in some susceptible individuals.

In addition to targeting possible reflux and rhinitis, medications and treatments specific to reducing neural sensitivity are important in the management of severe cough associated with rhinitis. The tricyclic antidepressant amitriptyline at 10 mg has been shown to be superior to codeine in a post-viral neural hypersensitivity cough [75]. Gabapentin also has demonstrated efficacy in chronic cough [76] by reducing cough frequency and severity and improving quality of life. Speech therapy may be helpful in teaching cough suppression exercises [77].

Summary

Cough associated with rhinitis often is associated with neural hypersensitivity and reduced threshold of activation, but other disease processes such as GERD and asthma may also be involved. Treatment of only one condition can result in the failure of resolving the cough.

References

1. Hamizan AW, Christensen JM, Ebenzer J, Oakley G, Tattersall J, Sacks R, et al. Middle turbinate edema as a diagnostic marker of inhalant allergy. Int Forum Allergy Rhinol. 2017;7(1):37–42. https://doi.org/10.1002/alr.21835.
2. Fokkens WJ, Lund VJ, Mullol J, Bachert C, Alobid I, Baroody F, et al. EPOS 2012: European position paper on rhino-sinusitis and nasal polyps 2012. A summary for otorhinolaryngologists. Rhinology. 2012;50(1):1–12. https://doi.org/10.4193/Rhino50E2.
3. Mbarek C, Akrout A, Khamassi K, Ben Gamra O, Hariga I, Ben Amor M, et al. Recurrent upper respiratory tract infections in children and allergy. A cross-sectional study of 100 cases. Tunis Med. 2008;86(4):358–61.
4. Ulanovski D, Barenboim E, Raveh E, Grossman A, Azaria B, Shpitzer T. Sinusitis in pilots of different aircraft types: is allergic rhinitis a predisposing factor? Am J Rhinol. 2008;22(2):122–4.
5. Southwood JE, Hoekzema CR, Samuels TL, Wells C, Poetker DM, Johnston N, et al. The impact of pepsin on human nasal epithelial cells in vitro: a potential mechanism for extraesophageal reflux induced chronic rhinosinusitis. Ann Otol Rhinol Laryngol. 2015;124(12):957–64. https://doi.org/10.1177/0003489415593556.
6. Pinnock CB, Graham NM, Mylvaganam A, Douglas RM. Relationship between milk intake and mucus production in adult volunteers challenged with rhinovirus-2. Am Rev Respir Dis. 1990;141(2):352–6.
7. Rimmer J, Hellgren J, Harvey RJ. Simulated postnasal mucus fails to reproduce the symptoms of postnasal drip in rhinitics but only in healthy subjects. Rhinology. 2015;53(2):129–34.
8. Brusch AM, Clarke RC, Platt PR, Phillips EJ. Exploring the link between pholcodine exposure and neuromuscular blocking agent anaphylaxis. Br J Clin Pharmacol. 2014;78(1):14–23. https://doi.org/10.1111/bcp.12290.

9. Bisgaard H, Study Group on Montelukast and Respiratory Syncytial Virus. A randomized trial of montelukast in respiratory syncytial virus postbronchiolitis. Am J Respir Crit Care Med. 2003;167(3):379–83.

10. Wang K, Birring SS, Taylor K, Fry NK, Hay AD, Moore M, et al. Montelukast for postinfectious cough in adults: a double-blind randomised placebo-controlled trial. Lancet Respir Med. 2014;2(1):35–43. https://doi.org/10.1016/S2213-2600(13)70245-5.

11. Macpherson LJ, Geierstanger BH, Viswanath V, Bandell M, Eid SR, Hwang S, et al. The pungency of garlic: activation of TRPA1 and TRPV1 in response to allicin. Curr Biol. 2005;15(10):929–34.

12. Nilius B, Appendino G. Spices: the savoury and beneficial science of pungency. Rev Physiol Biochem Pharmacol. 2013;164:1–76. https://doi.org/10.1007/112_2013_11.

13. Widdicombe JG. Neurophysiology of the cough reflex. Eur Respir J. 1995;8:1193–202.

14. Shannon R, Baekey DM, Morris KF, Nuding SC, Segers LS, Lindsey BG. Production of reflex cough by brainstem respiratory networks. Pulm Pharmacol Ther. 2004;17:369–76.

15. Mazzone SB, Cole LJ, Ando A, Egan GF, Farrell MJ. Investigation of the neural control of cough and cough suppression in humans using functional brain imaging. J Neurosci. 2011;31(8):2948–58.

16. Mazzone SB. An overview of the sensory receptors regulating cough. Cough. 2005;1:2.

17. Canning BJ, Reynolds SM, Mazzone SB. Multiple mechanisms of reflex bronchospasm in guinea pigs. J Appl Physiol. 2001;91:2642–53.

18. Mario Polverin M, Francesca Polverino F, Marco Fasolino M, Filippo Andò F, Antonio Alfieri A, De Blasio F. Anatomy and neuro-pathophysiology of the cough reflex arc. Multidiscip Respir Med. 2012;7:5.

19. Mazzone SB, Undem BJ. Cough sensors. V. Pharmacological modulation of cough sensors. Handb Exp Pharmacol. 2009;187:99–127.

20. Song WJ, Chang YS, Morice AH. Changing the paradigm for cough: does 'cough hypersensitivity' aid our understanding? Asia Pac Allergy. 2014;4:3–13.

21. Caterina MJ, Schumacher MA, Tominaga M, Rosen TA, Levine JD, Julius D. The capsaicin receptor: a heat-activated ion channel in the pain pathway. Nature. 1997;389:816–24.

22. Henrich F, Magerl W, Klein T, Greffrath W, Treede RD. Capsaicin-sensitive C- and A-fibre nociceptors control long-term potentiation-like pain amplification in humans. Brain. 2015;138(Pt 9):2505–20.

23. Shim WS, Tak MH, Lee MH, Kim M, Kim M, Koo JY, et al. TRPV1 mediates histamine-induced itching via the activation of phospholipase A2 and 12-lipoxygenase. J Neurosci. 2007;27(9):2331–7.

24. Lee LY, Gu Q. Role of TRPV1 in inflammation-induced airway hypersensitivity. Curr Opin Pharmacol. 2009;9(3):243–9.

25. Nilius B, Owsianik G. The transient receptor potential family of ion channels. Genome Biol. 2011;12:218.

26. Tominaga M, Caterina MJ, Malmberg AB, Rosen TA, Gilbert H, Skinner K, et al. The cloned capsaicin receptor integrates multiple pain-producing stimuli. Neuron. 1998;21:531–43.

27. Bessac BF, Sivula M, von Hehn CA, Escalera J, Cohn L, Jordt SE. TRPA1 is a major oxidant sensor in murine airway sensory neurons. J Clin Invest. 2008;118(5):1899–910.

28. Bandell M, Story GM, Hwang SW, Viswanath V, Eid SR, Petrus MJ, et al. Noxious cold ion channel TRPA1 is activated by pungent compounds and bradykinin. Neuron. 2004;41:849–57.

29. Enyedi P, Czirják G. Molecular background of leak K+ currents: two-pore domain potassium channels. Physiol Rev. 2010;90:559–605.

30. Sluka KA, Winter OC, Wemmie JA. Acid-sensing ion channels: a new target for pain and CNS diseases. Curr Opin Drug Discov Devel. 2009;12:693–704.

31. Reznikov LR, Meyerholz DK, Adam RJ, Abou Alaiwa M, Jaffer O, Michalski AS, et al. Acid-sensing ion channel 1a contributes to airway hyperreactivity in mice. PLoS One. 2016;11(11):e0166089. https://doi.org/10.1371/journal.pone.0166089.

32. Hattori M, Gouaux E. Molecular mechanism of ATP binding and ion channel activation in P2X receptors. Nature. 2012;485:207–12.

33. G B, Brouns I, Adriaensen D, Timmermans JP. Purinergic signaling in the airways. Pharmacol Rev. 2012;64(4):834–68.

34. Groneberg DA, Niimi A, Dinh QT, Cosio B, Hew M, Fischer A, Chung KF. Increased expression of transient receptor potential vanilloid-1 in airway nerves of chronic cough. Am J Respir Crit Care Med. 2004;170(12):1276–80.

35. O'Connell F, Thomas VE, Pride NB, Fuller RW. Capsaicin cough sensitivity decreases with successful treatment of chronic cough. Am J Respir Crit Care Med. 1994;150:374–80.

36. Grace MS, Belvisi MG. TRPA1 receptors in cough. Pulm Pharmacol Ther. 2011;24(3):286–8. https://doi.org/10.1016/j.pupt.2010.11.002.

37. El-Hashim AZ, Jaffal SM. Nerve growth factor enhances cough and airway obstruction via TrkA receptor- and TRPV1-dependent mechanisms. Thorax. 2009;64:791–7.

38. Diogenes A, Akopian AN, Hargreaves KM. NGF up-regulates TRPA1: implications for orofacial pain. J Dent Res. 2007;86:550–5.

39. Ji RR, Samad TA, Jin SX, Schmoll R, Woolf CJ. p38 MAPK activation by NGF in primary sensory neurons after inflammation increases TRPV1 levels and maintains heat hyperalgesia. Neuron. 2002;36:57–68.

40. Kobayashi H, Gleich GJ, Butterfield JH, Kita H. Human eosinophils produce neurotrophins and secrete nerve growth factor on immunologic stimuli. Blood. 2002;99:2214–20.

41. Raap U, Deneka N, Bruder M, Kapp A, Wedi B. Differential upregulation of neurotrophin receptors and functional role of neurotrophins on peripheral blood eosinophils of patients with atopic dermatitis,

allergic rhinitis and nonatopic healthy controls. Clin Exp Allergy. 2008;38:1493–8.

42. Khan AA, Diogenes A, Jeske NA, Henry MA, Akopian A, Hargreaves KM. Tumor necrosis factor alpha enhances the sensitivity of rat trigeminal neurons to capsaicin. Neuroscience. 2008;155:503–9.

43. Alenmyr L, Herrmann A, Högestätt ED, Greiff L, Zygmunt PM. TRPV1 and TRPA1 stimulation induces MUC5B secretion in the human nasal airway in vivo. Clin Physiol Funct Imag. 2011;31(6):435–44. https://doi.org/10.1111/j.1475-097X.2011.01039.x.

44. Bianchi ME. DAMPs, PAMPs and alarmins: all we need to know about danger. J Leukoc Biol. 2007;81:1–5.

45. Saenz SA, Taylor BC, Artis D. Welcome to the neighborhood: epithelial cell-derived cytokines license innate and adaptive immune responses at mucosal sites. Immunol Rev. 2008;226:172–90. https://doi.org/10.1111/j.1600-065X.2008.00713.x.

46. Wilson SR, Thé L, Batia LM, Beattie K, Katibah GE, McClain SP, et al. The epithelial cell-derived atopic dermatitis cytokine TSLP activates neurons to induce itch. Cell. 2013;155(2):285–95. https://doi.org/10.1016/j.cell.2013.08.057.

47. Hensellek S, Brell P, Schaible HG, Brauer R, Segond v BG. The cytokine TNFalpha increases the proportion of DRG neurones expressing the TRPV1 receptor via the TNFR1 receptor and ERK activation. Mol Cell Neurosci. 2007;36:381–91.

48. Wessler IA, Kirkpatrick CJ, Rack K. Non-neuronal acetylcholine, a locally acting molecule, widely distributed in biological systems: expression and function in humans. Pharmacol Ther. 1998;77:59–79.

49. Remheimer T, Baumgartner D, Oelert H, Racke K, Wessler I. Acetylcholine inhibits ionophore-induced histamine release from human bronchi via stimulation of muscarinic receptors. Naunyn Schmiedebergs Arch Pharmacol. 1996;353(Suppl):R79.

50. Remheimer T, Baumgsrtner D, Hohle K-D, Racke K, Wessler I. Acetylcholine inhibits histamine release from human isolated bronchi via stimulation of muscaric receptors. Am J Respir Crit Care Med. 1997;156:389–95.

51. Reinheimer T, Münch M, Bittinger F, Racké K, Kirkpatrick CJ, Wessler I. Glucocorticoids mediate reduction of epithelial acetylcholine content in the airways of rats and humans. Eur J Pharmacol. 1998;349:277–84.

52. Lee LY, Burki NK, Gerhardstein DC, Gu Q, Kou YR, Xu J. Airway irritation and cough evoked by inhaled cigarette smoke: role of neuronal nicotinic acetylcholine receptors. Pulmonary Pharmacol Ther. 2007;20(4):355–64.

53. Kichko TI, Lennerz J, Eberhardt M, Babes RM, Neuhuber W, Kobal G, et al. Bimodal concentration-response of nicotine involves the nicotinic acetylcholine receptor, transient receptor potential vanilloid type 1, and transient receptor potential ankyrin 1 channels in mouse trachea and sensory neurons.

J Pharmacol Exp Ther. 2013;347(2):529–39. https://doi.org/10.1124/jpet.113.205971.

54. Hecker A, Mikulski Z, Lips KS, Pfeil U, Zakrzewicz A, Wilker S, et al. Pivotal advance: up-regulation of acetylcholine synthesis and paracrine cholinergic signaling in intravascular transplant leukocytes during rejection of rat renal allografts. J Leukoc Biol. 2009;86(1):13–22. https://doi.org/10.1189/jlb.1107722.

55. Skok MV. To channel or not to channel? Functioning of nicotinic acetylcholine receptors in leukocytes. J Leukoc Biol. 2016;86(1):1–3.

56. Chen C-Y, Joad JP, Bric J, Bonham AC. Central mechanisms I: plasticity of central pathways. Handb Exp Pharmacol. 2009;187:187–201.

57. Canning BJ. Afferent nerves regulating the cough reflex: mechanisms and mediators of cough in disease. Otolaryngol Clin N Am. 2010;43(1):15–vii. https://doi.org/10.1016/j.otc.2009.11.012.

58. Ashley Woodcock A, Young EC, Smith JA. New insights in cough. Br Med Bull. 2010;96(1):61–73. https://doi.org/10.1093/bmb/ldq034.

59. Wong IW, Rees G, Greiff L, Myers JC, Jamieson GG, Wormald PJ. Gastroesophageal reflux disease and chronic sinusitis: in search of an esophageal-nasal reflex. Am J Rhinol Allergy. 2010;24(4):255–9. https://doi.org/10.2500/ajra.2010.24.3490.

60. Braunstahl GJ, Overbeek SE, Fokkens WJ, Kleinjan A, McEuen AR, Walls AF, et al. Segmental broncho-provocation in allergic rhinitis patients affects mast cell and basophil numbers in nasal and bronchial mucosa. Am J Respir Crit Care Med. 2001;164(5):858–65.

61. Braunstahl GJ, Kleinjan A, Overbeek SE, Prins JB, Hoogsteden HC, Fokkens WJ. Segmental bronchial provocation induces nasal inflammation in allergic rhinitis patients. Am J Respir Crit Care Med. 2000 Jun;161(6):2051–7.

62. Braunstahl GJ, Fokkens WJ, Overbeek SE, KleinJan A, Hoogsteden HC, Prins JB. Mucosal and systemic inflammatory changes in allergic rhinitis and asthma: a comparison between upper and lower airways. Clin Exp Allergy. 2003;33(5):579–87.

63. Braunstahl GJ, Overbeek SE, Kleinjan A, Prins JB, Hoogsteden HC, Fokkens WJ. Nasal allergen provocation induces adhesion molecule expression and tissue eosinophilia in upper and lower airways. J Allergy Clin Immunol. 2001;107(3):469–76.

64. Irwin RS, Baumann MH, Bolser DC, Boulet L-P, Braman SS, Brightling CE, et al. Diagnosis and management of cough executive summary: ACCP evidence-based clinical practice guidelines. Chest. 2006;129(1 Suppl):1S–23S.

65. Schindlbeck NE, Heinrich C, Huber RM, Müller-Lissner SA. Effects of albuterol (salbutamol) on esophageal motility and gastroesophageal reflux in healthy volunteers. JAMA. 1988;260(21):3156–8.

66. Rachelefsky GS, Goldberg M, Katz RM, Boris G, Gyepes MT, Shapiro MJ, et al. Sinus disease in children with respiratory allergy. J Allergy Clin Immunol. 1978;61(5):310–4.

67. Bjermer L. The nose as an air conditioner for the lower airways. Allergy. 1999;54(Suppl 57):26–30.

68. Chong LY, Head K, Hopkins C, Philpott C, Glew S, Scadding G, Burton MJ, et al. Saline irrigation for chronic rhinosinusitis. Cochrane Database Syst Rev. 2016;(4):CD011995. https://doi.org/10.1002/14651858.CD011995.pub2.

69. Takahama K, Tetsuya Shirasaki T. Central and peripheral mechanisms of narcotic antitussives: codeine-sensitive and -resistant coughs. Cough. 2007;3:8.

70. Millqvist E, Ternesten-Hasséus E, Bende M. Inhalation of menthol reduces capsaicin cough sensitivity and influences inspiratory flows in chronic cough. Respir Med. 2013;107(3):433–8. https://doi.org/10.1016/j.rmed.2012.11.017.

71. Galeotti N, Di Cesare Mannelli L, Mazzanti G, Bartolini A, Ghelardini C. Menthol: a natural analgesic compound. Neurosci Lett. 2002;322(3):145–8.

72. Karashima Y, Damann N, Prenen J, Talavera K, Segal A, Voets T, Nilius B. Bimodal action of menthol on the transient receptor potential channel TRPA1. J Neurosci. 2007;27(37):9874–84.

73. Fokkens W, Peter Hellings P, Segboer C. Capsaicin for rhinitis. Curr Allergy Asthma Rep. 2016;16:60. https://doi.org/10.1007/s11882-016-0638-1.

74. Adeleye IA, Opiah L. Antimicrobial activity of extracts of local cough mixtures on upper respiratory tract bacterial pathogens. West Indian Med J. 2003;52(3):188–90.

75. Jeyakumar A, Brickman TM, Haben M. Effectiveness of amitriptyline versus cough suppressants in the treatment of chronic cough resulting from postviral vagal neuropathy. Laryngoscope. 2006;116(12):2108–12.

76. Gibson PG, Vertigan AE. Gabapentin in chronic cough. Pulm Pharmacol Ther. 2015;35:145–8. https://doi.org/10.1016/j.pupt.2015.06.007.

77. Ryan NM. Gibson PG recent additions in the treatment of cough. Thoracic Dis. 2014;6(Suppl 7):S739–47.

Pamela Tongchinsub and Tara F. Carr

Case Presentation 1

A 40-year-old otherwise healthy male presents with a 3-year history of progressive left sided nasal congestion. He reports difficulty breathing through the left nostril and associated headaches. He has been treated with intranasal corticosteroids, intranasal antihistamines, and sinus washes without symptomatic improvement. He denies right-sided nasal symptoms except for occasional clear rhinorrhea. Several years ago, he sustained an injury to his nasal bridge after being hit in the face with a football. He opted not to seek medical care for his injury and instead had a friend reset his nose. He denies itchy nose, watery eyes, or frequent sneezing.

On examination, there is misalignment between his nasal tip and nasal bridge. The nasal contour is crooked and shifted towards the left. Direct visualization with a nasal speculum reveals bilateral patent nares, but the left nasal cavity is noticeably smaller than the right. Mucous membranes are moist and turbinates are normal in color and size. No masses or polyps are seen. Further examination with rhinoscopy

P. Tongchinsub · T. F. Carr (✉)
Department of Medicine, University of Arizona,
Banner-University Medical Center-Tucson,
Tucson, AZ, USA
e-mail: pana@email.arizona.edu;
tcarr@deptofmed.arizona.edu

reveals a markedly deviated septum towards the left.

Anatomic Abnormalities

Static anatomic abnormalities include nasal septal deviation, nasal septal perforation, turbinate hypertrophy, and atrophic rhinitis (Table 10.1). These disorders can be relatively easy to distinguish by history and physical examination. Treatment options range from conservative medical management to surgical correction. Choice of therapy will be driven by severity of the problem as well as the degree to which these disorders are causing clinical symptoms [1].

The nasal septum is a bony and cartilaginous wall that separates the nasal cavity into two nostrils. A normal nasal septum lies midline and gives rise to two symmetrical nares, but is susceptible to physical distortion due to its soft connective tissue composition. A deviated septum is defined by a lateral displacement of the septum towards one side of the nasal cavity and is present in up to 62% of the population [2]. Mild septal deviation is common in the general population and is usually asymptomatic [3]. When severe, a deviated septum most commonly presents with nasal obstruction or congestion and progresses slowly over time. Obstruction is most often unilateral, affecting the side towards which the septum is displaced, but may be bilateral if the

Table 10.1 Structural causes of rhinitis symptoms

Classification	Common causes
Anatomic abnormalities	Deviated nasal septum
	Nasal septal perforation
	Nasal turbinate hypertrophy
	Atrophic rhinitis
Space-occupying lesions	Benign tumors
	Malignant tumors
	Granulomatous disease
	Nasal polyposis
	Adenoidal hypertrophy

deviation is sigmoidal. Other symptoms may include snoring, difficulty breathing through the nose, and headaches. Septal deviation can worsen perception of symptoms from other causes of rhinitis, including allergic and nonallergic rhinitis and predispose patients to chronic sinusitis.

Deviated septa are most commonly acquired from physical trauma or injury, including sports injuries and motor vehicle accidents. However, they can also occur as a congenital abnormality in 20% of otherwise normal neonates [4].

Septal deviation can be diagnosed by physical examination or imaging. Physical examination, including rhinoscopy, is recommended as the first-line method for diagnosis due to lack of risk, expense, and radiation. External examination of the nasal contour may reveal misalignment between the nasal tip and the nasal bridge. Direct visualization with anterior rhinoscopy, which allows for visualization and comparison of the inferior and middle turbinates, or nasal endoscopy, which can better visualize the superior turbinates and posterior nasal structures, allows for comparison of asymmetry between bilateral structures. This will identify both the deviated septum and the laterality of deviation. Evaluation by cross-sectional imaging either with computed tomography (CT) scan or magnetic resonance imaging (MRI) can easily identify bony abnormalities, including nasal septum deformities. However, CT scan is generally not recommended as a first-line diagnostic procedure to evaluate for septal deviation as studies have shown that there is little correlation between septal deviation findings on CT scan and clinical significance of nasal obstruction [5]. Asymptomatic or minimally

symptomatic nasal septal deviation can contribute to intolerance of nasal corticosteroid sprays used to treat other causes of rhinitis. In this case, patients should be directed to aim the spray nozzle towards the ipsilateral ear to avoid septal irritation. Symptomatic nasal septal deviation can be corrected surgically through a septoplasty. Patients may expect significant subjective improvement in nasal obstructive symptoms with this treatment [6, 7].

Nasal septal perforation may also contribute to rhinitis symptoms as a structural abnormality [8]. A nasal septum perforation is a patency within the septal wall that creates an unnatural passageway between the two nostrils. Perforations generally develop from external insults to the nasal septal cartilage. Various chemical, physical, and iatrogenic insults have been implicated in nasal septum perforations, most commonly as a complication of septoplasty. Other insults include intranasal cocaine use, exposure to industrial chemicals, piercings and foreign bodies, improper use of nasal sprays, trauma due to picking, rheumatologic diseases (e.g., granulomatosis with polyangiitis, systemic lupus erythematosus), infectious disease (e.g., tuberculosis, syphilis), and atrophic rhinitis [9].

With normal respiration, in the presence of septal perforation, there is significant airflow through the perforated septum, disrupting normal nasal airflow and causing turbulence. Septal perforations therefore commonly present with the sensations of nasal obstruction and/or congestion. Turbulent airflow through the perforation can also cause chronic purulent discharge, excessive drying and nasal crusting, recurrent epistaxis, and high-pitched whistling noises during breathing, especially if the perforation is small.

Diagnosis of septal perforation can be made on physical examination with direct visualization by a nasal speculum, rhinoscope, otoscope, or endoscope. The clinician may promptly identify the through-and-through hole in the nasal septum that allows for light passage to and visualization of structures within the contralateral nare. It is recommended to insert an illuminated otoscope into each nare and assess for light in the contralateral nostril. In the absence of a known physical or chemical insult, workup for a systemic disorder should be considered, particularly if there is prominent crusting or progression of the size of the perforation.

Avoidance of contributing factors should be encouraged for all patients. Conservative management may be adequate to relieve patient symptoms but does not necessarily prevent progression of disease. Nasal saline washes and intranasal lubricants may help to reduce crusting, dryness, and rhinorrhea. Small perforations may heal spontaneously, particularly in the absence of ongoing septal irritation. For larger perforations that are symptomatic, surgical intervention may be required. The type of intervention will depend on location and size of the perforation. A septal button is a small device which may be utilized to treat perforations less than two centimeters in diameter, cover the perforation, and relieve associated symptoms [10]. Surgical correction through cartilage or tissue flaps may be considered. Surgical failure is more likely in patients with inadequate blood supply to the perforation site and in the setting of tissue scarring.

The turbinates are a group of bilateral, symmetrical curvaceous bony structures that protrude from the lateral wall of the nose into the nasal cavity and are overlaid with mucosal tissue. They are responsible for maintaining optimal airflow, humidification, warming, and filtering of inhaled air [1]. Middle turbinate enlargement is commonly due to pneumatization of the bone, also known as a concha bullosa. The inferior turbinates can enlarge due to hypertrophy of the soft tissue overlying the bony structures, or due to the developmental influence of other structural abnormalities such as deviated septum or concha bullosa [11]. Soft-tissue hypertrophy occurs most commonly secondary to chronic allergic rhinitis, although recurrent upper respiratory infections, vasomotor rhinitis, pregnancy or hormonal changes, and environmental irritants are also implicated.

Turbinate hypertrophy can cause physical obstruction of the nasal passage, resulting in a sense of nasal blockage and localized nasal or facial fullness. Patients may report worsening symptoms during sleep, as the inferior turbinates

enlarge while supine due to normal neural reflexes. Diagnosis of inferior turbinate hypertrophy can be made by direct visualization with an otoscope/rhinoscope, but the middle turbinates are better visualized by endoscopy.

Medical management with intranasal corticosteroids and intranasal antihistamines is the first-line therapy for inferior turbinate hypertrophy, to reduce the mucosal hypertrophy and address underlying disorders. Surgical reduction of inferior turbinate hypertrophy can address the underlying deformity, and is usually reserved for cases refractory to medical management [12, 13].

Atrophic rhinitis is a noninflammatory process associated with the loss of normal secretory and humidifying functions of the nose that leads to progressive atrophy of the nasal mucosa [14, 15]. Atrophic rhinitis is classified into primary and secondary forms. Primary (idiopathic) atrophic rhinitis is associated with *Klebsiella ozaenae* microbial colonization. This disorder is predominantly seen in young to middle-aged patients, particularly female adolescents, in developing countries with warm climates [16]. Primary atrophic rhinitis causes foul-smelling nasal discharge, halitosis, and abnormally enlarged nasal cavities. Other common signs and symptoms include nasal crusts, purulent discharge, anosmia, and epistaxis. Nasal cavity examination shows shiny, thin, pale mucosa covered by thick, yellow-brown-green crusts with possible bloody or purulent discharge.

Secondary atrophic rhinitis is common in developed countries and is mainly seen in patients with an extensive history of sinonasal surgery, trauma, irradiation, or other inflammatory conditions (e.g., granulomatous diseases) [17]. Secondary atrophic rhinitis primarily presents with nasal congestion, daily nasal crusting, and dryness. Other reported symptoms include episodic anosmia, persistent postnasal drip, and recurrent epistaxis. Some patients with associated underlying inflammatory conditions may also have thick mucus discharge in the initial stages of secondary atrophic rhinitis prior to the destruction and loss of mucus-secreting glandular cells that result in nasal dryness. Physical examination reveals thin, erythematous mucosa. Compared with primary atrophic rhinitis, patients with secondary atrophic rhinitis have lesser degrees of nasal bleeding, dryness, and widening of the nasal cavity.

Diagnosis of atrophic rhinitis should be suspected based on history but can be made with the combination of physical examination, imaging, and when necessary biopsy [17]. Rhinoscopy or endoscopy may show reduced turbinates, crusting, and an enlarged nasopharyngeal space. Computed tomography can reveal a combination of bony resorption, mucosal thickening and atrophy, enlargement of the nasal cavities with destruction of the lateral nasal walls, and hypoplasia of the sinuses [18]. If performed, nasal biopsy reveals a spectrum of histologic changes including damage to the pseudostratified epithelium, squamous metaplasia, and loss of goblet cells.

Currently, there are no studies that compare the long-term efficacy of various treatment modalities and management is primarily symptomatic [19]. Most commonly recommended therapies include daily or twice-daily nasal saline irrigation followed by lubrication of nasal mucosa with water-based personal lubricants. Superimposed bacterial infections can be treated with systemic antibiotics (considering those with activity against *Klebsiella ozaenae*) and topical antibiotic creams or by adding antibiotics to the saline irrigation solution. Lastly, surgical debridement can be considered for cases refractory to medical management, although routine surgical intervention is not recommended as controlled trials have not yet been performed to assess their efficacy.

In the presented case 1, a deviated nasal septum was diagnosed by direct visualization of the structure. The patient had previously failed medical management, including treatment of underlying and contributing causes of rhinitis, so he elected surgical management. Endoscopic septoplasty surgically corrected the septum, restoring normal nasal function and thereby resolving the patient's symptoms.

Case Presentation 2

A 13-year-old previously healthy male presents to clinic with 6 months of bilateral persistent progressive nasal congestion. He has difficulty breathing through his nose, which is worse when he lies down. His mother reports that he began snoring loudly during sleep. He also reports a loss of sense of smell and mucoid nasal drainage. He has a history of occasional bloody noses that have become more frequent and occurs on both sides. His symptoms do not vary with pollen seasons or environmental exposures and have worsened despite medical management with intranasal corticosteroids and intranasal antihistamines.

On physical exam, he is noticeably mouth breathing. Nasal rhinoscopy shows patent nares with normal-sized, non-boggy turbinates. His nasal mucosa is moist and pink. There are no visible polyps or papillomas. The septum is midline and there is no septal trauma or granuloma. Nasal endoscopy reveals a mass in the superior nasal cavity.

Space-Occupying Lesions

Space-occupying lesions are important but rare structural causes of rhinitis symptoms (see Table 10.1). Tumors, polyps, granulomas, and adenoidal hypertrophy can be identified with visualization on endoscopy, rhinoscopy, or cross-sectional imaging. Biopsy is necessary to rule out malignancy in most cases, and surgical resection is usually necessary for symptom control.

Both benign and malignant tumors can develop in the nasopharyngeal cavity and paranasal sinuses. Common benign tumors include inverted papillomas, nasal cavity hemangiomas, and juvenile nasal angiofibromas. Primary malignant nasal cavity tumors are rare and make up 1% of all malignant tumors and 3% of head and neck tumors [20]. The most common malignant tumor in the nasal cavity is squamous cell carcinoma. Other tumors include adenocarcinomas, adenoid cystic carcinomas, olfactory neuroblastomas, and melanomas [21].

In general, nasal congestion and discharge are common in benign nasal airway tumors. Symptoms may be unilateral or bilateral. Inverted papillomas are found on the lateral wall of the nasal mucosa. Juvenile nasal angiofibromas are found in the nasopharynx and present with a triad of epistaxis, nasal obstruction, and nasal drainage [22, 23]. They are most commonly found in adolescent males and make up 0.05% of head and neck tumors.

Unilateral nasal congestion with localized pain or bloody discharge is a sign of ominous pathology in the nasal, paranasal, or nasopharyngeal cavities. Evaluation for malignant nasal cavity tumors is recommended for elderly patients who complain of unilateral epistaxis and nasal pain. Nasal cavity malignancies tend to cause visual changes, facial pain, and bleeding while paranasal sinus malignancies are associated with dental pain and epistaxis. Ear pain, neurological changes, and asymmetry of the neck or face may also be noted.

Direct visualization, often requiring endoscopy, and imaging are used to identify the presence of nasal cavity masses, but biopsy is necessary to differentiate between benign and malignant tumors. Computed tomography or magnetic resonance imaging will define the parameters of the lesion, and assess the extent of bony erosion or involvement of the surrounding tissues. Management of nasal tumors will include a multidisciplinary team including surgical excision by otolaryngologists and, when malignant, management by medical and radiation oncologists.

A granuloma is a type of space-occupying granulation tissue that is formed typically after direct trauma or inflammation of the tissue, or related to neoplasm [24], and is generally progressive and destructive. Direct trauma can occur through foreign body or caustic substance exposure. Inflammation that contributes to granuloma formation may result from acute or chronic infection with bacteria (mycobacterium, syphilis), fungus (histoplasmosis), parasite (leishmaniasis), or virus (Epstein-Barr virus). Vasculitides that affect the innate tissue structure include the anti-neutrophil cytoplasmic antibodies—associated vasculitides and sarcoidosis. The most common malignancy causing granuloma formation is natural killer cell/T-cell lymphoma, an extranodal lymphoma related to Epstein-Barr virus infection, and which causes midline granuloma disease.

Granuloma can present differently, depending on the underlying cause. Foreign bodies may present as purulent or foul-smelling nasal discharge with a friable mucosa. NK cell lymphoma affecting the nasal cavity has a broad presentation but is rapidly progressive and can present with EBV positivity, signs of tissue necrosis, and angioinvasion. Granuloma can be progressively destructive of surrounding soft tissues and bony structures.

Direct visualization is the best method for visualization of nasal cavity granulomas. Tissue biopsy can confirm the presence of granuloma and evaluate for neoplasia. Testing for systemic diseases is warranted when clinically suspected and may include measurement of anti-neutrophil cytoplasmic antibodies, peripheral blood eosinophil counts, titers for Epstein-Barr virus, erythrocyte sedimentation rate, and C-reactive protein levels. Treatment of the granuloma will depend on the underlying cause and will include surgical and medical management. Nonsurgical treatment options of midline granulomas depend on the presence of systemic involvement. For NK cell lymphoma, treatment typically involves radiation and chemotherapy with consideration of monoclonal antibody therapy for refractory cases. For localized granulomas due to trauma or foreign bodies, topical or intralesional corticosteroids are considered first-line treatment options.

In contrast, nasal polyps are benign semitranslucent edematous inflammatory growths of the nasal and paranasal mucosa and do not require biopsy for diagnosis. Polyps develop from the ethmoid and maxillary sinuses, and can be unilateral or bilateral. In adults, nasal polyps are frequently associated with anosmia, aspirin sensitivity, and asthma, but can occur independently [25]. Nasal polyps are uncommon in children but can be seen in those with cystic fibrosis. Although the pathogenesis of chronic rhinosinusitis with nasal polyposis is unclear, polyps contain prominent lymphocytic and/or eosinophilic cellular infiltration, leukotrienes, and mucin [26]. Polyps in children with cystic fibrosis are typically associated with a neutrophilic cellular infiltration.

Chronic rhinosinusitis with nasal polyposis presents symptomatically with a triad of unilateral or bilateral obstruction of nasal passages, anosmia, and rhinorrhea. Physical examination with rhinoscopy or endoscopy shows semitranslucent, grapelike masses within the nasal cavity that may extend to the anterior nasal vault. Due to structural similarities, unilateral nasal polyps should be differentiated from inverted papillomas and occasionally malignant tumors. Adjunctive imaging with coronal computed tomography can be performed to determine the extent of disease and evaluate underlying concomitant sinusitis, particularly for patients who are symptomatic and considering surgical intervention.

Nasal polyps can be managed medically or surgically. Oral corticosteroids are the most effective known medical therapy for reducing large or obstructing polyps and intranasal corticosteroids are useful for reducing smaller polyps and indicated as a long-term therapy for nasal polyps. Other medical treatments include leukotriene-modifying agents including 5-lipoxygenase inhibitors and leukotriene receptor antagonists, but are less effective in treating nasal polyps compared to corticosteroids. Surgical removal of polyps is the treatment of choice for recurring nasal polyps that are not adequately treated or controlled with medical management. However, recurrence rates may be as high as 60%.

Adenoidal hypertrophy may also contribute to rhinitis symptoms. The adenoid is a mass of lymphatic tissue that is situated above the uvula in the posterior wall of the nasopharynx, at the junction of the nose and throat. Adenoidal hypertrophy is caused by recurrent viral or bacterial infection that results in enlargement of this lymphoid tissue. While lymphoid tissue is typically only enlarged during acute active infection, adenoidal tissue can remain enlarged due to chronic infection or after recurrent infections. A common cause of chronic adenoidal infection causing adenoidal hypertrophy is the Epstein-Barr virus (EBV) [27, 28].

Adenoidal hypertrophy most commonly occurs in young children. These patients will present with bilateral nasal congestion associated with mouth breathing, hyponasal speech, and snoring. Symptoms may be more noticeable at night when sleeping or in supine position. If severe, patients may also exhibit abnormal sleep cycles due to nasopharyngeal obstruction causing sleep-disordered breathing and contributing to obstructive sleep apnea (OSA). In addition, enlarged adenoids can obstruct the torus tubarius (the nasopharyngeal opening of the auditory canal) resulting in recurrent otitis media.

The best method for evaluation of adenoid size is by direct visualization via endoscopy by an otolaryngologist. Endolateral neck radiographs may also capture adenoidal hypertrophy, facilitating diagnosis, but imaging is not a recommended first-line method for evaluation and diagnosis of adenoidal hypertrophy in order to minimize iatrogenic radiation exposure in small children. Adenoidectomy is the definitive treatment of adenoidal hypertrophy. Occasionally, adenoid hypertrophy can recur postoperatively requiring repeat surgical intervention [29].

In case 2, due to the presence of a nasal mass, a biopsy of the lesion was performed, which confirmed histologically the presence of a juvenile nasal angiofibroma. The patient underwent a complete surgical excision of the tumor. Postoperatively, he reported improvement in all of his symptoms including sense of smell and nasal congestion. Periodic endoscopic surveillance has thus far seen no evidence of tumor recurrence.

Clinical Pearls and Pitfalls

- Structural abnormalities of the nose and paranasal sinuses can contribute to rhinitis symptoms and severity.
- In general, structural problems of the nasopharynx cause symptoms of unilateral or bilateral nasal obstruction or congestion.
- Patients should be assessed for structural abnormalities if symptoms suggest such, or if they fail to respond to usual treatments.
- Visualization of the nasopharynx via rhinoscopy and/or endoscopy may easily identify

structural lesions. Cross-sectional imaging can identify the extent of disease.

- Biopsy of mass lesions is often necessary to rule out malignant or systemic disease.
- Surgical correction of anatomic abnormalities and space-occupying lesions may be required to restore structural functionality and reduce symptoms in patients.

References

1. Neskey D, Eloy JA, Casiano RR. Nasal, septal, and turbinate anatomy and embryology. Otolaryngol Clin N Am. 2009;42(2):193–205. vii
2. Lloyd GA. CT of the paranasal sinuses: study of a control series in relation to endoscopic sinus surgery. J Laryngol Otol. 1990;104(6):477–81.
3. Salihoglu M, Cekin E, Altundag A, Cesmeci E. Examination versus subjective nasal obstruction in the evaluation of the nasal septal deviation. Rhinology. 2014;52(2):122–6.
4. Harugop AS, Mudhol RS, Hajare PS, Nargund AI, Metgudmath VV, Chakrabarti S. Prevalence of nasal septal deviation in new-borns and its precipitating factors: a cross-sectional study. Indian J Otolaryngol Head Neck Surg. 2012;64(3):248–51.
5. Ardeshirpour F, McCarn KE, McKinney AM, Odland RM, Yueh B, Hilger PA. Computed tomography scan does not correlate with patient experience of nasal obstruction. Laryngoscope. 2016;126(4):820–5.
6. Corey CL, Most SP. Treatment of nasal obstruction in the posttraumatic nose. Otolaryngol Clin N Am. 2009;42(3):567–78.
7. Gandomi B, Bayat A, Kazemei T. Outcomes of septoplasty in young adults: the nasal obstruction septoplasty effectiveness study. Am J Otolaryngol. 2010;31(3):189–92.
8. Wallace DV, Dykewicz MS, Bernstein DI, Blessing-Moore J, Cox L, Khan DA, et al. The diagnosis and management of rhinitis: an updated practice parameter. J Allergy Clin Immunol. 2008;122(2 Suppl):S1–84.
9. Lanier B, Kai G, Marple B, Wall GM. Pathophysiology and progression of nasal septal perforation. Ann Allergy Asthma Immunol. 2007;99(6):473–9. quiz 80–1, 521
10. Taylor RJ, Sherris DA. Prosthetics for nasal perforations: a systematic review and meta-analysis. Otolaryngol Head Neck Surg. 2015;152(5):803–10.
11. Tomblinson CM, Cheng MR, Lal D, Hoxworth JM. The impact of middle turbinate concha bullosa on the severity of inferior turbinate hypertrophy in patients with a deviated nasal septum. AJNR Am J Neuroradiol. 2016;37(7):1324–30.
12. Teichgraeber JF, Gruber RP, Tanna N. Surgical management of nasal airway obstruction. Clin Plast Surg. 2016;43(1):41–6.
13. Ye T, Zhou B. Update on surgical management of adult inferior turbinate hypertrophy. Curr Opin Otolaryngol Head Neck Surg. 2015;23(1):29–33.
14. Shah K, Guarderas J, Krishnaswamy G. Empty nose syndrome and atrophic rhinitis. Ann Allergy Asthma Immunol. 2016;117(3):217–20.
15. deShazo RD, Stringer SP. Atrophic rhinosinusitis: progress toward explanation of an unsolved medical mystery. Curr Opin Allergy Clin Immunol. 2011;11(1):1–7.
16. Bunnag C, Jareoncharsri P, Tansuriyawong P, Bhothisuwan W, Chantarakul N. Characteristics of atrophic rhinitis in Thai patients at the Siriraj Hospital. Rhinology. 1999;37(3):125–30.
17. Ly TH, deShazo RD, Olivier J, Stringer SP, Daley W, Stodard CM. Diagnostic criteria for atrophic rhinosinusitis. Am J Med. 2009;122(8):747–53.
18. Pace-Balzan A, Shankar L, Hawke M. Computed tomographic findings in atrophic rhinitis. J Otolaryngol. 1991;20(6):428–32.
19. Mishra A, Kawatra R, Gola M. Interventions for atrophic rhinitis. Cochrane Database Syst Rev. 2012;(2):CD008280.
20. Osguthorpe JD. Sinus neoplasia. Arch Otolaryngol Head Neck Surg. 1994;120(1):19–25.
21. Turner JH, Reh DD. Incidence and survival in patients with sinonasal cancer: a historical analysis of population-based data. Head Neck. 2012;34(6):877–85.
22. Makhasana JA, Kulkarni MA, Vaze S, Shroff AS. Juvenile nasopharyngeal angiofibroma. J Oral Maxillofac Pathol. 2016;20(2):330.
23. Yi Z, Fang Z, Lin G, Lin C, Xiao W, Li Z, et al. Nasopharyngeal angiofibroma: a concise classification system and appropriate treatment options. Am J Otolaryngol. 2013;34(2):133–41.
24. Laudien M. Orphan diseases of the nose and paranasal sinuses: pathogenesis—clinic—therapy. GMS Curr Top Otorhinolaryngol Head Neck Surg. 2015;14:Doc04.
25. Peters AT, Spector S, Hsu J, Hamilos DL, Baroody FM, Chandra RK, et al. Diagnosis and management of rhinosinusitis: a practice parameter update. Ann Allergy Asthma Immunol. 2014;113(4):347–85.
26. Stevens WW, Lee RJ, Schleimer RP, Cohen NA. Chronic rhinosinusitis pathogenesis. J Allergy Clin Immunol. 2015;136(6):1442–53.
27. Al-Salam S, Dhaheri SA, Awwad A, Daoud S, Shams A, Ashari MA. Prevalence of Epstein-Barr virus in tonsils and adenoids of United Arab Emirates nationals. Int J Pediatr Otorhinolaryngol. 2011;75(9):1160–6.
28. Mowry SE, Strocker AM, Chan J, Takehana C, Kalantar N, Bhuta S, et al. Immunohistochemical analysis and Epstein-Barr virus in the tonsils of transplant recipients and healthy controls. Arch Otolaryngol Head Neck Surg. 2008;134(9):936–9.
29. Lesinskas E, Drigotas M. The incidence of adenoidal regrowth after adenoidectomy and its effect on persistent nasal symptoms. Eur Arch Otorhinolaryngol. 2009;266(4):469–73.

Cerebrospinal Fluid Rhinorrhea

11

Andrew C. Rorie and Jill A. Poole

Case Presentation 1

A 26-year-old female presents during the month of April with complaints of rhinorrhea, nasal congestion, postnasal drainage, sneezing, and nasal pruritus. She also indicates that she is 8 weeks pregnant with her first child. Her symptoms have been ongoing since childhood, but historically present only during the spring and fall and were relieved with cetirizine 10 mg daily. Over the past 8 months she has developed perennial symptoms of copious, watery rhinorrhea that seems to be predominantly left sided. She also notes postnasal drainage that is more apparent when she lies down to sleep. She has a medical history notable for cystic fibrosis with nasal polyposis and recurrent sinusitis that has required several endoscopic sinus surgeries with the most recent occurring when she was 25 years old. She has lived in a 70-year-old home without a basement for the past 8 years. She has an indoor cat, but has been around cats her entire life without increased clinical symptoms.

Physical examination reveals a normal exam of the eyes, ears, and throat. The inferior nasal turbinates are slightly enlarged and the mucosa appears slightly pale. There is no evidence of

A. C. Rorie · J. A. Poole (✉)
Department of Medicine, University of Nebraska Medical Center, Omaha, NE, USA
e-mail: arorie@unmc.edu; japoole@unmc.edu

nasal polyposis but there is evidence of clear rhinorrhea. Skin prick testing demonstrated good positive and negative controls along with positive skin prick test reactions to a number of tree and weed pollens. All other aeroallergens tested were negative including molds, feather, cockroach, cat, mouse, and dust mites.

The patient is started on cetirizine 10 mg daily, budesonide two sprays each nostril daily, montelukast 10 mg daily, and ipratropium 0.06% nasal, two sprays every 6 h for rhinorrhea. She returns for follow-up visit 4 weeks later and reports no improvement in the rhinorrhea and postnasal drainage despite taking medications as directed.

Diagnosis/Assessment

The differential diagnosis of this patient with clear rhinorrhea is broad and includes, but is not limited to, gustatory rhinitis, seasonal allergic rhinitis, cerebrospinal fluid leak, rhinitis of pregnancy, and atrophic rhinitis. Patients with gustatory rhinitis typically present with a primary symptom of clear rhinorrhea, as does the patient in the clinical vignette. However, in gustatory rhinitis the rhinorrhea is triggered shortly after eating, which is not described by this patient. Nearly any food has been reported to cause this phenomenon, but hot and spicy foods are the most common agitators [1]. Allergic rhinitis is likely the cause of her prior history of seasonal rhinitis that has been present since her childhood. This is further supported by positive skin testing to tree and weed pollen. Skin testing, however, failed to demonstrate sensitization to a perennial allergen that would explain her new year-round symptoms. More importantly, allergic rhinitis does not present with a primary symptom of unilateral copious, watery rhinorrhea.

The most common cause of rhinitis in pregnancy is preexisting rhinitis; however, a minority of pregnant patients will develop vasomotor (or pregnancy) rhinitis. This is a result of hormones associated with pregnancy, namely estrogen and progesterone, which have direct and indirect effects on nasal physiology [2]. Although this patient is pregnant, her symptoms began prior to her pregnancy. Pregnancy rhinitis typically does not occur until the second trimester. Atrophic rhinitis commonly occurs in the elderly population or those who live in regions of the world with lengthy warm seasons. These patients have symptoms of nasal crusting and halitosis, which is not a complaint of this patient [3].

The best explanation for the rhinorrhea in this patient is a cerebrospinal fluid (CSF) leak. Although she does have a component of seasonal allergic rhinitis, this alone does not explain her primary complaints of predominately unilateral, perennial, copious rhinorrhea that is exacerbated when lying supine. These symptoms paired with her history of multiple endoscopic sinus surgeries should raise concern for the possibility of an iatrogenic CSF leak.

CSF rhinorrhea is a rare phenomenon that requires a high index of suspicion. Although this is an uncommon etiology of a common clinic presentation, rhinorrhea, it must not go undiagnosed as it could result in catastrophic infectious and neurological sequela. The differential diagnosis of rhinorrhea is broad; however, there are historical clues that should prompt one to consider a CSF etiology. These patients will classically complain of unilateral rhinorrhea which is watery, clear, and salty in taste. The rhinorrhea typically occurs intermittently but can be continual. It may be described as copious or minimal. Although there may be concomitant

perennial or seasonal allergic rhinoconjunctivitis, CSF rhinorrhea does not cause lacrimation, ocular pruritus, nasal pruritus, or sneezing. The rhinorrhea can be exacerbated by the Valsalva maneuver or bending forward and cause postnasal drip when lying supine. CSF rhinorrhea is not improved with oral antihistamines, intranasal corticosteroids or antihistamines, and anticholinergics [4].

Development of CSF rhinorrhea results from an anomalous communication between the subarachnoid space and the sinonasal tract. The etiology of CSF leaks can be divided into traumatic and nontraumatic origins. The most common is traumatic (approximately 90% of cases), which can be further subclassified as secondary to head trauma (74%) or iatrogenic from intracranial or otolaryngological surgery (15%) [5]. The majority of these patients will be symptomatic within 2 days of the trauma; however, in as many as 5%, the presentation may be delayed up to 3 months [6]. The initial delay in rhinorrhea may be related to local hemorrhage sealing the defect. The rare patients who have a delayed presentation which occurs months or even years past the initial trauma may occur due to atrophy of granulation tissue or perhaps bony fragments that erode the dura [7]. Due to this potential delay in symptoms, it is essential to take a thorough history of prior trauma or surgical procedures in order to generate a proper differential diagnosis.

Nontraumatic CSF leaks account for only 10% of CSF rhinorrhea and without the obvious history of trauma or surgery it creates more of a challenge for making the correct diagnosis. Nontraumatic CSF leaks are subdivided into normal-pressure and high-pressure CSF leaks. Examples of high-pressures leaks include intracranial space-occupying lesions, hydrocephalus, and idiopathic intracranial hypertension (IIH). The causes of normal pressure CSF leaks may be due to infections, encephalocele, cholesteatoma, arachnoid granulations, and empty sella syndrome [4, 6]. Another type of CSF leak which is both nontraumatic and normal pressure is idiopathic or spontaneous.

When a CSF leak is suspected, the first step should be confirming the presence of CSF followed by localization of the leak. The "ring sign" may be an initial clue into the possibility of a CSF leak particularly in a trauma patient. When CSF is mixed with blood it can leave behind the appearance of a ring or halo on white linens. However, the ring or halo sign can also be observed when other clear fluids are mixed with blood [8]. Thus, due to the poor specificity of the "ring sign" it should not be used for the diagnosis of a CSF leak.

There have historically been three primary options for analysis of the rhinorrhea fluid: assessing for the presence of glucose, beta-2 transferrin, and beta-trace protein. Testing for glucose in rhinorrhea can be quickly analyzed by using a glucose strip because it is rapid and inexpensive. Unfortunately, this method has performed poorly in studies and is no longer recommended due to low sensitivity, specificity, and poor positive predictive value. The reported specificity has ranged from 0 to 45%, and sensitivity 80 to 100%, and positive predictive value is 0.57 [9, 10]. The poor specificity can be explained by several studies demonstrating the presence of glucose in the airway secretions of healthy volunteers, patients with acute viral rhinitis, mechanically ventilated patients, and subjects with hyperglycemia [11, 12].

The test of choice for confirming the presence of CSF is beta-2 transferrin which is a glycoprotein formed only in the CSF by neuraminidase [9, 13, 14]. In a study by Warnecke et al. [9], 205 patients with a suspected CSF leak were tested for beta-2 transferrin. They reported that 35 patients had positive testing and 34 of those were considered true positives, which was confirmed by radionucleotide cisternography or direct intraoperative visualization. In addition, they concluded that beta-2 transferrin has a sensitivity of 97%, specificity of 98%, positive predictive value of 97%, and a negative predictive value of 99%. Similar findings have been reported in other studies [15]. Rarely will patients have ample rhinorrhea to collect in the office, and therefore patients will be required to collect nasal secretions at home. Concerns about beta-2

transferrin stability at varying storage conditions have been evaluated [16]. These studies demonstrated that there was no alteration in the accuracy of beta-2 transferrin detection between storing CSF samples for 1 week at room temperature and refrigeration [16]. Beta-2 transferrin testing is a noninvasive diagnostic tool with high sensitivity and specificity that is also cost effective at approximately $37.90 [13], making it the test of choice for CSF rhinorrhea.

Another option that may be used more frequently outside of the United States is beta-trace protein detection. Similar to beta-2 transferrin, beta-trace protein is also present in high concentrations in the CSF. The sensitivity and specificity of beta-trace protein for CSF rhinorrhea have been reported to range from 91–100% to 86–100%, respectively [13, 17–21]. This protein is also detectable in the serum, but at significantly lower concentrations as compared to the CSF. However, due to its presence in the blood, wide application for the accuracy of this test has been raised. It was reported that renal insufficiency and bacterial meningitis significantly increased CSF levels of beta-trace protein, and therefore beta-trace protein should not be used in these specific clinical situations [22].

Clinical Pearls and Pitfalls

- CSF leak diagnosis requires a thorough history and high index of suspicion.
- Common presentation is with copious, unilateral rhinorrhea that may exhibit positional worsening.
- The test of choice for diagnosis is collection of nasal fluid for beta-2 transferrin.

Case Presentation 2

A 78-year-old male veteran is seen by his primary care physician in June for altered mental status. The patient has a history of psoriasis, hypertension, and hyperlipidemia which are all well controlled. Several weeks prior he was involved in a motor vehicle accident where his vehicle was struck from behind resulting in a whiplash injury. In addition, he struck his face on the steering wheel which caused bruising and pain but no lacerations or loss of consciousness. It was recommended that he go to the hospital after the accident for evaluation but he declined saying "I've been through a lot worse than this and lived to tell about it." Over the next few days he continued to experience a dull achy pain and muscle spasms in his neck. Plain films of his cervical spine were ordered by his PCP which were normal. He was referred for physical therapy for the neck pain which had been helpful.

Approximately 10 days after the accident he began to notice an increase in rhinorrhea without sneezing, nasal pruritus, nasal congestion, or ocular symptoms. His physical exam revealed normal vital signs, and he was alert and oriented. There were additionally no abnormalities on examination of his eyes, ears, or throat, and cranial nerve function was intact. However, he had clear unilateral rhinorrhea from the left nares and mild bilateral periorbital ecchymosis. His doctor thought that he may have developed new environmental allergies and ordered serum-specific IgE testing to common aeroallergens in his geographical area. These tests in addition to complete environmental allergy skin prick tests performed by an allergy specialist were negative. He was diagnosed as having nonallergic rhinitis and started on fluticasone propionate.

The patient was brought in by his wife who indicates that he has not been acting like himself the past 24 h and may have a fever. She also says "he has always been tough as nails but on the drive over he was yelling with pain every time I hit the smallest bump. I just don't know what's got into him." On physical exam his temperature is 103.6°, heart rate 126, respirations 22, and blood pressure 108/74. He is alert, but not oriented and toxic appearing. He is asked to lay supine on the exam table and when his neck is flexed there is also immediate flexion of his hips and knees and he yells "ouch."

The patient is admitted to the intensive care unit for sepsis and empirically treated for bacterial meningitis. As expected the CSF cultures from his lumbar puncture collected at the time of admission have grown *Streptococcus pneumoniae*. An astute internal medicine resident notices that the patient continues to have unilateral rhinorrhea and questions the possibility of a CSF leak. The clear rhinorrhea fluid is collected and sent for beta-2 transferrin which comes back as positive (detected) and a high-resolution CT scan of the paranasal sinuses ordered to localize the leak.

Diagnosis/Assessment

Once the CSF leak has been confirmed by the presence of beta-2 transferrin the next step is imaging studies for evaluation of leak localization. Numerous imaging studies are available such as high-resolution CT, contrast-enhanced CT cisternography, magnetic resonance imaging, radionuclide cisternography, and contrast-enhanced magnetic resonance cisternogram that can be utilized for specific clinical scenarios (Fig. 11.1). These latter studies have the potential to demonstrate visualization of active CSF leaks through dural disruption (Fig. 11.2). However, several of these modalities are more invasive due to the requirement of intrathecal injection of contrast media or radioactive tracers.

The initial imaging study most frequently recommended is high-resolution CT (see Fig. 11.1) of the paranasal sinuses and mastoids due to its high sensitivity [7, 15, 23–25]. In the setting of a positive beta-2 transferrin it has been reported that HRCT has a sensitivity of 88–95% [23–25]. One of the advantages of this imaging strategy is that there does not need to be an active CSF leak to identify a defect, unlike other imaging modalities. Another advantage is that the HRCT provides the surgeon with exceptional visualization of the osseous sinonasal anatomy which is advantageous for image-guided interventions. The disadvantage of this study arises when multiple areas of osseous defects are visualized as it can be challenging to determine which defect(s) is the source of the leak.

Contrast-enhanced CT cisternography is less frequently used in present day due to inferior

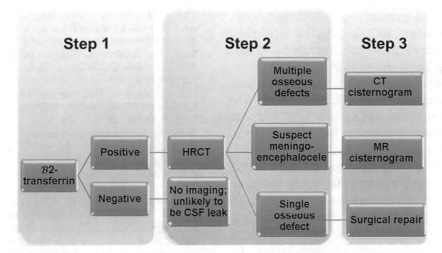

Fig. 11.1 Algorithm for evaluation of CSF leak. *β2 Transferrin* beta-2 transferrin; *HRCT* high-resolution computed tomography; *CSF* cerebrospinal fluid; *CT* cisternogram, computed tomography cisternogram; *MR cisternogram* magnetic resonance cisternogram. Adapted from [7], Copyright 2017, with permission from Elsevier

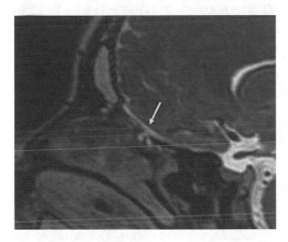

Fig. 11.2 Magnetic resonance cisternogram (MRC) demonstrating a cerebral spinal fluid (CSF) leak. MRC uses heavily T2-weighted images to delineate the contrast between cerebrospinal fluid and skull base. In this sagittal image there are multiple tracts (arrow) demonstrating a CSF leak along the cribriform plate [7]

sensitivity as compared to other modalities [15, 23, 25–31]. The low sensitivity of these studies is likely due to the fact that there must be an active CSF leak to visualize the pooling of contrast at the site of the defect [7]. This study is also more invasive as it requires an intrathecal iodinated contrast injection through a lumbar puncture. This study also results in a higher dose of radiation due to multiple scans being required.

A strategy in patients with a slow or intermittent leak that has not been successfully visualized by other imaging modalities may be a contrast-enhanced magnetic resonance cisternogram (MRC) [7]. A potential benefit of MRC is the lack of ionizing radiation. The obvious concern about this technique is the intrathecal use of gadolinium that is administered via lumbar puncture. It should be noted that the intrathecal administration of gadolinium is not approved by the US Food and Drug Administration (FDA). This however has been used in select institutions worldwide and has been reported to be safely used in low doses in patients with normal renal function [32, 33].

Radionuclide cisternography involves intrathecal injection of technetium-99 or indium-111 via lumbar puncture. Pledgets (small cotton nasal tampons) are positioned throughout the nasal cavity for several hours and upon removal are measured for the radioactive tracer. The level of tracer in the pledgets is compared to baseline serum levels, and a positive study is considered when the ratio of pledgets to serum levels is 2:1 or 3:1 [7]. However, this study would only be considered a confirmatory study for CSF leak because it rarely provides accurate information for leak localization, which limits its clinical utility.

There are potential serious complications associated with CSF leaks including meningitis, brain abscesses, persistent neurological deficits, and death. These critical sequelae underscore the importance of diagnosing a CSF leak. It has been reported that an untreated CSF leak increases the risk of developing meningitis by 10% per year [23]. Historically there has been controversy in the use of prophylactic antibiotics in patients with CSF leaks. This has primarily been an issue with small sample-sized studies not reproducibly showing prophylactic antibiotics to be beneficial. A meta-analysis by Brodie and colleagues [34] challenged this potential treatment by reporting in six studies involving 324 patients that the incidence of meningitis was 2.5% in those treated with antibiotics compared to 10.3% in the untreated group ($P = 0.006$). Up to 30% of CSF leaks may spontaneously resolve during the initial 3 weeks but given the potential catastrophic complications these patients should be referred to neurosurgery or otolaryngology immediately [7].

Clinical Pearls and Pitfalls

- The most common cause of a CSF leak is related to trauma.
- The development of CSF rhinorrhea may be delayed after the inciting traumatic event.
- If a CSF leak is not properly diagnosed it may result in serious complications such as meningitis.

References

1. Jovancevic L, Georgalas C, Savovic S, Janjevic D. Gustatory rhinitis. Rhinology. 2010;48(1):7–10.
2. Orban N, Maughan E, Bleach N. Pregnancy-induced rhinitis. Rhinology. 2013;51(2):111–9.
3. Banks TA, Gada SM. Atrophic rhinitis. Allergy Asthma Proc. 2013;34(2):185–7.
4. Ku MJ, Rao YA, Silverman BA, Schneider AT. Unusually persistent rhinorrhea in a patient with allergic rhinitis. Ann Allergy Asthma Immunol. 2004;93(1):23–8.
5. Swift AC, Foy P. Advances in the management of CSF rhinorrhoea. Hosp Med. 2002;63(1):28–32.
6. Zlab MK, Moore GF, Daly DT, Yonkers AJ. Cerebrospinal fluid rhinorrhea: a review of the literature. Ear Nose Throat J. 1992;71(7):314–7.
7. Reddy M, Baugnon K. Imaging of cerebrospinal fluid rhinorrhea and otorrhea. Radiol Clin N Am. 2017;55(1):167–87.
8. Dula DJ, Fales W. The 'ring sign': is it a reliable indicator for cerebral spinal fluid? Ann Emerg Med. 1993;22(4):718–20.
9. Warnecke A, Averbeck T, Wurster U, Harmening M, Lenarz T, Stover T. Diagnostic relevance of beta2-transferrin for the detection of cerebrospinal fluid fistulas. Arch Otolaryngol Head Neck Surg. 2004;130(10):1178–84.
10. Chan DT, Poon WS, IP CP, Chiu PW, goh KY. How useful is glucose detection in diagnosing cerebrospinal fluid leak? The rational use of CT and Beta-2 transferrin assay in detection of cerebrospinal fluid fistula. Asian J Surg. 2004;27(1):39–42.
11. Philips BJ, Meguer JX, Redman J, Baker EH. Factors determining the appearance of glucose in upper and lower respiratory tract secretions. Intensive Care Med. 2003;29(12):2204–10.
12. Wood DM, Brennan AL, Philips BJ, Baker EH. Effect of hyperglycaemia on glucose concentration of human nasal secretions. Clin Sci (Lond). 2004;106(5):527–33.
13. Oakley GM, Alt JA, Schlosser RJ, Harvey RJ, Orlandi RR. Diagnosis of cerebrospinal fluid rhinorrhea: an evidence-based review with recommendations. Int Forum Allergy Rhinol. 2016;6(1):8–16.
14. Knight JA. Advances in the analysis of cerebrospinal fluid. Ann Clin Lab Sci. 1997;27(2):93–104.
15. Zapalac JS, Marple BF, Schwade ND. Skull base cerebrospinal fluid fistulas: a comprehensive diagnostic algorithm. Otolaryngol Head Neck Surg. 2002;126(6):669–76.
16. Marshall AH, Jones NS, Robertson IJ. An algorithm for the management of CSF rhinorrhoea illustrated by 36 cases. Rhinology. 1999;37(4):182–5.
17. Bleier BS, Debnath I, O'Connell BP, Vandergrift WA 3rd, Palmer JN, Schlosser RJ. Preliminary study on the stability of beta-2 transferrin in extracorporeal cerebrospinal fluid. Otolaryngol Head Neck Surg. 2011;144(1):101–3.
18. Arrer E, Meco C, Oberascher G, Piotrowski W, Albegger K, Patsch W. beta-Trace protein as a marker for cerebrospinal fluid rhinorrhea. Clin Chem. 2002;48(6 Pt 1):939–41.
19. McCudden CR, Senior BA, Hainsworth S, Oliveira W, Silverman LM, Bruns DE, et al. Evaluation of high resolution gel beta(2)-transferrin for detection of cerebrospinal fluid leak. Clin Chem Lab Med. 2013;51(2):311–5.
20. Bachmann G, Nekic M, Michel O. Clinical experience with beta-trace protein as a marker for cerebrospinal fluid. Ann Otol Rhinol Laryngol. 2000;109(12 Pt 1):1099–102.
21. Petereit HF, Bachmann G, Nekic M, Althaus H, Pukrop R. A new nephelometric assay for beta-trace

protein (prostaglandin D synthase) as an indicator of liquorrhoea. J Neurol Neurosurg Psychiatry. 2001;71(3):347–51.

22. Schnabel C, Di Martino E, Gilsbach JM, Riediger D, Gressner AM, Kunz D. Comparison of beta2-transferrin and beta-trace protein for detection of cerebrospinal fluid in nasal and ear fluids. Clin Chem. 2004;50(3):661–3.

23. Mostafa BE, Khafagi A. Combined HRCT and MRI in the detection of CSF rhinorrhea. Skull Base. 2004;14(3):157–62. discussion 162

24. Algin O, Hakyemez B, Gokalp G, Ozcan T, Korfali E, Parlak M. The contribution of 3D-CISS and contrast-enhanced MR cisternography in detecting cerebrospinal fluid leak in patients with rhinorrhoea. Br J Radiol. 2010;83(987):225–32.

25. Shetty PG, Shroff MM, Sahani DV, Kirtane MV. Evaluation of high-resolution CT and MR cisternography in the diagnosis of cerebrospinal fluid fistula. AJNR Am J Neuroradiol. 1998;19(4):633–9.

26. Stone JA, Castillo M, Neelon B, Mukherji SK. Evaluation of CSF leaks: high-resolution CT compared with contrast-enhanced CT and radionuclide cisternography. AJNR Am J Neuroradiol. 1999;20(4):706–12.

27. Sillers MJ, Morgan CE, el Gammal T. Magnetic resonance cisternography and thin coronal computerized tomography in the evaluation of cerebrospinal fluid rhinorrhea. Am J Rhinol. 1997;11(5):387–92.

28. Goel G, Ravishankar S, Jayakumar PN, Vasudev MK, Shivshankar JJ, Rose D, et al. Intrathecal gadolinium-enhanced magnetic resonance cisternography in cerebrospinal fluid rhinorrhea: road ahead? J Neurotrauma. 2007;24(10):1570–5.

29. Eberhardt KE, Hollenbach HP, Deimling M, Tomandl BF, Huk WJ. MR cisternography: a new method for the diagnosis of CSF fistulae. Eur Radiol. 1997;7(9):1485–91.

30. Ozgen T, Tekkok IH, Cila A, Erzen C. CT cisternography in evaluation of cerebrospinal fluid rhinorrhea. Neuroradiology. 1990;32(6):481–4.

31. Payne RJ, Frenkiel S, Glikstein R, Mohr G. Role of computed tomographic cisternography in the management of cerebrospinal fluid rhinorrhea. J Otolaryngol. 2003;32(2):93–100.

32. Aydin K, Terzibasioglu E, Sencer S, Sencer A, Suoglu Y, Karasu A, et al. Localization of cerebrospinal fluid leaks by gadolinium-enhanced magnetic resonance cisternography: a 5-year single-center experience. Neurosurgery. 2008;62(3):584–9. discussion 584–9

33. Arbelaez A, Medina E, Rodriguez M, Londono AC, Castillo M. Intrathecal administration of gadopentetate dimeglumine for MR cisternography of nasoethmoidal CSF fistula. Am J Roentgenol. 2007;188(6):W560–4.

34. Brodie HA. Prophylactic antibiotics for posttraumatic cerebrospinal fluid fistulae. A meta-analysis. Arch Otolaryngol Head Neck Surg. 1997;123(7):749–52.

Alan P. Baptist and Sharmilee M. Nyenhuis

Case Presentation 1

J.J. is a 66-year-old woman who presents to an allergy/immunology specialist with complaints of nasal congestion, sneezing, and clear nasal drainage for the past 10 years. Over the past year her symptoms have gotten worse, which prompted her to make an appointment with an allergist. She has had two sinus infections this year that required one course of antibiotics and 5 missed days of work. Her symptoms are present all year round but are worse in the winter. Other triggers of her symptoms include exposure to strong odors, including cleaning products and air fresheners. She has tried antihistamines (diphenhydramine 25 mg and chlorpheniramine 4 mg) for her symptoms with some relief but rarely uses these as they cause drowsiness and dry mouth.

The patient's past medical history includes hypertension and urinary incontinence for which she takes atenolol 25 mg daily and solifenacin 5 mg daily, respectively. She denies any surgeries

in the past. The patient lives in a house with her husband, who smokes five cigarettes per day in his car, and about 18 months ago she adopted her daughter's dog, who lives inside their home. She states that she has trouble with dogs who have fur and are heavy shedders but has no trouble with her daughter's dog, which has hair and is a non-shedder. There is carpet throughout the home, and there is ongoing construction of new homes around her and she feels that the increased dust often triggers her symptoms. The patient's home has not had any recent flooding nor is there visible indoor mold. She works as a paralegal in a law firm but notices no difference in her symptoms at home versus work unless exposed to triggers that cause symptoms which are more difficult for her to avoid.

On physical exam, pertinent positive findings were ocular conjunctival injection bilaterally, clear mucoid drainage in both nasal passages, pale and congested turbinates bilaterally, and cobblestoning of the posterior oropharynx indicative of postnasal drainage.

Allergy skin prick testing (SPT) revealed an adequate histamine response and a 3 mm wheal/10 mm flare reaction to dog by SPT. Intracutaneous testing revealed a 4 mm wheal/12 mm flare reaction to both species of dust mites (*Dermatophagoides pteronyssinus* and *Dermatophagoides farinae*). All other aeroallergens tested were negative. Her creatinine was 0.9 mg/dL, and her glomerular filtration rate was 55 mL/min.

A. P. Baptist (✉)
Department of Allergy and Clinical Immunology, University of Michigan, Ann Arbor, MI, USA
e-mail: abaptist@med.umich.edu

S. M. Nyenhuis
Division of Pulmonary, Critical Care, Sleep and Allergy, Department of Medicine, University of Illinois Hospital and Health Sciences System, Chicago, IL, USA
e-mail: snyenhui@uic.edu

© Springer International Publishing AG, part of Springer Nature 2018
J. A. Bernstein (ed.), *Rhinitis and Related Upper Respiratory Conditions*,
https://doi.org/10.1007/978-3-319-75370-6_12

Based on the clinical history, physical exam findings, and allergy testing, the patient was diagnosed with persistent mixed rhinitis based on her perennial allergic rhinitis symptoms triggered by dogs and dust mites and nonallergic (vasomotor) rhinitis symptoms triggered by odorants and chemical irritants. Allergen avoidance measures were reviewed with the patient in detail and she was started on a nasal corticosteroid spray (fluticasone one spray in each nostril twice a day) in conjunction with loratadine 10 mg daily.

Diagnosis/Assessment

The approach to rhinitis in older adults must consider the clinical symptoms of the patient, response to testing, and knowledge of the different types of rhinitis commonly found in older adults. Rhinitis is categorized broadly into allergic rhinitis and nonallergic rhinitis. While allergic rhinitis is often thought of as a disease affecting only the young, it is becoming increasingly common in older adults [1].

Allergic Rhinitis

Although the peak incidence of allergic rhinitis (AR) is during adulthood, AR is prevalent among older people affecting approximately 5.4–10.7% of patients above 65 years old, as in the case presented above [2–4]. Allergic rhinitis is characterized by intermittent or persistent symptoms of nasal congestion, rhinorrhea, nasal/ocular pruritus, sneezing, and postnasal drainage. The Allergic Rhinitis and Its Impact on Asthma (ARIA) Report defines "intermittent" symptoms that are present less than 4 days per weeks or less than 4 consecutive weeks [5]. "Persistent" symptoms are present more than 4 days per week and for more than 4 consecutive weeks [5]. These symptoms are a result of IgE-mediated allergic inflammation in the nasal mucosa triggered by various allergens. Triggering allergens may be seasonal or perennial. The seasonal allergens include pollen and mold, while perennial allergens include dust mites, pet dander, and pests (cockroach, mice).

In addition to the nasal symptoms of AR, patients may also have generalized symptoms that include fatigue, mood changes, depression, anxiety, impairments of work, and cognitive function [6]. Many of these symptoms may also occur with aging, but it is important to recognize that these symptoms could also be related to moderate or severe AR or secondary to the therapies used to treat rhinitis. Furthermore, AR is associated with a diminished quality of life, although the impact that both the nasal and nonnasal symptoms have on the quality of life of older adults is still poorly elucidated [7].

A key component to diagnosing AR is objective evidence of allergen sensitivity. Allergy skin testing (prick and in some cases intracutaneous) or serum testing for specific IgE is used to assess allergen sensitization to environmental allergens. Allergen sensitization, as well as total IgE, has been shown to diminish with age [8–10]. However, evaluating for allergen sensitivity remains important in older adults, as between 25 and 41% have evidence of sensitization, as the patient did in this case [8, 10]. The clinical diagnosis of AR is confirmed by the onset of symptoms after exposure to the sensitizing allergen.

Local Allergic Rhinitis

While this patient did have evidence of AR by skin testing, there have been recent reports of a subset of rhinitis patients with positive nasal provocation to allergens despite negative skin prick tests [11–13]. It has been hypothesized that these patients have local AR (LAR). Bozek and colleagues recently examined the prevalence of LAR in older adults (mean age 65.8 years old) and found that LAR and AR are common in this population (21% and 40%, respectively) [14]. *Dermatophagoides pteronyssinus* was the main sensitizing aeroallergens in older adults with LAR and AR [14]. Further studies are needed to gain a better understanding of the immunopathology, practical diagnostic tests, and management of LAR in older adults.

Nonallergic Rhinitis

Nonallergic rhinitis (NAR) is characterized by symptoms of nasal congestion, rhinorrhea, and postnasal drainage that are not the result of IgE-dependent events [15]. The diagnosis of NAR is based on clinical history and exclusion of other causes of rhinitis. The symptoms of NAR may be persistent, intermittent, seasonal (climatic), and/or elicited by recognized triggers. These triggers include but are not limited to cold air, changes in temperature or barometric pressure, strong odors, pollutants, chemicals, and exercise. In the case presented, the patient did have worsening of symptoms with exposure to strong odors and chemicals.

As allergic sensitization decreases with age, it is often assumed that rhinitis in older adults is nonallergic [8]. Jessen examined the prevalence of NAR in adults and found a U-shaped relationship with age with the lowest prevalence occurring in middle-aged (50–60 years old) persons and an increase after age 60 [16]. Other studies have found little relationship between age and self-reported nonallergic symptoms [17, 18]. Overall, AR remains common in older adults but nonallergic causes of rhinitis appear to be more prevalent with age [19]. Further studies are necessary to determine the true prevalence in older adults.

Mixed Rhinitis

Allergic and nonallergic rhinitides frequently coexist (at least 35%) as in this case. This condition (NAR and AR) is called mixed rhinitis and has multiple triggers (e.g., pollens, change in weather, strong odors) [20]. The clinical presentation of mixed rhinitis can be variable and is characterized by intermittent or persistent rhinitis symptoms that are not fully explained by specific IgE sensitization and not completely responsive to medications designed to treat AR (Fig. 12.1). Despite the often similar clinical presentation, it is important to assess for the presence of both by trigger identification. Recognition of co-occurrence of these two common conditions will help clinicians provide the most effective and appropriate treatment and help impact the morbidity associated with both diseases.

Atrophic Rhinitis

Atrophic rhinitis is a rhinitis subtype that is more prevalent in older adult populations [21]. This type of rhinitis is manifested by symptoms of congestion, nasal crusting, and fetor. Decreased blood flow to the nasal mucosa contributes to the local atrophy and leads to the enlargement of nasal space with paradoxical nasal congestion [21]. Atrophic rhinitis is often complicated by bacterial colonization and often actual infections, frequently with *Klebsiella ozaenae* [22].

Management/Outcome

Allergic Rhinitis

The main non-pharmacologic treatment option for AR is avoidance of offending allergens. In some cases, avoidance may reduce or eliminate the patient's symptoms. Older adults may have difficulty implementing avoidance measures due to physical limitations of regular cleaning, financial constraints, or communal living situations. Older adults living in communal living situations such as nursing homes or assisted living may have little control to make changes in their environmental surroundings.

Antihistamines, specifically second-generation H1-antagonists, are standard treatment for mild AR. Their easy availability (over the counter) and in most cases low cost account for their high use. This class of medication can be effective for controlling ocular and nasal pruritus, rhinorrhea, and sneezing, but is less effective for improving nasal congestion [23]. First-generation H1-antagonists should be avoided in older adults when possible as they have adverse effects on the central nervous system and interact with other medications. Additionally, studies have shown that first-generation antihistamines can affect driving performance, disturb the normal sleep cycle, and impact cognition, which can further worsen conditions prevalent in the geriatric population [24, 25]. In contrast, second-generation H1-antagonists are generally safe in older adults with rhinitis, but dose adjustment must be made for patients with renal failure. In this case, as the creatinine clearance was >30 mL/min, no dose adjustment was made for loratadine.

Fig. 12.1 Type of rhinitis seen in the elderly

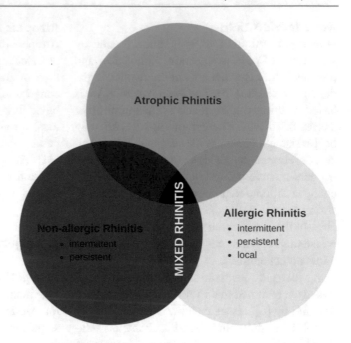

Intranasal antihistamines are an alternative to oral antihistamines. They are as effective as oral antihistamines but are more effective at reducing nasal congestion. The main adverse effects from intranasal antihistamines include bitter taste, sedation, headache, and application-site irritation. Azelastine, a topical antihistamine, has been found to be well tolerated in older adults with rhinitis [26, 27].

Intranasal corticosteroids (INS) are the first-line therapy for moderate/severe persistent AR [23]. They are effective in reducing all rhinitis symptoms including nasal congestion, anterior and posterior rhinorrhea, and nasal pruritus. They are generally effective and well tolerated in older adults [28]. These agents have negligible systemic corticosteroid absorption and the most common side effects include epistaxis, nasal dryness, and mucosal crusting. Patients should be instructed on the proper use of nasal sprays specifically angling them away from the nasal septum and be monitored periodically to assess for these adverse effects.

Allergen immunotherapy (AIT) is the only treatment that can modify the natural course of AR during its initial stages. Subcutaneous IT (SCIT) can be considered an effective therapeutic option in otherwise healthy older adults with short disease duration whose symptoms cannot be adequately controlled by medications alone [29, 30]. Recent studies demonstrate the efficacy of sublingual IT (SLIT) in older adults [31]. Bozek and colleagues found that SLIT reduces symptoms, drug consumption, and progression of the disease in both young and older adults allergic to house dust mites and grass pollen with persistent AR and mild bronchial asthma [32, 33]. If the patient presented in this case does not respond well to second-generation antihistamines and intranasal corticosteroids alone or in combination with intranasal antihistamines, SCIT could be considered. An alternative would be SLIT for dust mites which was recently approved by the FDA. Her current use of a beta-blocker would need to be taken into consideration, as beta-blockers can make systemic reactions to allergen immunotherapy more severe and difficult to treat. Therefore, a cautious attitude should be adopted toward starting AIT) in patients who require use of beta-blocker agents. In those circumstances where an alternative agent to a selective beta-blocker can't be substituted and AIT is believed to be essential, the patient's values and preferences should be considered in conjunction with the risks and benefits of treatment in the decision-making process [34].

Nonallergic Rhinitis

Evidence-based guidance for the treatment of NAR in older adults is lacking. The treatment of NAR typically includes the use of intranasal corticosteroids (INCSs), intranasal antihistamines, intranasal anticholinergics, oral decongestants, and nasal lavage. Intranasal corticosteroids are recommended for the treatment of persistent NAR. They have shown to improve nasal congestion compared to intranasal anticholinergics (i.e., ipratropium bromide) in a randomized controlled trial [35]. Oral second-generation antihistamines have little role in the treatment of NAR. There has been no randomized controlled study which has examined the use of oral second-generation antihistamines alone in the treatment of NAR [35]. One study from 1982 used a first-generation antihistamine in combination with a decongestant and found an improvement in NAR symptoms with this regimen [36]. While the first-generation antihistamines do carry some anticholinergic properties, which might improve anterior and posterior rhinorrhea, it is likely the decongestant was providing more benefit in relieving nasal congestion. Second-generation antihistamines exhibit little to no anticholinergic properties, which is why they have a decreased benefit in NAR. However, if dosed properly at bedtime, first-generation antihistamines like chlorpheniramine maleate or diphenhydramine HCl can be used to control persistent postnasal drainage and are frequently well tolerated without significant side effects.

The intranasal antihistamine, azelastine, has been shown to be effective in NAR due to the anti-inflammatory and neuroinflammatory blockade properties that it exhibits [37, 38]. A noninferiority study found that olopatadine was as effective as azelastine in treating NAR but this compound is a more selective H1-antihistamine and its mechanistic effectiveness in NAR is less understood [39, 40]. Studies that have compared topical antihistamines (azelastine, olopatadine) to INCSs (fluticasone) have found no superiority of either drug in the treatment of NAR [41, 42]. Furthermore, when intranasal antihistamines and INCSs have been used concurrently, patients obtained greater symptomatic relief than with the use of either drug alone [43–45]. Although oral decongestants are effective in treating nasal congestion, few studies have examined the use of oral decongestants for the treatment of NAR. Two randomized controlled studies using phenylpropanolamine found a decrease in nasal congestion and rhinorrhea though this drug has since been removed from the market to risk of thromboembolic events [35]. No studies using pseudoephedrine in NAR have been reported. Further, the use of oral decongestants in older adults should be used cautiously due to the side effects of increased heart rate, anxiety, insomnia, urinary retention, and dry mouth and avoided in patients with uncontrolled hypertension, coronary heart disease, cerebrovascular disease, and prostatism [46]. Recently, several studies have found that topical decongestants can be used for extended periods of time (longer than 3–5 days) without the development of rhinitis medicamentosa when used in conjunction with an INCS. This approach may be useful in controlling more difficult-to-control congestion especially in older patients with chronic rhinitis where oral decongestants should be avoided [47, 48].

Anticholinergics such as ipratropium bromide have demonstrated efficacy in reducing anterior rhinorrhea in several randomized controlled trials [35]. Despite its potent effect on rhinorrhea, it has little effect on nasal congestion. This class of medications is best used when the main rhinitis symptom is rhinorrhea as in gustatory or cold air-induced rhinitis. Finally, similar to AR, environmental control measures should be taken to reduce irritant indoor triggers such as tobacco smoke and strong odors and to avoid being outdoors during times of extremes in temperature, humidity, or high air pollution when possible.

Mixed Rhinitis

Currently, no treatment is specifically approved by the US Food and Drug Administration (FDA) for the treatment of mixed rhinitis. The standard approach has been to treat patients with this condition similarly to patients with allergic or nonallergic rhinitis as was in the case presented

[23]. However, many times these patients have difficult-to-treat rhinitis and require more complex treatment regiments including nasal irrigation with saline and combination INCS and intranasal antihistamines.

Atrophic Rhinitis

Treatment of primary and secondary atrophic rhinitis involves reducing crusting and alleviating the foul odor by instituting a regimen of nasal hygiene, such as saline irrigation and crust debridement, and the use of topical and/or systemic antibiotics when purulent secretions or an acute infection is present [49].

Clinical Pearls and Pitfalls

- Allergic rhinitis is a prevalent condition in adulthood and may affect up to 10% of adults ≥65 years old.
- Allergic rhinitis may be mixed with nonallergic rhinitis in many cases (up to 50%).
- While there is a reduction in specific IgE and number of positive skin tests with age, it is important to do allergy testing in the evaluation of rhinitis in older adults to assess for an allergic component. Although less common in older patients, sensitization to new allergens can occur over time.
- Selection of medications for rhinitis treatment should take into account that older adults may be more susceptible to adverse effects of some of these medications.
- Review current medications used to treat comorbid conditions at each clinical encounter.
- Consider writing out treatment plans as memory may be an issue in older adults.
- Environmental controls for patients with nonallergic rhinitis should target *irritant triggers* such as tobacco smoke, strong odors, and extremes in temperature and humidity.
- Consideration of nasal lavage is important in older adults, especially those with atrophic

rhinitis—a condition more common among older adults than younger age groups.

Case Presentation 2

A 74-year-old woman presents to the clinic with a chief concern of "a nose that runs all of the time." She has noted symptoms for most of her life, but it has significantly worsened over the past 5 years. She does state that cold air can exacerbate the symptoms, and that they will also somewhat worsen in the fall. Along with rhinorrhea, the patient feels that there is occasional associated nasal congestion and "perhaps" some nasal pruritus, but has not noted sneezing paroxysms nor ocular symptoms. She has tried medications in the past, though cannot remember what those medications were and cannot remember if they were effective. When pressed, she mentions that she is using some "home remedies" now, but they don't seem very effective. She does have a history of hypothyroidism, obesity, GERD, hypertension, and depression, for which she takes a beta-blocker, calcium channel blocker, proton pump inhibitor, thyroid replacement medication, and a tricyclic antidepressant. When asked about her social history, she notes that she has never smoked, rarely drinks alcohol, and lives with her 86-year-old husband in a one-bedroom apartment with a cat.

Epidemiology of Rhinitis in the Elderly

The true impact of rhinitis in the elderly has been difficult to fully ascertain, as older adults have historically been excluded from many large epidemiological studies on rhinitis. For example, both NHANES III and the European SAPALDIA study (which each had over 8000 participants) excluded anyone over the age of 60 when analyzing rhinitis outcomes and prevalence [50]. Allergic rhinitis may decrease with age, as older literature has suggested a prevalence of

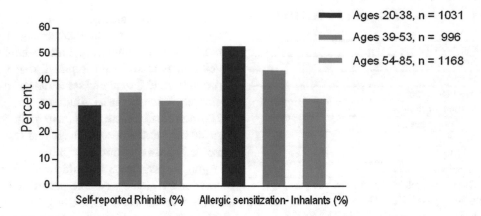

Fig. 12.2 Self-reported rhinitis and allergic sensitization among participants in the NHANES 2005–2006 study. Data from [46]

approximately 12% [51]. However, more recent literature suggests that this figure significantly underestimates the current rhinitis prevalence rate [1]. Results from the NHANES 2005–2006 study found that the self-reported prevalence of rhinitis was approximately 32% among those between the ages of 54 and 89, which was no different than younger adult populations (Fig. 12.2) [52]. However, in that study adults aged 54–89 had significantly lower rates of allergic sensitization compared to younger age groups (though approximately 33% of older adults were positive for inhalant allergen sensitivity on skin testing). Overall, it appears that NAR increases with age, and the highest prevalence is seen in the elderly [53].

Differential Diagnosis of Rhinitis

It is important, especially in the older adult, to examine for comorbidities that may cause or contribute to rhinitis. The differential is varied from granulomatous diseases such as Wegener's granulomatosis and sarcoidosis to nasal polyposis, hypothyroidism, cerebrospinal fluid leak, and malignancy (Table 12.1). Many medications that are widely used in older adults such as antihypertensives, psychotropics, alpha-adrenergic antagonists, and phosphodiesterase-5 inhibitors can cause a drug-induced rhinitis (Table 12.2). As noted in the case above,

the patient is on a number of medications that can contribute to rhinitis.

Special Considerations in Older Adults

Age-Related Nasal Changes

With normal aging, several changes occur in the nasal anatomy and physiology that may impact the presence and severity of rhinitis symptoms. Structural changes include loss of nasal tip support due to weakening of fibrous connective tissue at the upper and lower lateral cartilages, along with collagen fiber atrophy, which also leads to a dropped nasal tip [54, 55]. Furthermore, fragmentation and weakening of septal cartilage and nasal columella retraction cause changes in the nasal cavity [56]. These changes may decrease nasal airflow and symptoms of nasal congestion often found in older adults.

In addition to structural changes in the nose, mucosal changes are found with normal aging. The mucosal epithelium becomes atrophic and dry. A decrease in mucosal blood flow has been found with increasing age [56]. The decreased blood flow can contribute to decreased humidification of the nasal passages as the submucosal vessels are not able to warm and moisten the inspired air sufficiently [56]. The decreased humidification of the nose leads to dryness, crusting, and irritation.

Table 12.1 Differential diagnosis for rhinitis in older adults[a]

- Allergic rhinitis
  - Intermittent
  - Persistent
- Nonallergic rhinitis
  - Vasomotor rhinitis
  - Gustatory rhinitis
  - Infectious
  - NARES
- Occupational rhinitis
  - Caused by protein and chemical allergens, immunoglobulin E (IgE) mediated
  - Caused by chemical respiratory sensitizers, immune mechanism uncertain
  - Work-aggravated rhinitis
- Other rhinitis syndromes
  - Hormonally induced
  - Drug induced
  - Atrophic rhinitis
- Rhinitis associated with inflammatory-immunologic disorders
  - Granulomatous infections
  - Wegener's granulomatosis
  - Sarcoidosis
  - Midline granuloma
  - Churg-Strauss
  - Relapsing polychondritis
  - Amyloidosis
- Cerebrospinal fluid leak
- Nasopharyngeal malignancy

[a]Adapted from data in Wallace DV, Dykewicz MS, Bernstein DI, et al. The diagnosis and management of rhinitis, an updated practice parameter. J Allergy Clin Immunol 2008;122(Suppl):S1–84

Table 12.2 Medications that can cause or contribute to rhinitis

- ASA/NSAIDs
- Alpha-blockers (doxazosin, terazosin)
- ACE inhibitors
- Beta-blockers (carvedilol, labetalol, nadolol)
- Calcium channel blockers
- Diuretics
- Oxymetazoline
- Oral contraceptives
- Phosphodiesterase 5 inhibitors (sildenafil, tadalafil, vardenafil)
- Psychotropics (risperidone, chlorpromazine, amitriptyline)
- Phentolamine

There are also changes in the viscoelastic properties of nasal mucus that account for the excessively thick mucus in older adults [57]. Thick mucus mixed with impaired mucociliary function leads to the rhinitis symptoms of chronic postnasal drainage, nasal drainage, and cough [57]. Additionally, there is an increase in cholinergic activity in the nose with age that causes an increase in postnasal drainage [58].

Aging is associated with decreases in olfaction, with the greatest decline occurring usually after the seventh decade. Seiberling demonstrated that both the sense of smell and ability to distinguish two smells diminish with age [59]. Diminished olfaction is also commonly found in rhinitis patients. One study found that 71% of patients with dysosmia had evidence of allergic sensitization [60]. The dysosmia that occurs in allergic rhinitis is attributed to obstruction of the nasal passages, though Pinto demonstrated that inflammation of the olfactory cleft might be the cause [61].

Immunosenescence and Rhinitis

Immunosenescence describes the change in the function of immune cells with aging. With normal aging, the thymus rapidly involutes, resulting in a decline in total T cells (CD3+) involving both CD4+ and CD8+ subsets. In addition, there is a decrease in naïve T cells and an increase in the production of memory T cells. Despite the increase in memory T cells, their responses and T cell proliferative responses to antigens and mitogens are diminished [62–64].

Finally, with aging, an increase in FOXP3+ CD4+ regulatory T cells exerting suppressive effects on T cell function along with a shift in cytokine pattern from T-helper type 1 (Th1) to Th2 also has been described [65, 66]. These changes in cytokine patterns may explain late-onset rhinitis and the decreases in T cell response may be associated with the increase in infections found in older adults

Impact of Comorbidities

As people age, the number of medical conditions and medications to manage these conditions increases. In the United States, 40% of those above the age of 65 use five or more prescription medications on a daily basis [67]. Patients with multiple chronic medical problems have several challenges including interactions between conditions, difficulties in determining which medical problem is primarily active when the symptoms are similar, decreased compliance with multiple medications, and conflicting recommendations in self-care management [68]. In the case above, the patient has five comorbidities and five additional medications, all of which need to be considered in order to provide optimal care.

Medication and self-management costs can increase exponentially in elderly patients with multiple comorbidities, and therefore certain conditions may receive suboptimal care due to a lower prioritization by the individual [69]. Previous research has demonstrated that physicians also often ignore and underdiagnose rhinitis [70]. While rhinitis is typically not a life-threatening condition, it can significantly affect the quality of life [6], and is deserving of care among older adults.

A few specific comorbidities deserve special mention when considering rhinitis in the elderly. Depression has been associated with anosmia, rhinitis, and chronic sinonasal disease in a number of studies [71–74]. Theories for the association include sleep disturbance, inflammatory cytokine upregulation, and common etiologic pathogenic factors. Depression and depressive syndromes have an extremely high prevalence among the elderly population, with rates ranging from 15 to 35% [75, 76]. One study found that compared to placebo, treatment of depression and/or anxiety with escitalopram improved nasal symptoms [77]. It is also important to note that multiple psychiatric medications can cause nasal drying or rhinitis, and therefore knowledge of the side effects of drugs that each patient is taking (even when prescribed by another physician) is critically important.

A second common comorbidity among the elderly is gastroesophageal reflux disease (GERD). The prevalence of this condition is thought to increase with age [78], and among the elderly up to 22% of individuals have GERD [79]. A 10-year prospective cohort study found that those with nocturnal GERD were 60% more likely to develop rhinitis symptoms [80]. Another recent study that included subjects up to the age of 75 also found a link between GERD and rhinitis symptoms [81]. The exact underlying mechanisms of the GERD-rhinitis association, and whether treatment of GERD will improve rhinitis symptoms in the elderly, deserve further investigation.

Sleep disturbances, and in particular obstructive sleep apnea (OSA), are also common in older adults. Similar to GERD, OSA symptoms increase with age. Among adults over the age of 70, approximately 25% are thought to have OSA which is by far higher than any other age group [82]. Two recent studies evaluated the effects of AR treatment for OSA, and both found significant improvements in OSA symptomatology [83, 84]. Underlying mechanisms of this improvement were thought to be related to improvements in nasal inflammation with a resultant decrease in nasal obstruction. Although the mean age of the participants in these studies was approximately 49 years, the results may also be applicable to older adults—though again further studies are needed.

Limited Income/Poverty

Among older adults, poverty is common. Data from the US Census Bureau found that approximately 10% of older adults lived below the poverty line [85]. This number has been increasing over the past 10 years due to a variety of factors such as increased medical costs, loss of pension or retirement benefits, spending down assets to qualify for Medicaid and state-sponsored supplemental insurance coverage, and economic recessions requiring spending of retirement savings [86]. Currently, multiple antihistamines and intranasal corticosteroids have moved from prescription to over-the-counter (OTC) status. One study examining this switch for antihistamines found a 65% decrease in medication utilization [87], and similar decreases in utilization have been seen in other prescription-to-OTC medication changes. Studies have not been conducted to examine the impact of prescription-to-OTC changes on rhinitis quality of life and symptom control associated with decreased utilization. It is important for the physician caring for older adults with rhinitis to inquire about their ability to afford both prescription and OTC medications, and to offer prescription assistance programs or a social work referral when appropriate.

Complementary and Alternative Medicine for Rhinitis Among the Elderly

Complementary and alternative medicine (CAM) is defined as a group of diverse medical and healthcare systems, practices, and products that are not generally considered part of the conventional allopathic medical practices. Patients often use CAM therapy because of low cost, concerns of medication side effects, belief that adverse effects are not encountered with CAM therapy, and effectiveness (though such claims are often not based on clinical trials) [88]. Examples of CAM used for allergic disease include herbal therapies, traditional Chinese medicine, acupuncture, nasal powders, and others.

Overall CAM use has been increasing steadily, and 40% of the US population has used some form of CAM therapy [89]. Similarly, high levels of CAM use for rhinitis have also been seen in both children and adults [90, 91]. Older adults are often more likely than younger adults to use CAM therapy [92], though this has not been examined specifically for rhinitis therapy. Additionally, older adults with atopic conditions such as asthma rarely tell their physician about CAM use and physicians typically do not ask [93]. Although CAM use is typically thought to be safe by patients, adverse event monitoring is typically poor, and interactions with allopathic medications can occur. It is therefore important for the physician caring for the older adult with rhinitis to assess CAM utilization, and to work with the patient on a strategy that is both patient centered and effective.

Dementia, Memory Loss, and Medication Compliance in Older Adults

One cornerstone in the management of a chronic disease such as AR is compliance with a daily medical regimen. Unfortunately, memory loss due to conditions such as dementia and neurovascular complications can make such a task difficult. Dementia and/or memory loss are common among older adults. For adults over the age of 60, approximately 13% note some degree of memory loss [94]; among those over 85, the rate of dementia is a staggering 37% [95]. Additionally, the number of people in the United States with Alzheimer's dementia is expected to increase dramatically over the next 30 years as the population ages [96].

Although the different methods of screening an older adult for memory loss and dementia are beyond the scope of this chapter, once such a patient is identified there are steps the physician can do to help maximize medication compliance. These steps include prescribing as few medicines as possible, tailoring dose regimens to personal habits, and coordinating all drug dosing schedules as feasible [97]. The healthcare provider must assess the patient's level of self-efficacy and particular living situation when searching for the optimal medication adherence strategy and at times may need to enlist a family member or other individual to accommodate medication delivery. Along with memory loss, other factors can affect compliance. Poor coordination, hand weakness, and arthritis may influence the ability to use nasal sprays or open medicine bottles or pill boxes. Healthcare providers should review the use of nasal sprays at each visit to ensure proper use.

Clinical Pearls and Pitfalls

- Rhinitis symptoms are common affecting approximately 32% of older adults.
- Nonallergic (including gustatory) and atrophic rhinitides are more common among older adults than younger populations. Determining

the rhinitis subtype can help to provide the most appropriate therapy.

- Age-related nasal changes and immunosenescence contribute to atrophic rhinitis.
- Comorbidities can affect the presentation of rhinitis, cause medication interactions, and impact compliance. The provider needs to be aware of each comorbidity, and how it may affect rhinitis management.
- Poverty is common among older adults, and can affect the ability of patients to afford and adhere to therapeutic recommendations.
- Older adults are more likely to use complementary and alternative medication, and rarely provide this information to their physician nor does the physician routinely inquire about CAM use.
- Dementia and memory loss are see in 13% of patients above age 60 which affects the ability of a patient to manage a chronic disease like rhinitis. Screening for memory loss may be appropriate.
- Medication side effects are far more common in older adults. The provider should be aware of adverse drug effects for each medication a patient is taking and prescribe the fewest number to maximize clinical outcomes while minimizing side effects.

References

1. Slavin RG. Special considerations in treatment of allergic rhinitis in the elderly: role of intranasal corticosteroids. Allergy Asthma Proc. 2010;31(3):179–84.
2. Bakos N, Schöll I, Szalai K, Kundi M, Untersmayr E, Jensen-Jarolim E. Risk assessment in elderly for sensitization to food and respiratory allergens. Immunol Lett. 2006;107(1):15–21.
3. Pinto JM, Jeswani S. Rhinitis in the geriatric population. Allergy Asthma Clin Immunol. 2010;6(1):10.
4. Bauchau V, Durham SR. Prevalence and rate of diagnosis of allergic rhinitis in Europe. Eur Respir J. 2004;24(5):758–64.
5. Bachert C, van Cauwenberge P, Khaltaev N. Allergic rhinitis and its impact on asthma. In collaboration with the World Health Organization. Executive summary of the workshop report. 7–10 December 1999, Geneva, Switzerland. Allergy. 2002;57(9):841–55.
6. Ozdoganoglu T, Songu M, Inancli HM. Quality of life in allergic rhinitis. Ther Adv Respir Dis. 2012;6(1):25–39.
7. Bousquet PJ, Demoly P, Devillier P, Mesbah K, Bousquet J. Impact of allergic rhinitis symptoms on quality of life in primary care. Int Arch Allergy Immunol. 2013;160(4):393–400.
8. Warm K, Backman H, Lindberg A, Lundbäck B, Rönmark E. Low incidence and high remission of allergic sensitization among adults. J Allergy Clin Immunol. 2012;129(1):136–42.
9. Simola M, Holopainene E, Malmberg H. Changes in skin and nasal sensitivity to allergens and the course of rhinitis; a long-term follow-up study. Ann Allergy Asthma Immunol. 1999;82(2):152–6.
10. Busse PJ, Lurslurchachai L, Sampson HA, Halm EA, Wisnivesky J. Perennial allergen-specific immunoglobulin E levels among inner-city elderly asthmatics. J Asthma. 2010;47(7):781–5.
11. Alvares ML, Khan DA. Allergic rhinitis with negative skin tests. Curr Allergy Asthma Rep. 2011;11(2):107–14.
12. Rondon C, Canto G, Blanca M. Local allergic rhinitis: a new entity, characterization and further studies. Curr Opin Allergy Clin Immunol. 2010;10(1):1–7.
13. Klimek L, von Bernus L, Pfaar O. Local (exclusive) IgE production in the nasal mucosa. Evidence for local allergic rhinitis. HNO. 2013;61(3):217–23.
14. Bozek A, Ignasiak B, Kasperska-Zajac A, Scierski W, Grzanka A, Jarzab J. Local allergic rhinitis in elderly patients. Ann Allergy Asthma Immunol. 2015;114(3):199–202.
15. Dykewicz MS, Fineman S, Skoner DP, Nicklas R, Lee R, Blessing-Moore J, et al. Diagnosis and management of rhinitis: complete guidelines of the joint task force on practice parameters in allergy, asthma and immunology. Ann Allergy Asthma Immunol. 1998;81(5):478–518.
16. Jessen M, Janzon L. Prevalence of non-allergic nasal complaints in an urban and a rural population in Sweden. Allergy. 1989;44(8):582–7.
17. Olsson P, Berglind N, Bellander T, Stjärne P. Prevalence of self-reported allergic and non-allergic rhinitis symptoms in Stockholm: relation to age, gender, olfactory sense and smoking. Acta Otolaryngol. 2003;123(1):75–80.
18. Settipane GA, Klein DE. Non allergic rhinitis—demography of eosinophils in nasal smear, blood total eosinophil counts and IGE levels. N Engl Reg Allergy Proc. 1985;6(4):363–6.
19. Brandt D, Bernstein JA. Questionnaire evaluation and risk factor identification for nonallergic vasomotor rhinitis. Ann Allergy Asthma Immunol. 2006;96(4):526–32.
20. Settipane RA. Other causes of rhinitis: mixed rhinitis, rhinitis medicamentosa, hormonal rhinitis, rhinitis of the elderly, and gustatory rhinitis. Immunol Allergy Clin N Am. 2011;31(3):457–67.
21. Moore EJ, Kern EB. Atrophic rhinitis: a review of 242 cases. Am J Rhinol. 2001;15(6):355–61.
22. Ferguson JL, McCaffrey TV, Kern EB, Martin WJ 2nd. Effect of Klebsiella ozaenae on ciliary activity in vitro: implications in the pathogenesis of atrophic rhinitis. Otolaryngol Head Neck Surg. 1990;102(3):207–11.

23. Dykewicz MS, Fineman S, Joint Task SDP. Force Algorithm and Annotations for Diagnosis and Management of Rhinitis. Ann Allergy Asthma Immunol. 1998;81(5):474–7.

24. McCue JD. Safety of antihistamines in the treatment of allergic rhinitis in elderly patients. Arch Fam Med. 1996;5(8):464–8.

25. Holgate ST, Canonica GW, Simons FE, Taglialatela M, Tharp M, Timmerman H, et al. Consensus Group on New-Generation Antihistamines (CONGA): present status and recommendations. Clin Exp Allergy. 2003;33(9):1305–24.

26. Golden SJ, Craig TJ. Efficacy and safety of azelastine nasal spray for the treatment of allergic rhinitis. J Am Osteopath Assoc. 1999;99(7 Suppl):S7–12.

27. Peter G, Romeis P, Borbe HO, Büker KM, Riethmüller-Winzen H. Tolerability and pharmacokinetics of single and multiple doses of azelastine hydrochloride in elderly volunteers. Arzneimittelforschung. 1995;45(5):576–81.

28. Grossman J, Gopalan G. Efficacy and safety of mometasone furoate nasal spray in elderly subjects with perennial allergic rhinitis. J Allergy Clin Immunol. 123(2):S271.

29. Armentia A, Fernández A, Tapias JA, Méndez J, de la Fuente R, Sánchez-Palla P, Sanchís E. Immunotherapy with allergenic extracts in geriatric patients: evaluation of effectiveness and safety. Allergol Immunopathol (Madr). 1993;21(5):193–6.

30. Asero R. Efficacy of injection immunotherapy with ragweed and birch pollen in elderly patients. Int Arch Allergy Immunol. 2004;135(4):332–5.

31. Marogna M, Bruno ME, Massolo A, Falagiani P. Sublingual immunotherapy for allergic respiratory disease in elderly patients: a retrospective study. Eur Ann Allergy Clin Immunol. 2008;40(1):22–9.

32. Bozek A, Ignasiak B, Filipowska B, Jarzab J. House dust mite sublingual immunotherapy: a double-blind, placebo-controlled study in elderly patients with allergic rhinitis. Clin Exp Allergy. 2013;43(2):242–8.

33. Bozek A, Kolodziejczyk K, Warkocka-Szoltysek B, Jarzab J. Grass pollen sublingual immunotherapy: a double-blind, placebo-controlled study in elderly patients with seasonal allergic rhinitis. Am J Rhinol Allergy. 2014;28(5):423–7.

34. Cox L, Nelson H, Lockey R, Calabria C, Chacko T, Finegold I, et al. Allergen immunotherapy: a practice parameter third update. J Allergy Clin Immunol. 2011;127(1 Suppl):S1–55.

35. Long A, McFadden C, DeVine D, Chew P, Kupelnick B, Lau J. Management of allergic and nonallergic rhinitis. Evid Rep Technol Assess (Summ). 2002;(54):1–6.

36. Broms P, Malm L. Oral vasoconstrictors in perennial non-allergic rhinitis. Allergy. 1982;37(2):67–74.

37. Banov CH, Lieberman P. Vasomotor rhinitis study groups. Efficacy of azelastine nasal spray in the treatment of vasomotor (perennial nonallergic) rhinitis. Ann Allergy Asthma Immunol. 2001;86(1):28–35.

38. Gawlik R, Jawor B, Rogala B, Parzynski S, DuBuske L. Effect of intranasal azelastine on substance P release in perennial nonallergic rhinitis patients. Am J Rhinol Allergy. 2013;27(6):514–6.

39. Kaliner MA. Nonallergic rhinopathy (formerly known as vasomotor rhinitis). Immunol Allergy Clin N Am. 2011;31(3):441–55.

40. Lieberman P, Meltzer EO, LaForce CF, Darter AL, Tort MJ. Two-week comparison study of olopatadine hydrochloride nasal spray 0.6% versus azelastinehydrochloride nasal spray 0.1% in patients with vasomotor rhinitis. Allergy Asthma Proc. 2011;32(2):151–8.

41. Kaliner MA. Azelastine and olopatadine in the treatment of allergic rhinitis. Ann Allergy Asthma Immunol. 2009;103(5):373–80.

42. Kaliner MA, Storms W, Tilles S, Spector S, Tan R, LaForce C, et al. Comparison of olopatadine 0.6% nasal spray versus fluticasone propionate 50 microg in the treatment of seasonal allergic rhinitis. Allergy Asthma Proc. 2009;30(3):255–62.

43. Ratner PH, Hampel F, Van Bavel J, Amar NJ, Daftary P, Wheeler W, et al. Combination therapy with azelastine hydrochloride nasal spray and fluticasone propionate nasal spray in the treatment of patients with seasonal allergic rhinitis. Ann Allergy Asthma Immunol. 2008;100(1):74–81.

44. Hampel F, Ratner P, Haeusler JM. Safety and tolerability of levocetirizine dihydrochloride in infants and children with allergic rhinitis or chronic urticaria. Allergy Asthma Proc. 2010;31(4):290–5.

45. LaForce CF, Carr W, Tilles SA, Chipps BE, Storms W, Meltzer EO, et al. Evaluation of olopatadine hydrochloride nasal spray, 0.6%, used in combination with an intranasal corticosteroid in seasonal allergic rhinitis. Allergy Asthma Proc. 2010;31(2):132–40.

46. Tan R, Corren J. Optimum treatment of rhinitis in the elderly. Drugs Aging. 1995;7(3):168–75.

47. Meltzer EO, Bernstein DI, Prenner BM, Berger WE, Shekar T, Teper AA. Mometasone furoate nasal spray plus oxymetazoline nasal spray: short-term efficacy and safety in seasonal allergic rhinitis. Am J Rhinol Allergy. 2013;27(2):102–8.

48. Vaidyanathan S, Williamson P, Clearie K, Khan F, Lipworth B. Fluticasone reverses oxymetazoline-induced tachyphylaxis of response and rebound congestion. Am J Respir Crit Care Med. 2010;182(1):19–24.

49. Little D. Geriatric Rhinitis: under-diagnosed and undertreated. Geriatr Aging. 2005;8(5):52–3.

50. Mims JW. Epidemiology of allergic rhinitis. Int Forum Allergy Rhinol. 2014;4(Suppl 2):S18–20.

51. Enright PL, Kronmal RA, Higgins MW, Schenker MB, Haponik EF. Prevalence and correlates of respiratory symptoms and disease in the elderly. Cardiovascular Health Study. Chest. 1994;106(3):827–34.

52. Shargorodsky J, Garcia-Esquinas E, Galán I, Navas-Acien A, Lin SY. Allergic sensitization, rhinitis and tobacco smoke exposure in US adults. PLoS One. 2015;10(7):e0131957.

53. Georgitis JW. Prevalence and differential diagnosis of chronic rhinitis. Curr Allergy Asthma Rep. 2001;1(3):202–6.

54. Reiss M, Reiss G. Rhinitis in old age. Praxis (Bern 1994). 2002;91(9):353–8.

55. Patterson CN. The aging nose: characteristics and correction. Otolaryngol Clin N Am. 1980;13(2):275–88.

56. Bende M. Blood flow with 133Xe in human nasal mucosa in relation to age, sex and body position. Acta Otolaryngol. 1983;96(1–2):175–9.

57. Edelstein DR. Aging of the normal nose in adults. Laryngoscope. 1996;106(9 Pt 2):1–25.

58. Dumas JA, Newhouse PA. The cholinergic hypothesis of cognitive aging revisited again: cholinergic functional compensation. Pharmacol Biochem Behav. 2011;99(2):254–61.

59. Seiberling KA, Conley DB. Aging and olfactory and taste function. Otolaryngol Clin N Am. 2004;37(6):1209–28. vii

60. Apter AJ, Mott AE, Frank ME, Clive JM. Allergic rhinitis and olfactory loss. Ann Allergy Asthma Immunol. 1995;75(4):311–6.

61. Sivam A, Jeswani S, Reder L, Wang J, DeTineo M, Taxy J, et al. Olfactory cleft inflammation is present in seasonal allergic rhinitis and is reduced with intranasal steroids. Am J Rhinol Allergy. 2010;24(4):286–90.

62. Flurkey K, Stadecker M, Miller RA. Memory T lymphocyte hyporesponsiveness to non-cognate stimuli: a key factor in age-related immunodeficiency. Eur J Immunol. 1992;22(4):931–5.

63. Murasko DM, Nelson BJ, Silver R, Matour D, Kaye D. Immunologic response in an elderly population with a mean age of 85. Am J Med. 1986;81(4):612–8.

64. Naylor K, Li G, Vallejo AN, Lee WW, Koetz K, Bryl E, et al. The influence of age on T cell generation and TCR diversity. J Immunol. 2005;174(11):7446–52.

65. Lages CS, Suffia I, Velilla PA, Huang B, Warshaw G, Hildeman DA, et al. Functional regulatory T cells accumulate in aged hosts and promote chronic infectious disease reactivation. J Immunol. 2008;181(3):1835–48.

66. Sandmand M, Bruunsgaard H, Kemp K, Andersen-Ranberg K, Pedersen AN, Skinhøj P, et al. Is ageing associated with a shift in the balance between type 1 and type 2 cytokines in humans? Clin Exp Immunol. 2002;127(1):107–14.

67. National Center for Health Statistics. Health, United States, 2012: With special feature on emergency care. Hyattsville, MD: Library of Congress Catalog Number 76–641496; 2013.

68. Bayliss EA, Steiner JF, Fernald DH, Crane LA, Main DS. Descriptions of barriers to self-care by persons with comorbid chronic diseases. Ann Fam Med. 2003;1(1):15–21.

69. Schoenberg NE, Leach C, Edwards W. "It's a toss up between my hearing, my heart, and my hip": prioritizing and accommodating multiple morbidities by vulnerable older adults. J Health Care Poor Underserved. 2009;20(1):134–51.

70. Nolte H, Nepper-Christensen S, Backer V. Unawareness and undertreatment of asthma and allergic rhinitis in a general population. Respir Med. 2006;100(2):354–62.

71. Katotomichelakis M, Simopoulos E, Tzikos A, Balatsouras D, Tripsianis G, Danielides G, et al. Demographic correlates of anxiety and depression symptoms in chronic sinonasal diseases. Int J Psychiatry Med. 2014;48(2):83–94.

72. Audino P, La Grutta S, Cibella F, La Grutta S, Melis MR, Bucchieri S, et al. Rhinitis as a risk factor for depressive mood in pre-adolescents: a new approach to this relationship. Pediatr Allergy Immunol. 2014;25(4):360–5.

73. Nanayakkara JP, Igwe C, Roberts D, Hopkins C. The impact of mental health on chronic rhinosinusitis symptom scores. Eur Arch Otorhinolaryngol. 2013;270(4):1361–4.

74. Wasan A, Fernandez E, Jamison RN, Bhattacharyya N. Association of anxiety and depression with reported disease severity in patients undergoing evaluation for chronic rhinosinusitis. Ann Otol Rhinol Laryngol. 2007;116(7):491–7.

75. Barry LC, Allore HG, Guo Z, Bruce ML, Gill TM. Higher burden of depression among older women: the effect of onset, persistence, and mortality over time. Arch Gen Psychiatry. 2008;65(2):172–8.

76. Beekman AT, Copeland JR, Prince MJ. Review of community prevalence of depression in later life. Br J Psychiatry. 1999;174:307–11.

77. Erkul E, Cingi C, Özçelik Korkmaz M, Çekiç T, Çukurova I, Yaz A, et al. Effects of escitalopram on symptoms and quality of life in patients with allergic rhinitis. Am J Rhinol Allergy. 2012;26(5):e142–6.

78. Becher A, Dent J. Systematic review: ageing and gastro-oesophageal reflux disease symptoms, oesophageal function and reflux oesophagitis. Aliment Pharmacol Ther. 2011;33(4):442–54.

79. Achem SR, DeVault KR. Gastroesophageal reflux disease and the elderly. Gastroenterol Clin N Am. 2014;43(1):147–60.

80. Schioler L, Ruth M, Jõgi R, Gislason T, Storaas T, Janson C, et al. Nocturnal GERD—a risk factor for rhinitis/rhinosinusitis: the RHINE study. Allergy. 2015;70(6):697–702.

81. Hellgren J, Olin AC, Toren K. Increased risk of rhinitis symptoms in subjects with gastroesophageal reflux. Acta Otolaryngol. 2014;134(6):615–9.

82. Duran J, Esnaola S, Rubio R, Iztueta A. Obstructive sleep apnea-hypopnea and related clinical features in a population-based sample of subjects aged 30 to 70 yr. Am J Respir Crit Care Med. 2001;163(3 Pt 1):685–9.

83. Acar M, Cingi C, Sakallioglu O, San T, Fatih Yimenicioglu M, Bal C. The effects of mometasone furoate and desloratadine in obstructive sleep apnea syndrome patients with allergic rhinitis. Am J Rhinol Allergy. 2013;27(4):e113–6.

84. Lavigne F, Petrof BJ, Johnson JR, Lavigne P, Binothman N, Kassissia GO, et al. Effect of topical corticosteroids on allergic airway inflammation and disease severity in obstructive sleep apnoea. Clin Exp Allergy. 2013;43(10):1124–33.

85. DeNavas-Walt C, Proctor BD, Smith JC. Income, poverty, and health insurance coverage in the United States: 2012. U.S. Census Bureau. Washington, DC: U.S. Government Printing Office; 2013. p. 60–245.
86. Banerjee S. Time trends in poverty for older Americans between 2001–2009. Washington, DC: Employee Benefit Research Institute; 2012. p. 20.
87. Andrade SE, Gurwitz JH, Fish LS. The effect of an Rx-to-OTC switch on medication prescribing patterns and utilization of physician services: the case of H2-receptor antagonists. Med Care. 1999;37(4):424–30.
88. Mainardi T, Kapoor S, Bielory L. Complementary and alternative medicine: herbs, phytochemicals and vitamins and their immunologic effects. J Allergy Clin Immunol. 2009;123(2):283–94. quiz 295–6
89. Barnes PM, Bloom B, Nahin RL. Complementary and alternative medicine use among adults and children: United States. Natl Health Stat Report. 2007;2008(12):1–23.
90. Kemper KJ, Vohra S, Walls R. Task force on complementary and alternative medicine; provisional section on complementary, holistic, and integrative medicine. American Academy of Pediatrics. The use of complementary and alternative medicine in pediatrics. Pediatrics. 2008;122(6):1374–86.
91. Kapoor S, Bielory L. Allergic rhinoconjunctivitis: complementary treatments for the 21st century. Curr Allergy Asthma Rep. 2009;9(2):121–7.
92. McFadden KL, Hernandez TD, Ito TA. Attitudes toward complementary and alternative medicine influence its use. Explore (NY). 2010;6(6):380–8.
93. Baptist AP, Deol BB, Reddy RC, Nelson B, Clark NM. Age-specific factors influencing asthma management by older adults. Qual Health Res. 2010;20(1):117–24.
94. Centers for Disease Control and Prevention. Self-reported increased confusion or memory loss and associated functional difficulties among adults aged >/= 60 years—21 States, 2011. MMWR Morb Mortal Wkly Rep. 2013;62(18):347–50.
95. Mathillas J, Lovheim H, Gustafson Y. Increasing prevalence of dementia among very old people. Age Ageing. 2011;40(2):243–9.
96. Hebert LE, Weuve J, Scherr PA, Evans DA. Alzheimer disease in the United States (2010-2050) estimated using the 2010 census. Neurology. 2013;80(19):1778–83.
97. Arlt S, Lindner R, Rösler A, von Renteln-Kruse W. Adherence to medication in patients with dementia: predictors and strategies for improvement. Drugs Aging. 2008;25(12):1033–47.

Sino-Nasal Sarcoidosis

13

Robert P. Baughman, Allen Seiden,
and Elyse E. Lower

Case Presentation 1

DW was a 41-year-old black female when she developed eye pain and was found to have anterior uveitis. As part of her evaluation, she had a chest X-ray which demonstrated bilateral hilar adenopathy and diffuse lung filtrates. She was diagnosed as having sarcoidosis on clinical grounds. She was not dyspneic and denied cough. Her iritis was treated with topical steroids and within 6 months she was tapered off steroid drops.

She then started having recurrent sinus symptoms. Initially this was felt to be allergic rhinitis and she was treated with intranasal steroids. Three years later, she developed severe pain behind and below her right eye. She underwent an MRI and was found to have complete opacification of her right maxillary sinus (Fig. 13.1a, b). She was seen by an ophthalmologist, who diagnosed her as having dacrocystitis, with compression of her nasolacrimal duct. She first had surgical intervention to clear her ethmoid and maxillary sinuses. Pathologic examination of the surgical specimen revealed non-caseating granulomas. After recovery, a nasolacrimal stent was placed by her ophthalmologist. Confirmation of placement of the stent beyond the inflammation was made by the otolaryngologist in the operating room.

Postoperatively the patient was placed on prednisone 40 mg a day. Over the next 6 months, attempts to reduce the dose below 20 mg a day led to recurrence of pain and bleeding from her sinuses. She was started on methotrexate and after 6 months she was able to reduce her prednisone to 10 mg a day.

Two years later, she began having recurrent sinus infections. These usually responded to antibiotics and prolonged courses of high-dose prednisone. She developed macular papular lesions on her cheeks and nasal alae. She also had new papular lesions on her arms. A biopsy of one of the arm lesions again found granulomas consistent with sarcoidosis.

She was felt to have refractory sarcoidosis with sinus disease and *lupus pernio*. The antitumor necrosis factor (TNF) antibody infliximab was initiated. The patient received 5 mg/kg initially, then 2 weeks later, and then once a month. She has done well on the combination of infliximab, methotrexate, and low-dose prednisone. She has been maintained on 5 mg-a-day prednisone and has not required increased prednisone for more than a year.

R. P. Baughman (✉) · E. E. Lower
Department of Internal Medicine, University of Cincinnati Medical Center, Cincinnati, OH, USA
e-mail: bob.baughman@uc.edu

A. Seiden
Department of Otolaryngology, Head and Neck Surgery, University of Cincinnati Academic Medical Center, Cincinnati, OH, USA

© Springer International Publishing AG, part of Springer Nature 2018
J. A. Bernstein (ed.), *Rhinitis and Related Upper Respiratory Conditions*,
https://doi.org/10.1007/978-3-319-75370-6_13

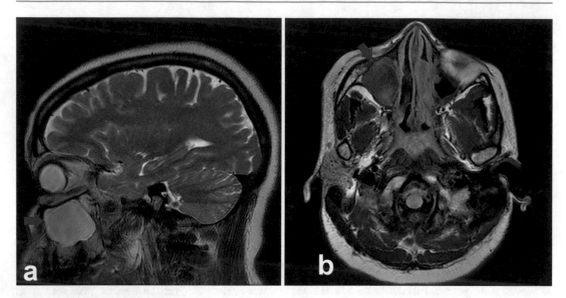

Fig. 13.1 MRI imaging demonstrating right ethmoid opacification (arrow). (**a**) Sagittal view. (**b**) Axial plane

Case Presentation 2

MC is a black female who at the age of 39 was complaining of sinus congestion and a sore on the roof of her mouth. She was referred to an otolaryngologist because of refractory sinus disease. He noted on exam that her hard palate was perforated. She denied cocaine or other drug use. A sinus biopsy found non-caseating granulomas. Her antineutrophil cytoplasmic antibody (ANCA) test was repeatedly negative. She was referred to our sarcoidosis clinic. On exam, she was noted to have extensive purplish, raised lesions of the entire nose. She also had lesions on both cheeks and was diagnosed as having *lupus pernio*. Her chest X-ray demonstrated upper lobe fibrosis consistent with Scadding stage 4 sarcoidosis. She was initially treated with prednisone and methotrexate with only modest response.

Because of insurance issues, she was not seen for 3 years. She was referred back to clinic because of respiratory distress. She had been taken off her methotrexate for unclear reasons and was on only 5 mg-a-day prednisone when she had developed acute stridor. She was found to have recurrence of pan sinusitis (Fig. 13.2a) as well as laryngeal infiltration and upper airway narrowing (Fig. 13.2b) by what proved to be her

sarcoidosis. She was only marginally better on 40 mg prednisone.

She was then started on adalimumab since her insurance would not cover infliximab. After 3 months, she started improving and eventually she was weaned to 10 mg-a-day prednisone and maintained on adalimumab 40 mg weekly.

After 2 years, she developed left hip and upper leg pain. On MRI, she was found to have an infiltrative lesion. A percutaneous needle aspirate of the bone lesion was consistent with a low-grade liposarcoma. She had surgical resection of the lesion. Because of concerns about potential carcinogenicity of adalimumab, the drug was discontinued.

Over the next 2 years, she has had no evidence of recurrence of her tumor. However, her sinus disease and facial lesions returned within 3 months of stopping the adalimumab. She was initially controlled with prednisone alone. However, as she gained more weight with the prednisone, she asked for another steroid-sparing regimen. She was begun on repository corticotrophin injection (RCI) 40 units twice. For the past year, she has been maintained on RCI alone, that with no oral prednisone.

Comments on two cases: Both of these cases had sinus disease and *lupus pernio*. This skin lesion is highly specific for sarcoidosis. It is also

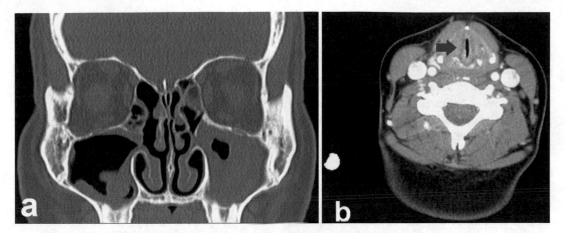

Fig. 13.2 CT scan coronal plane of sarcoidosis patient. (**a**) Sinus disease and retention cyst. (**b**) Upper airway narrowing (arrow)

commonly associated with sinus sarcoidosis. In some series of *lupus pernio*, around half of the patients had symptomatic sarcoidosis of the sinus [1, 2]. Dacrocystis is another condition associated with sinus sarcoidosis. In sarcoidosis patients with dacrocystitis, stenting alone is unlikely to work. That is because there is a high risk for granulomatous reaction to the stent. In case one, immunosuppressive therapy was able to control the disease. Both of these cases had refractory disease requiring third-line therapy. Anti-TNF antibodies can be quite effective in chronic conditions, including *lupus pernio* [3]. Unfortunately, the second case developed a liposarcoma while receiving were adalimumab. The patient is currently stable on another third-line treatment, RCI.

General Discussion

Sino-nasal sarcoidosis is one of the many manifestations of sarcoidosis of the upper respiratory tract (SURT) [4, 5]. Nasal and sino-nasal disease is the most common manifestation of SURT, but the larynx, oral cavity, and tongue can also be affected [5, 6]. Sinus symptoms are common in sarcoidosis patients. In one prospective study, nearly 40% of patients complained of nasal symptoms that had lasted for more than 3 weeks [7]. Half of these patients

continued to have symptoms despite nasal steroids and short-course antibiotic therapy. However, biopsy confirmation of sino-nasal sarcoidosis was made in only 4% of all patients in the study.

Etiology and Epidemiology of Sarcoidosis

Sarcoidosis is a granulomatous disease of unknown etiology [8]. The defining feature of sarcoidosis is the granuloma. One proposed model of sarcoidosis is exposure to an antigen, usually through inhalation [9]. This antigen activates several cells including macrophages and dendritic cells through the Toll-like receptor-2 (TLR-2). The dendritic cell transports the antigen across the epithelium to the lymph node, where it is processed with differentiation and clonal expression of T helper cells (Th1 and Th17). The antigen also stimulates macrophages to release tumor necrosis factor (TNF). TNF crosses the epithelial layer where it activates tissue macrophages and natural killer (NK) cells. Stimulated NK cells release interferon gamma (IFN-γ) which upregulates the tissue macrophages. The activated macrophages and clonal Th1/Th17 cells form the core of the granuloma. Other cells in the granuloma include T regulatory cells (Treg) and B cells (B cells). Key cytokines involved in the granuloma formation include MCP-1, CCL20, and CXCL10.

For most sarcoidosis patients, the granuloma resolves over the first few years. However, persistence of granulomas leads to chronic disease. Several features have been associated with persistent granulomas. The most important may be the upregulation of Th17.1 cells [10, 11], programmed death cells (PD-1) [12], and Treg cells [13]. Certain cytokines have been associated with chronic disease, including CXCL9 [14] and interleukin 8 (IL-8) [15, 16]. Persistent production of TNF by alveolar macrophages has also been found in patients with chronic sarcoidosis [17]. These observations have led to treatment strategies focused on these potential targets.

The antigen which stimulates the inflammatory response of sarcoidosis remains unknown. Several potential ligands for TL2-R have been studied. Antibodies for mycobacterial proteins mKatG [18], ESAT-6 [19], and *M. tuberculosis* heat-shock proteins (Mtb-hsp) [20] have been reported in a significant number of sarcoidosis patients, mostly from North America. However, no studies to date have been able to identify mycobacteria that are causing the antibody reaction. Studies from Japan and China have found evidence for propionibacterium including *P. acnes* in over half of the cases they studied [21, 22]. Inhaled particles have also been reported to cause a sarcoidosis-like reaction. Some first responders to the World Trade Center attack developed a sarcoidosis-like reaction, including multi-organ disease [23]. These observations support the hypothesis that sarcoidosis is due to multiple antigens. What makes sarcoidosis sarcoidosis is the reaction to the antigen(s) (Fig. 13.3).

Sarcoidosis is a worldwide disease. Table 13.1 summarizes the estimated incidence and prevalence of sarcoidosis for some countries across the world [24–26]. In the United Sates, several studies have noted that the disease is more frequent in African-American women [25, 27, 28]. Figure 13.4 demonstrates the prevalence rate per 100,000 population for African-American and Caucasian women and men in one recent study of over thirty-two million Americans [25]. In this study, sarcoidosis was more frequently observed in women than men for all races studied, including Asian and Hispanics.

Clinical Presentation and Diagnosis of Sino-Nasal Sarcoidosis

Nasal congestion is the most common feature in patients with sino-nasal sarcoidosis [5, 29, 30]. In a prospective study of 159 sarcoidosis patients, 60 (38%) had nasal symptoms (usually congestion) for at least 3 weeks [7]. Twenty-seven still had symptoms after 3 weeks of nasal steroids and oral antibiotics. Of these, six were found to have biopsy-confirmed sino-nasal sarcoidosis. Epistaxis was noted in 10–30% of cases [5, 29, 30]. In one series of 12 cases of biopsy-confirmed sino-nasal sarcoidosis, anosmia was noted in five, crusting in eight, and polyps in four cases [29]. Other areas in the upper airway can be involved in sino-nasal sarcoidosis. These include the larynx, oral cavity, and tongue [5, 6].

At the University of Cincinnati Sarcoidosis clinic, we have seen 2000 patients with sarcoidosis in the past 6 years. Of these, 64 (3.2%) had sino-nasal sarcoidosis. This was the most common manifestation of SURT in our clinic, with an additional 39 patients having upper airway or parotid involvement without documented sino-nasal disease. Table 13.2 summarizes the clinical features and the frequency of other organ involvement, using standard organ involvement criteria [31]. Patients with sino-nasal involvement were younger at the time of diagnosis of sarcoidosis than those without sino-nasal involvement. There was no difference in the race or gender for those with or without sino-nasal involvement. Lung and eye involvement were reported with equal frequency in both groups. Skin involvement was more common in those with sino-nasal disease, often on the face (Fig. 13.5a). In this group, 20% of patients with sino-nasal disease had *lupus pernio* (Fig. 13.5b).

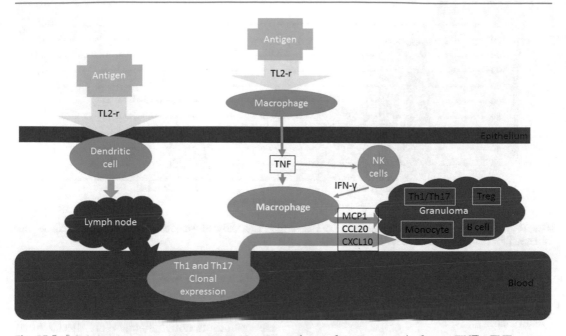

Fig. 13.3 Inhaled antigen comes into contact with cells at the epithelial layer. Activation of both macrophages and dendritic cells occurs through the Toll-like receptor-2 (TLR-2). The dendritic cell transports the antigen across the epithelium to the lymph node, where it is processed and differentiation and clonal expression of T helper cells (Th1 and Th17) occur. The antigen also stimulates macrophages on the surface of the epithelium and leads to the release of tumor necrosis factor (TNF). TNF crosses epithelial layer where it activates tissue macrophages and natural killer (NK) cells. NK releases interferon-gamma (IFN-γ) which upregulates the tissue macrophages. The activated macrophages and clonal Th1/Th17 cells form the core of the granuloma. Other cells in the granuloma include T regulatory cells (Treg) and B cells (B cells). Key cytokines involved in the granuloma formation include MCP-1, CCL20, and CXCL10

Table 13.1 Estimated incidence and prevalence of sarcoidosis[a]

Country	Population (millions)	Incidence per 100,000	Total new cases per year	Prevalence per 100,000	Total cases
China[a]	1312	0.56	7349	2.1	27,190
India[a]	1131	4.57	51,669	16.9	191,176
United States[b]	247[c]	8.8	21,736	60	148,200
Japan[a]	127	1.3	1657	4.7	5990
Germany[a]	82	4	3118	14	11,537
France[a]	61	3	1649	10	6101
United Kingdom[a]	60	5	4000	27	16,270
Sweden[d]	8[c]	11.5	920	160	12,800

[a]Estimated by Denning et al. [24]
[b]Reported by Baughman et al. [25]
[c]Only for those aged 18 or older
[d]Reported by Arkema et al. [26]

Diagnosis of Sino-Nasal Sarcoidosis

Many patients with documented sino-nasal sarcoidosis have been diagnosed prior to the diagnosis of sino-nasal involvement. Sarcoidosis patients present with a wide range of symptoms, including no symptoms at all. In up to a third of cases, patients are detected based on an abnormal chest X-ray or laboratory test [32]. Symptoms from sarcoidosis depend on what organ is affected. Table 13.3 summarizes the symptoms,

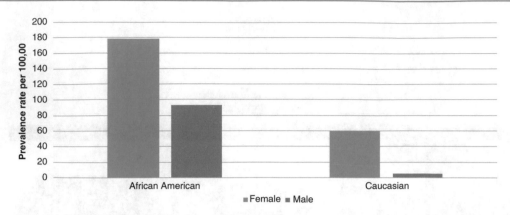

Fig. 13.4 Prevalence rate for sarcoidosis in the United States for African-Americans and Caucasians. Higher rate observed for female versus male for both races [25]

Table 13.2 Clinical features of sino-nasal sarcoidosis at University of Cincinnati sarcoidosis clinic

Feature	Number
Total number	64 (3.2%)[a]
Age at the time of diagnosis, years (median [range])	37 (21–60)[b]
Female:male	46:17
African-American:Caucasian	34:28
Lung involvement	58 (90.6%)[c]
Skin involvement	38 (59.4%)[d]
Lupus pernio	13 (20.3%)[e]
Eye involvement	24 (37.5%)
Other upper airway involvement	
Larynx	1
Parotid	2
Tongue	1
Supraglottic	1

[a]Of a total of 2000 patients seen in clinic
[b]Significantly younger than sarcoidosis patients without sino-nasal involvement ($p = 0.0001$)
[c]Percent of all sino-nasal sarcoidosis cases
[d]Skin involvement significantly more frequent than sarcoidosis patients without sino-nasal involvement (Chi square = 34.4, $p < 0.0001$)
[e]Lupus pernio significantly more frequent than sarcoidosis patients without sino-nasal involvement (Chi square = 63.5, $p < 0.0001$)

physical findings, and laboratory tests for various manifestations of the disease. Criteria have been established for identifying various organ involvement [33].

Criteria have also been developed to define sino-nasal involvement in sarcoidosis [33]. A patient with known sarcoidosis elsewhere who has granulomatous changes on direct fiber-optic nasal endoscopy or imaging studies (Fig. 13.6) is felt to have at least probable sino-nasal sarcoidosis. Patients with chronic sinusitis are felt to have at least possible sino-nasal sarcoidosis. Patients with a positive sinus or nasal biopsy demonstrating non-caseating granulomas are highly probable to have sino-nasal sarcoidosis.

Patients with sino-nasal sarcoidosis can have a range of symptoms, including no specific complaints [5, 30, 34], although nasal congestion and rhinorrhea are reported in most cases. Crusting and/or epistaxis occur in about a quarter of patients. Anosmia, purulent rhinorrhea, and facial pain can also occur. Local examination will often demonstrate hypertrophy and/or a purplish hue due to the granulomatous inflammation. Figure 13.6 shows an endoscopic view of a patient with sino-nasal sarcoidosis.

Figure 13.7 shows our approach to evaluation of patients with possible sino-nasal disease [7]. Patients with nasal congestion or other symptoms are treated with nasal steroids and/or antibiotics. If symptoms persist for more than 3 weeks, a CT scan is performed. If the scan is suggestive of sinus disease, the patient is considered for referral to an otolaryngologist for possible endoscopy and biopsy. If the CT scan is normal, the patient may receive a longer course of therapy. If the

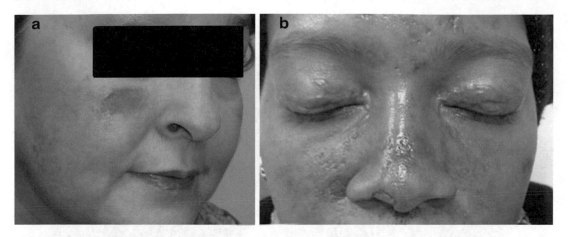

Fig. 13.5 Sarcoidosis lesions of patients with sino-nasal sarcoidosis. (**a**) Lesion on cheek. (**b**) Nasal and periocular lesion of patient with *lupus pernio*. Both patients provided written informed consent for publication of their photographs

Table 13.3 Common symptoms, physical findings, and laboratory tests in sarcoidosis

	Symptom	Physical finding	Laboratory test
Lung	Cough	Hilar adenopathy	Hilar adenopathy
	Dyspnea	Symmetrical upper lobe disease	Symmetrical upper lobe disease
	Chest pain	Peribronchial thickening on CT scan	Peribronchial thickening on CT scan
	Wheezing		Restriction and/or obstruction on PFTs
Eye	Pain	Iritis	Reduced visual fields
	Photophobia	Pars planitis	
	Blindness	Optic neuritis	
Neuro	Seventh cranial nerve paralysis		Gadolinium enhancement on MRI
	Unilateral weakness		Lymphocytic meningitis
	Seizure		
Cardiac	Palpitations		Ventricular arrhythmias
	Edema		Complete heart block
			Reduced left ventricular ejection fraction
			Late gadolinium enhancement on cardiac MRI
			Patchy enhanced uptake of cardiac PET scan
Skin	Lesions on face, arms, legs	Macular papular lesion	
		Lupus pernio	
		Papules in areas of scarring or tattoos	
Liver	Abdominal pain	Enlarged liver and/or spleen	Hepato/splenomegaly on imaging
Others			Increased serum or urine calcium with elevated vitamin D 1,25
			Elevated ACE level

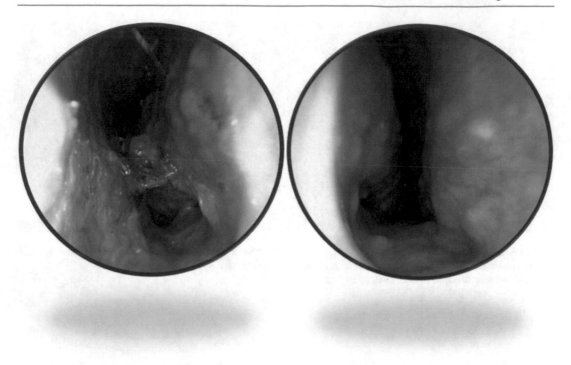

Fig. 13.6 Nasal endoscopic view of a patient with sino-nasal sarcoid. Submucosal nodules are evident on the nasal septum and inferior turbinate, and even the nasal floor

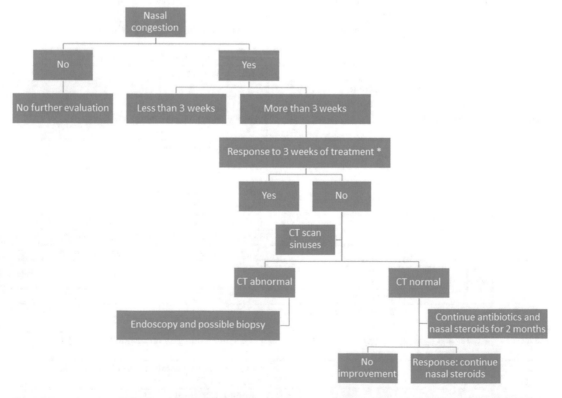

Fig. 13.7 University of Cincinnati Sarcoidosis Clinic approach to evaluation of patients with possible sino-nasal disease [7]. *Treatment with nasal steroids and/or oral antibiotics

patient is still requiring therapy after 2 months, they are referred for evaluation.

CT scanning is the most common imaging modality to detect sino-nasal disease, with abnormalities seen in most cases [30, 34]. Mucosal hypertrophy and/or opacification occurs in almost all cases of sino-nasal involvement. Turbinate or septal nodularity is present in about a third of cases (see Fig. 13.6), and bone lesions including erosions and osteoneogenesis is present in over a third of cases [30, 34].

There are some additional features that heighten the likelihood of sino-nasal sarcoidosis. *Lupus pernio* are papular lesions on the cheeks and nose, especially the nares [35]. In general, lupus pernio is seen in less than 2% of all sarcoidosis patients [36]. It is more frequent in patients of African descent, but can be seen in Caucasians [2, 3, 35]. There is strong association between *lupus pernio* and sino-nasal disease [1, 2].

Another important association is dacrocystitis. The drainage of the tear duct into the sinus can be blocked and lead to significant morbidity. This can be treated surgically with a dacryocystorhinostomy, although recurrent obstruction may occur [37]. Patients with dacrocystitis often have adnexal lesions [38]. In these patients, a CT scan may demonstrate lacrimal gland involvement as well as significant sinus disease (Fig. 13.8).

Table 13.4 lists the differential diagnosis of granulomatous sinus disease. In addition to routine pathologic examination, special stains should be performed to look for evidence of lymphoma or infection. In addition, testing for antineutrophil cytoplasmic antibody (ANCA) should be performed. Further characterization of ANCA should be done to distinguish between cytoplasmic (c-ANCA) and perinuclear (p-ANCA). Systemic granulomatosis disease with polyangiitis (GPA), formerly known as Wegener's disease, is strongly associated with a positive c-ANCA. On the other hand, a positive p-ANCA test has been reported in various inflammatory diseases, including Churg-Strauss.

The serum angiotensin-converting enzyme (ACE) has limited sensitivity and specificity in part because of genetic polymorphisms of the ACE enzyme [39] and because of the effect of corticosteroid therapy [40] on levels. However, a significantly elevated ACE level can be helpful in confirming the diagnosis of sarcoidosis. Over half of patients with active sarcoidosis will have an ACE level greater than 20% of the upper limit of normal. Patients with an ACE level that high have a greater than 90% chance of having sarcoidosis [41].

Management

The management of sino-nasal disease is usually a stepwise process. Figure 13.9 is the approach we employ in management of patients at our clinic. Initial therapy is topical, with use of nasal corticosteroids to control inflammation. If that is unsuccessful, we will use oral corticosteroids, usually prednisone.

In general, oral corticosteroid therapy for sarcoidosis is a long-standing intervention. Short-course treatments of up to 3 weeks are reserved for acute events [42, 43]. The rationale for long-term treatment with corticosteroids is because of the high rate of relapse of sarcoidosis when treatment is withdrawn [5, 30]. Once systemic therapy is initiated for sarcoidosis, about half of patients will require systemic therapy for more than 2 years [44, 45]. Some features, such as *lupus pernio*, are associated with the need for systemic treatment for 5 years or longer [46]. The goal with oral corticosteroid therapy is to reduce the patient to the lowest possible dose that maintains a clinical remission [47]. For most sarcoidosis patients, a maintenance dose of prednisone of less than 10 mg daily or its equivalent is associated with minimal adverse effects and is generally well tolerated [48].

For those patients unable to tolerate maintenance-dose prednisone or who have progressive disease despite corticosteroid therapy, antimetabolite therapy is a steroid-sparing alternative. Methotrexate is the most widely studied and used treatment as a second-line therapy for sarcoidosis [25, 49]. Table 13.5 summarizes several reported series as well as our own experience with various systemic therapies to treat sino-nasal sarcoidosis. For most studies, methotrexate was the most widely used steroid-sparing agent. Table 13.6 compares the various systemic treatments for sarcoidosis, including dosage and toxicity. Specific recommendations have been made for administrating and monitoring methotrexate therapy in sarcoidosis patients [50]. Azathioprine and leflunomide have been used less frequently to treat sarcoidosis. However, these drugs appear

to be about as effective as methotrexate [51–53]. Mycophenolate has recently been reported as an effective steroid-sparing agent in sarcoidosis [54, 55]. All four of these agents seem to work about two-thirds of the time as steroid sparing. The use of an individual agent depends on the experience of the clinician and potential or real toxicity for the individual patient.

The antimalarial drugs hydroxychloroquine and chloroquine appear to be most effective for treatment of cutaneous disease [56]. They are not as effective for more aggressive forms of sarcoidosis, such as *lupus pernio* [3]. For sino-nasal sarcoidosis, they are often used as an adjunct to other treatments (see Table 13.5). Their toxicity is relatively low, although patients need to undergo routine ocular screening [57].

Monoclonal antibodies to tumor necrosis factor (anti-TNF) have changed the outcome of many patients with chronic sarcoidosis. Infliximab, a chimeric monoclonal antibody, has been the most widely used anti-TNF drug. In advanced pulmonary sarcoidosis, it was found to be significantly better than placebo treatment [58]. It was also found to be more likely to induce complete resolution of *lupus pernio* than any other drug combination [3]. Adalimumab has also been reported as effective in treating sarcoidosis, including *lupus pernio* [59, 60]. Not all

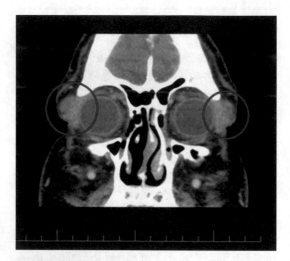

Fig. 13.8 Coronal CT scan demonstrating bilateral lacrimal gland involvement (red circles) in a sarcoidosis patient with dacrocystitis who also has left maxillary sinus disease

Table 13.4 Differential diagnosis of sino-nasal disease[a]

Disease	Differentiating features	Comments
Sarcoidosis	Multi-organ disease	Elevated ACE
Infectious rhinitis	Positive culture and/or special stains	Actinomycosis, Aspergillosis, Blastomycosis, Histoplasmosis, Mucomycosis, leprosy, syphilis
Granulomatosis with polyangiitis	Necrotizing vasculitis, associated with lung and renal disease	ANCA positive, especially c-ANCA
Churg-Strauss syndrome	Necrotizing granulomas with vasculitis, bronchial asthma, eosinophilia	ANCA positive, especially p-ANCA
Polymorphic reticulosis	Angiocentric lymphoid infiltrate	
Berylliosis	Non-caseating granulomas limited to lung, skin, and sinuses	Positive beryllium lymphocyte stimulation test Exposure to beryllium
Tuberculosis	Caseating granulomas	Positive smears and culture for *M. tuberculosis*
Lymphoma	Immunohistochemistry demonstrating clonal B or T cell infiltration	

[a]Adapted from Zeitlin et al. [7]

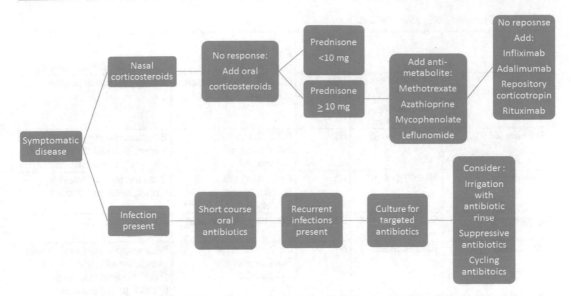

Fig. 13.9 A stepwise approach to management of sino-nasal sarcoidosis. Treatment is for the underlying sarcoidosis (top half of the flowchart) as well as management of any infection. Prednisone is the most commonly used oral corticosteroid in our clinic. Surgical management of residual scarring is usually reserved until after inflammation is controlled

Table 13.5 Systemic therapy for sino-nasal sarcoidosis

	University of Cincinnati Sarcoidosis Clinic 2016	Aloulah et al. (2013) [34]	Kirsten et al. (2013) [29]	Aubart et al. (2006) [30]	Zeitlin et al. (2000) [7]
Number of patients	64	38	12	20	18
No therapy	4	14	0	0 [b]	0
Prednisone [a]	60	24	12	18	13
Methotrexate	52	NC	NC	8	13
Azathioprine	12	NC	NC	2	3
Leflunomide	15	NC	NC	0	0
Mycophenolate	2	NC	NC	0	0
Hydroxychloroquine/ chloroquine	16	NC	NC	14	4
Infliximab	16	NC	NC	0	0
Adalimumab	2	NC	NC	0	0
Rituximab	2	NC	NC	0	0
Repository corticotrophin	7	NC	NC	0	0
Surgery[c]	NC	4	1	7	4

NC no comment
[a]Patients may have received more than one treatment
[b]Other treatments include thalidomide, cyclophosphamide, pentoxifylline, and cyclosporine
[c]Excludes biopsy

anti-TNF agents are equally effective in treating sarcoidosis. Adalimumab appears to be less potent than infliximab [61]. A recent randomized trial failed to demonstrate a benefit of golimumab versus placebo [62]. Moreover, these drugs are associated with significant potential toxicity. Guidelines have been developed for use of these drugs in patients with sarcoidosis [63].

Rituximab is a monoclonal antibody against B cells. While originally developed to treat lym-

Table 13.6 Systemic therapy for sarcoidosis

Drug	Dosage	Estimated efficacy (%)	Recommended monitoring	Common/significant toxicity
Prednisone	Initial 20–40 mg daily Maintenance 5–10 mg daily	>90	Glucose, blood pressure, edema, osteoporosis	Toxicity is dose dependant
Methotrexate	5–15 mg weekly	60	CBC, liver, renal function every 2–3 months	Bone marrow suppression, nausea, hepatotoxicity up to 5%, rarely pulmonary toxicity
Azathioprine	50–200 g daily	60	CBC, liver, renal function every 2–3 months	Bone marrow suppression, nausea, rarely hepatotoxic
Mycophenolate	500–1500 twice a day	50	CBC every 2–3 months	Bloating, diarrhea
Leflunomide	10–20 mg daily	60	CBC, liver, renal function every 2–3 months	Bone marrow suppression, less nausea, hepatotoxicity up to 5%, very rare pulmonary toxicity, peripheral neuropathy
Hydroxychloroquine	200–400 mg daily	20	Eye examination every 6–12 months	Rarely heart block, dermatitis, hepatotoxicity
Infliximab	3–5 mg/kg initially, 2 weeks later than once every 4–6 weeks	85	Initial screening for latent tuberculosis, monitor for fungal infections	Allergic reactions including anaphylaxis, reactivation of tuberculosis, dermatitis, lupus-like reaction, skin cancer, worsening congestive heart failure, solid malignancy, lymphoma, demyelinating diseases
Adalimumab	40 mg every 1–2 weeks	80	Initial screening for latent tuberculosis, monitor for fungal infections	Less likely allergic reactions than infliximab, reactivation of tuberculosis, dermatitis, lupus-like reaction, skin cancer, worsening congestive heart failure, solid malignancy, lymphoma, demyelinating diseases
Rituximab	1000 mg initially, 2 weeks later and then maintenance every 1–6 months	70	Screen for prior viral infections, including hepatitis B and C, monitor immunoglobulin levels every 3–6 months	Reaction to infusion, viral infections, IgG deficiency
Repository corticotrophin injection	40–80 units twice a week	50–80	Glucose, blood pressure, edema, osteoporosis	Toxicity is usually on the day of injection, edema and increased anxiety are frequent, toxicity is dose dependant

phoma, it has been found to have significant immunomodulatory effects. The drug has been reported as effective in refractory pulmonary [64] and ocular [65] disease.

Repository corticotrophin injections (RCI) have recently been reported as effective in treating advanced sarcoidosis [66]. While an old therapy, it had been abandoned for many years in routine management of sarcoidosis because of cost and question of mechanism of action. The drug stimulated the melanocortin receptors (MCR), including MCR-2. The

MCR-2 is on the adrenal gland and stimulation leads to release of cortisol. However, there are several other MCRs, including some that regulate the immune system. Stimulation of these other MCR is felt to have benefit beyond just steroid effect of the drug [67]. Repository corticotrophin injection has been used in cases of refractory sarcoidosis who have failed conventional therapy and/or developed significant toxicity to various treatments [68].

Most patients with sarcoidosis can be managed medically [34]. As noted in Table 13.5, surgical intervention has been used in the management of sino-nasal sarcoidosis [29, 69]. While some cases may respond to surgery [69], relapses after surgery are common [7, 29, 30]. Endoscopic surgery may be effective in controlling symptoms [70], but it can be very difficult to control healing and prevent scarring. The risk for relapse can be reduced by aggressive use of immunosuppressive agents. However, immunosuppression will only reduce inflammation and has no impact on scar tissue. Once scarring occurs, surgery may prove effective in removing obstruction. Even extensive reconstruction surgery has been successfully performed when inflammation has been controlled [71].

Lawson et al. have proposed the classification of sino-nasal sarcoidosis as atrophic, hypertrophic, destructive, and nasal enlargement [72]. They reported good results with surgery only for the subgroup of patients with architectural changes. While these recommendations seem reasonable, they were based on a retrospective review of a limited number of cases and need to be confirmed prospectively.

For the therapy of sino-nasal sarcoidosis, one has to also consider infection. Abnormal sinus architecture from sarcoidosis represents the same challenge for the clinician as any other condition which affects the sinuses. Antibiotic regimens often progress in a stepwise fashion as depicted on the bottom half of Fig. 13.9 [73]. Cultures may provide evidence to support targeted therapy, especially for aspergillosis and atypical mycobacteria. Figure 13.10 demonstrates the CT scan of a patient with chronic ocular, pulmonary,

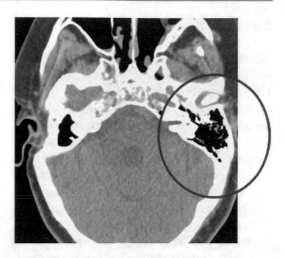

Fig. 13.10 Axial CT scan of head of a 70-year-old white female with chronic ocular, pulmonary, and sinus sarcoidosis for more than 12 years. Patient had developed headache and fever while on maintenance therapy of methotrexate 10 mg a week and infliximab 5 mg/kg once a month. Her CT scan demonstrated fluid collection in left maxillary sinus. Biopsy of sinus showed highly cellular inflammation with numerous acid-fast bacilli seen on special staining. Culture grew *M. avium* complex (MAC). Her infliximab was discontinued and she was placed on anti-mycobacterial therapy. While her sinus symptoms resolved, her optic neuritis flared and prednisone was reinstituted. After 1 year of anti-mycobacterial therapy, she is stable and without evidence of mycobacterial infection. However, she remains on 20 mg prednisone daily with 10 mg-a-week methotrexate

and sinus sarcoidosis treated at our institution. While on infliximab and methotrexate therapy, she had developed a chronic sinus infection. Cultures of her left maxillary sinus grew *M. avium*. Her sinus symptoms responded well to withdrawal of infliximab and anti-mycobacterial therapy. However, she had to be placed back on prednisone 20 mg to control her ocular disease.

In addition to targeted antibiotic therapy, nasal rinses with broad-spectrum antibiotics can be utilized. Gentamicin is commonly used, since topical application usually does not lead to toxicity. However, systemic absorption can still occur [74] and toxicity should be assessed for those on chronic therapy. Prolonged use of systemic antibiotics has shown benefit in some patients [75]. However, these antibiotic regimens have not been studied in sino-nasal sarcoidosis.

Conclusion

While sino-nasal sarcoidosis is an unusual form of sarcoidosis, it often leads to chronic disease. For some patients, local therapy may be sufficient. Systemic therapy follows a stepwise approach, with prednisone or similar oral corticosteroid the initial drug of choice. However, because of the need for long-term therapy, steroid-sparing alternatives should be considered early in the management of advanced sino-nasal disease. Antimetabolites are effective steroid-sparing agents. Newer modalities, including anti-TNF antibodies, have proved effective in treating refractory cases. Surgery is effective in addressing architectural changes due to scarring. It is most effective in patients in whom inflammation is controlled by immuno-suppression therapy.

References

1. Baughman RP, Judson MA, Teirstein AS, Moller DR, Lower EE. Thalidomide for chronic sarcoidosis. Chest. 2002;122:227–32.
2. Spiteri MA, Matthey F, Gordon T, Carstairs LS, James DG. Lupus pernio: a clinico-radiological study of thirty-five cases. Br J Dermatol. 1985;112(3):315–22.
3. Stagaki E, Mountford WK, Lackland DT, Judson MA. The treatment of lupus pernio: results of 116 treatment courses in 54 patients. Chest. 2009;135(2):468–76.
4. Baughman RP, Lower EE, Tami T. Upper airway. 4: sarcoidosis of the upper respiratory tract (SURT). Thorax. 2010;65(2):181–6.
5. Panselinas E, Halstead L, Schlosser RJ, Judson MA. Clinical manifestations, radiographic findings, treatment options, and outcome in sarcoidosis patients with upper respiratory tract involvement. South Med J. 2010;103(9):870–5.
6. Bouaziz A, Le SJ, Chapelon-Abric C, Varron L, Khenifer S, Gleizal A, et al. Oral involvement in sarcoidosis: report of 12 cases. QJM. 2012;105(8):755–67.
7. Zeitlin JF, Tami TA, Baughman R, Winget D. Nasal and sinus manifestations of sarcoidosis. Am J Rhinol. 2000;14(3):157–61.
8. Hunninghake GW, Costabel U, Ando M, Baughman R, Cordier JF, du Bois R, et al. ATS/ERS/WASOG statement on sarcoidosis. American Thoracic Society/European Respiratory Society/World Association of Sarcoidosis and other Granulomatous Disorders. Sarcoidosis Vasc Diffuse Lung Dis. 1999;16(Sep):149–73.
9. Broos CE, van Nimwegen M, Hoogsteden HC, Hendriks RW, Kool M, van den Blink B. Granuloma formation in pulmonary sarcoidosis. Front Immunol. 2013;4:437. https://doi.org/10.3389/fimmu.2013.00437.:437.
10. Broos CE, van NM, In 't Veen JC, Hoogsteden HC, Hendriks RW, van den Blink B, et al. Decreased cytotoxic T-lymphocyte antigen 4 expression on regulatory T cells and Th17 cells in sarcoidosis: double trouble? Am J Respir Crit Care Med. 2015;192(6):763–5.
11. Ramstein J, Broos CE, Simpson LJ, Ansel KM, Sun SA, Ho ME, et al. IFN-gamma-producing T-helper 17.1 cells are increased in sarcoidosis and are more prevalent than T-helper type 1 cells. Am J Respir Crit Care Med. 2016;193(11):1281–91.
12. Celada LJ, Rotsinger JE, Young A, Shaginurova G, Shelton D, Hawkins C, et al. Programmed death-1 inhibition of phosphatidylinositol 3-kinase/AKT/mechanistic target of rapamycin signaling impairs sarcoidosis CD4+ T cell proliferation. Am J Respir Cell Mol Biol. 2017;56(1):74–82.
13. Prasse A, Zissel G, Lutzen N, Schupp J, Schmiedlin R, Gonzalez-Rey E, et al. Inhaled vasoactive intestinal peptide exerts immunoregulatory effects in sarcoidosis. Am J Respir Crit Care Med. 2010;182(4):540–8.
14. Su R, Li MM, Bhakta NR, Solberg OD, Darnell EP, Ramstein J, et al. Longitudinal analysis of sarcoidosis blood transcriptomic signatures and disease outcomes. Eur Respir J. 2014;44(4):985–93.
15. Baughman RP, Keeton D, Lower EE. Relationship between interleukin-8 and neutrophils in the BAL fluid of sarcoidosis. Sarcoidosis. 1994;11:S217–20.
16. Loza MJ, Brodmerkel C, du Bois RM, Judson MA, Costabel U, Drent M, et al. Inflammatory profile and response to anti-TNF therapy in patients with chronic pulmonary sarcoidosis. Clin Vaccine Immunol. 2011;18:931–9.
17. Ziegenhagen MW, Benner UK, Zissel G, Zabel P, Schlaak M, Müller-Quernheim J. Sarcoidosis: TNF-alpha release from alveolar macrophages and serum level of sIL-2R are prognostic markers. Am J Respir Crit Care Med. 1997;156(5):1586–92.
18. Song Z, Marzilli L, Greenlee BM, Chen ES, Silver RF, Askin FB, et al. Mycobacterial catalase-peroxidase is a tissue antigen and target of the adaptive immune response in systemic sarcoidosis. J Exp Med. 2005;201(5):755–67.
19. Drake WP, Dhason MS, Nadaf M, Shepherd BE, Vadivelu S, Hajizadeh R, et al. Cellular recognition of Mycobacterium tuberculosis ESAT-6 and KatG peptides in systemic sarcoidosis. Infect Immun. 2007;75(1):527–30.
20. Dubaniewicz A, Trzonkowski P, Dubaniewicz-Wybieralska M, Dubaniewicz A, Singh M, Myśliwski A. Mycobacterial heat shock protein-induced blood T lymphocytes subsets and cytokine pattern: comparison

of sarcoidosis with tuberculosis and healthy controls. Respirology. 2007;12(3):346–54.

21. Eishi Y, Suga M, Ishige I, Kobayashi D, Yamada T, Takemura T, et al. Quantitative analysis of mycobacterial and propionibacterial DNA in lymph nodes of Japanese and European patients with sarcoidosis. J Clin Microbiol. 2002;40(Jan):198–204.

22. Zhou Y, Wei YR, Zhang Y, Du SS, Baughman RP, Li HP. Real-time quantitative reverse transcription-polymerase chain reaction to detect propionibacterial ribosomal RNA in the lymph nodes of Chinese patients with sarcoidosis. Clin Exp Immunol. 2015;181:511–7.

23. Izbicki G, Chavko R, Banauch GI, Weiden MD, Berger KI, Aldrich TK, et al. World Trade Center "sarcoid like" granulomatous pulmonary disease in New York City Fire Department rescue workers. Chest. 2007;131(5):1414–23.

24. Denning DW, Pleuvry A, Cole DC. Global burden of chronic pulmonary aspergillosis complicating sarcoidosis. Eur Respir J. 2013;41(3):621–6.

25. Baughman RP, Field S, Costabel U, Crystal RG, Culver DA, Drent M, et al. Sarcoidosis in America. Analysis based on health care use. Ann Am Thorac Soc. 2016;13(8):1244–52.

26. Arkema EV, Grunewald J, Kullberg S, Eklund A, Askling J. Sarcoidosis incidence and prevalence: a nationwide register-based assessment in Sweden. Eur Respir J. 2016;48(6):1690–9.

27. Rybicki BA, Major M, Popovich J Jr, Maliarik MJ, Iannuzzi MC. Racial differences in sarcoidosis incidence: a five year study in a health maintenance organization. Am J Epidemiol. 1997;145.234–41.

28. Dumas O, Abramovitz L, Wiley AS, Cozier YC, Camargo CA Jr. Epidemiology of sarcoidosis in a prospective cohort study of U.S. women. Ann Am Thorac Soc. 2016;13(1):67–71.

29. Kirsten AM, Watz H, Kirsten D. Sarcoidosis with involvement of the paranasal sinuses - a retrospective analysis of 12 biopsy-proven cases. BMC Pulm Med. 2013;13:59. https://doi.org/10.1186/1471-2466-13-59.:59-13.

30. Aubart FC, Ouayoun M, Brauner M, Attali P, Kambouchner M, Valeyre D, et al. Sinonasal involvement in sarcoidosis: a case-control study of 20 patients. Medicine (Baltimore). 2006;85(6):365–71.

31. Judson MA, Baughman RP, Teirstein AS, Terrin ML, Yeager H Jr. Defining organ involvement in sarcoidosis: the ACCESS proposed instrument. Sarcoidosis Vasc Diffuse Lung Dis. 1999;16:75–86.

32. Pietinalho A, Ohmichi M, Hiraga Y, Löfroos AB, Selroos O. The mode of presentation of sarcoidosis in Finland and Hokkaido, Japan. A comparative analysis of 571 Finnish and 686 Japanese patients. Sarcoidosis. 1996;13:159–66.

33. Judson MA, Costabel U, Drent M, Wells A, Maier L, Koth L, et al. The WASOG Sarcoidosis Organ Assessment Instrument: an update of a previous

clinical tool. Sarcoidosis Vasc Diffuse Lung Dis. 2014;31(1):19–27.

34. Aloulah M, Manes RP, Ng YH, Fitzgerald JE, Glazer CS, Ryan MW, et al. Sinonasal manifestations of sarcoidosis: a single institution experience with 38 cases. Int Forum Allergy Rhinol. 2013;3(7):567–72.

35. Baughman RP, Judson MA, Teirstein A, Lower EE, Lo K, Schlenker-Herceg R, et al. Chronic facial sarcoidosis including lupus pernio: clinical description and proposed scoring systems. Am J Clin Dermatol. 2008;9(3):155–61.

36. Neville E, Walker AN, James DG. Prognostic factors predicting the outcome of sarcoidosis: an analysis of 818 patients. Q J Med. 1983;208:525–33.

37. Garcia GH, Harris GJ. Sarcoid inflammation and obstruction of the nasolacrimal system. Arch Ophthalmol. 2000;118(5):719–20.

38. Demirci H, Christianson MD. Orbital and adnexal involvement in sarcoidosis: analysis of clinical features and systemic disease in 30 cases. Am J Ophthalmol. 2011;151(6):1074–80.

39. Tomita H, Ina Y, Sugiura Y, Sato S, Kawaguchi H, Morishita M, et al. Polymorphism in the angiotensin-converting enzyme (ACE) gene and sarcoidosis. Am J Respir Crit Care Med. 1997;156(1):255–9.

40. Baughman RP, Ploysongsang Y, Roberts RD, Srivastava L. Effects of sarcoid and steroids on angiotensin-converting enzyme. Am Rev Respir Dis. 1983;128:631–3.

41. Lieberman J, Nosal A, Schlessner A, Sastre-Foken A. Serum angiotensin-converting enzyme for diagnosis and therapeutic evaluation of sarcoidosis. Am Rev Respir Dis. 1979;120(2):329–35.

42. Baughman RP, Lower EE. Frequency of acute worsening events in fibrotic pulmonary sarcoidosis patients. Respir Med. 2013;107:2009–13.

43. McKinzie BP, Bullington WM, Mazur JE, Judson MA. Efficacy of short-course, low-dose corticosteroid therapy for acute pulmonary sarcoidosis exacerbations. Am J Med Sci. 2010;339(1):1–4.

44. Gottlieb JE, Israel HL, Steiner RM, Triolo J, Patrick H. Outcome in sarcoidosis. The relationship of relapse to corticosteroid therapy. Chest. 1997;111(3):623–31.

45. Baughman RP, Judson MA, Teirstein A, Yeager H, Rossman M, Knatterud GL, et al. Presenting characteristics as predictors of duration of treatment in sarcoidosis. QJM. 2006;99(5):307–15.

46. Baughman RP, Lower EE. Features of sarcoidosis associated with chronic disease. Sarcoidosis Vasc Diffuse Lung Dis. 2014;31(4):275–81.

47. Johns CJ, Michele TM. The clinical management of sarcoidosis: a 50-year experience at the Johns Hopkins hospital. Medicine. 1999;78:65–111.

48. Judson MA, Chaudhry H, Louis A, Lee K, Yucel R. The effect of corticosteroids on quality of life in a sarcoidosis clinic: the results of a propensity analysis. Respir Med. 2015;109(4):526–31.

49. Schutt AC, Bullington WM, Judson MA. Pharmacotherapy for pulmonary sarcoidosis: a Delphi consensus study. Respir Med. 2010;104(5):717–23.

50. Cremers JP, Drent M, Bast A, Shigemitsu H, Baughman RP, Valeyre D, et al. Multinational evidence-based World Association of Sarcoidosis and Other Granulomatous Disorders recommendations for the use of methotrexate in sarcoidosis: integrating systematic literature research and expert opinion of sarcoidologists worldwide. Curr Opin Pulm Med. 2013;19:545–61.

51. Vorselaars AD, Wuyts WA, Vorselaars VM, Zanen P, Deneer VHM, Veltkamp M, et al. Methotrexate versus azathioprine in second line therapy of sarcoidosis. Chest. 2013;144:805–12.

52. Sahoo DH, Bandyopadhyay D, Xu M, Pearson K, Parambil JG, Lazar CA, et al. Effectiveness and safety of leflunomide for pulmonary and extrapulmonary sarcoidosis. Eur Respir J. 2011;38:1145–50.

53. Baughman RP, Lower EE. Leflunomide for chronic sarcoidosis. Sarcoidosis Vasc Diffuse Lung Dis. 2004;21:43–8.

54. Hamzeh N, Voelker A, Forssen A, Gottschall EB, Rose C, Mroz P, et al. Efficacy of mycophenolate mofetil in sarcoidosis. Respir Med. 2014;108:1663–9.

55. Brill AK, Ott SR, Geiser T. Effect and safety of mycophenolate mofetil in chronic pulmonary sarcoidosis: a retrospective study. Respiration. 2013;86:376–83.

56. Jones E, Callen JP. Hydroxychloroquine is effective therapy for control of cutaneous sarcoidal granulomas. J Am Acad Dermatol. 1990;23(3 Pt 1):487–9.

57. Marmor MF, Kellner U, Lai TY, Lyons JS, Mieler WF, American Academy of Ophthalmology. Revised recommendations on screening for chloroquine and hydroxychloroquine retinopathy. Ophthalmology. 2011;118(2):415–22.

58. Baughman RP, Drent M, Kavuru M, Judson MA, Costabel U, du Bois R, et al. Infliximab therapy in patients with chronic sarcoidosis and pulmonary involvement. Am J Respir Crit Care Med. 2006;174(7):795–802.

59. Sweiss NJ, Noth I, Mirsaeidi M, Zhang W, Naureckas ET, Hogarth DK, et al. Efficacy results of a 52-week trial of adalimumab in the treatment of refractory sarcoidosis. Sarcoidosis Vasc Diffuse Lung Dis. 2014;31(1):46–54.

60. Judson MA. Successful treatment of lupus pernio with adalimumab. Arch Dermatol. 2011;147(11):1332–3.

61. Baughman RP. Tumor necrosis factor inhibition in treating sarcoidosis: the American experience. Revista Portuguesa de Pneumonologia. 2007;13:S47–50.

62. Judson MA, Baughman RP, Costabel U, Drent M, Gibson KF, Raghu G, et al. Safety and efficacy of ustekinumab or golimumab in patients with chronic sarcoidosis. Eur Respir J. 2014;44:1296–307.

63. Drent M, Cremers JP, Jansen TL, Baughman RP. Practical eminence and experience-based recommendations for use of TNF-alpha inhibitors in sarcoidosis. Sarcoidosis Vasc Diffuse Lung Dis. 2014;31(2):91–107.

64. Sweiss NJ, Lower EE, Mirsaeidi M, Dudek S, Garcia JG, Perkins D, et al. Rituximab in the treatment of refractory pulmonary sarcoidosis. Eur Respir J. 2014;43(5):1525–8.

65. Lower EE, Baughman RP, Kaufman AH. Rituximab for refractory granulomatous eye disease. Clin Ophthalmol. 2012;6:1613–8.

66. Baughman RP, Barney JB, O'Hare L, Lower EE. A retrospective pilot study examining the use of Acthar gel in sarcoidosis patients. Respir Med. 2016;110:66–72.

67. Berkovich R, Agius MA. Mechanisms of action of ACTH in the management of relapsing forms of multiple sclerosis. Ther Adv Neurol Disord. 2014;7(2):83–96.

68. Zhou Y, Lower EE, Li H, Baughman RP. Sarcoidosis patient with lupus pernio and infliximab-induced myositis: response to Acthar gel. Respir Med Case Rep. 2015;17:5–7.

69. Gulati S, Krossnes B, Olofsson J, Danielsen A. Sinonasal involvement in sarcoidosis: a report of seven cases and review of literature. Eur Arch Otorhinolaryngol. 2012;269(3):891–6.

70. Kay DJ, Har-El G. The role of endoscopic sinus surgery in chronic sinonasal sarcoidosis. Am J Rhinol. 2001;15(4):249–54.

71. Gurkov R, Berghaus A. Nasal reconstruction in advanced sinunasal sarcoidosis. Rhinology. 2009;47(3):327–9.

72. Lawson W, Jiang N, Cheng J. Sinonasal sarcoidosis: a new system of classification acting as a guide to diagnosis and treatment. Am J Rhinol Allergy. 2014;28(4):317–22.

73. Rudmik L, Soler ZM. Medical therapies for adult chronic sinusitis: a systematic review. JAMA. 2015;314(9):926–39.

74. Whatley WS, Chandra RK, MacDonald CB. Systemic absorption of gentamicin nasal irrigations. Am J Rhinol. 2006;20(3):251–4.

75. Head K, Chong LY, Piromchai P, Hopkins C, Philpott C, Schilder AG, et al. Systemic and topical antibiotics for chronic rhinosinusitis. Cochrane Database Syst Rev. 2016;4:CD011994. https://doi.org/10.1002/14651858.CD011994.pub2.

Rhinitis and Asthma

14

Merin Elizabeth Kuruvilla and David A. Khan

Case Presentation 1

A 35-year-old female patient presents for the evaluation of chronic rhinosinusitis with nasal polyps (CRSwNP) ongoing for about 10 years. Prior to this, she had no history of sinonasal symptoms. Since the onset of symptoms at the age of 25, she describes progressive and recalcitrant nasal congestion and loss of smell following a particularly severe viral upper respiratory infection (URI). Two years after the onset of rhinitis symptoms, she developed episodic chest tightness and wheeze triggered by URIs, and was diagnosed with asthma.

She eventually underwent endoscopic sinus surgery for refractory nasal congestion to remove/debulk her polyposis, but subsequently experienced rapid regrowth postoperatively. When questioned about triggers, she states that ingestion of ibuprofen on two separate occasions has induced nasal congestion, profuse rhinorrhea, and asthma exacerbation. Alcoholic beverages also reproduce these symptoms albeit to a lesser degree.

Her physical examination revealed grade III bilateral nasal polyps and an occasional expira-

tory wheeze on lung examination, with no other abnormal findings.

Lab work demonstrates peripheral eosinophilia at 700 cells/μL. Total IgE was elevated at 376 kU/L, although specific IgE testing to environmental allergens was negative.

Based on her clinical history, a diagnosis of aspirin-exacerbated respiratory disease (AERD) was made. She is presently on a baseline regimen of budesonide nasal irrigations, fluticasone/salmeterol controller inhaler, and montelukast daily. She declines aspirin (ASA) desensitization due to a history of severe peptic ulcer disease and reluctance to commit to long-term aspirin therapy.

Her clinical course continues to be punctuated by recurrent infectious episodes of acute sinusitis requiring antibiotics and systemic corticosteroids three to four times a year. High-dose corticosteroids transiently ameliorate chronic nasal congestion and restore sense of smell. She reports similarly poor control of asthma, with frequent daytime symptoms and nocturnal awakenings.

She presents today to discuss alternative therapeutic strategies for disease control.

M. E. Kuruvilla (✉)
Department of Allergy and Immunology, Emory University, Atlanta, GA, USA

D. A. Khan
Department of Allergy and Immunology, UT Southwestern Medical Center, Dallas, TX, USA

Discussion

AERD is characterized by asthma, chronic sinusitis with nasal polyps (CRSwNP), and respiratory reactions upon ingestion of cyclooxygenase (COX)-1 inhibitors. It generally develops de

© Springer International Publishing AG, part of Springer Nature 2018
J. A. Bernstein (ed.), *Rhinitis and Related Upper Respiratory Conditions*,
https://doi.org/10.1007/978-3-319-75370-6_14

novo in adulthood. Since the first description nearly a 100 years ago, the inciting event for its sudden development in healthy individuals is yet unknown.

Chronic pansinusitis is associated with nasal polyps (NPs) that often regrow rapidly despite repeated surgery. This is followed by development of late-onset, nonatopic asthma. Patients with both NPs and asthma seem to have a worse disease course with more severe nasal obstruction and loss of smell [1]. AERD in particular is characterized by especially severe olfactory impairment compared with other forms of NPs [2].

Pathogenesis

Although the mechanisms underlying AERD are not fully elucidated, the central defect appears to lie in dysregulated arachidonic acid (AA) metabolism. Prostaglandin E2 (PGE2) levels at baseline are markedly deficient along with its receptor EP2. PGE2 is critical in inhibiting the activation of mast cells and eosinophils and provides negative feedback to the 5-lipoxygenase (5-LOX) pathway. Its production is driven by COX-2, which is also constitutively diminished in AERD [3].

Aspirin is a potent COX-1 and COX-2 inhibitor. Through COX inhibition, AA metabolism is shifted from the COX to the 5-LOX pathway. This results in suppression of residual homeostatic PGE2, and removes negative checkpoints on cysteinyl leukotriene (CysLT) production from mast cells and eosinophils.

This increased cysLT production is mediated by leukotriene C4 synthase (LTC4S), and upregulated by both IL-4 and IFN-gamma [4]. Platelets have also been implicated in cysLT overproduction by adhering to eosinophils and neutrophils in AERD, and transcellular conversion of leukotriene A4 (LTA4) into CysLTs by platelet LTC4S [5]. The P2Y12 receptor facilitates the development of these platelet-leukocyte aggregates. Platelets also release thromboxane A2 (TXA2) that facilitates leukocyte recruitment.

CysLTs including leukotriene C4 (LTC4), LTD4, and LTE4 underlie much of the symptomatic component of AERD pathophysiology. The effect of cysLTs is augmented by cysLT receptor overexpression, making cells hyperresponsive to their action. LTE4 is the stable metabolite of this pathway. Urinary leukotriene E4 (LTE4) levels correlate with the severity of aspirin response, and may be a valid biomarker [6].

AERD is characterized by a high level of tissue and blood eosinophils, suggesting a type 2, Th2 immune response disorder. Epithelium-derived cytokines, including thymic stromal lymphopoietin (TSLP), IL-25, and IL-33, that initiate innate type 2 immune reactions are key mediators in AERD [7, 8]. These cytokines activate type 2 innate lymphoid cells (ILC2s) to express substantial quantities of type 2 cytokines, especially IL-5 and IL-13, propagating Th2 inflammation and eosinophilia. Their effect is further amplified by prostaglandin D2 (PGD2) and cysLTs.

Mast cell-derived PGD2 is another key effector molecule in AERD. Persistent ongoing production has been demonstrated in this population [9, 10]. Interaction of PGD2 with the chemoattractant receptor homologue expressed by Th2 cells (CRTH2) induces chemotaxis of eosinophils and Th2 cells. The severity of clinical reactions to aspirin challenge in patients with AERD also relates to the level of PGD2 production [9], and increased urinary levels of PGD2 metabolites are also characteristic of AERD.

Diagnosis

The diagnosis of AERD is contingent upon a positive challenge to ASA, lysine-ASA, or intranasal ketorolac [11]. Among patients with NPs and asthma referred for oral ASA challenge, 42% had a positive reaction. A clinical history of reactions to ASA or NSAIDs often yields important information and may obviate the need for a challenge. In the setting of a single prior ASA/NSAID respiratory reaction, the likelihood of a positive challenge was 80% and increased to 100% if that reaction was more severe requiring hospitalization [12].

Management

Asthma and sinusitis in AERD should be managed according to established guidelines. In addition, all patients should be prescribed leukotriene blocking medications, including leukotriene receptor antagonists (LTRAs such as montelukast) and/or 5-LOX inhibitors (zileuton).

ASA desensitization followed by chronic therapy with 325–650 mg once or twice daily has the potential to improve upper and lower airway disease [13, 14]. However, tolerance may be limited by gastrointestinal (GI) bleeding or dyspepsia. Following ASA desensitization, urine LTE4 levels gradually decline to basal levels with continued treatment. There appears to be a "PGD2 high" subset of AERD patients who are resistant to ASA desensitization. This is in contrast to subjects who tolerate desensitization who show markedly reduced levels of urinary PGD2 metabolites on high-dose aspirin therapy [9].

With increased understanding of disease mechanism, a host of investigational therapies are being applied towards AERD (Fig. 14.1). Several randomized, double-blind, placebo-controlled studies increasingly support the targeting of Th2 inflammatory pathways to improve outcome measures in CRSwNP patients, including AERD.

The humanized anti-IL-5 monoclonal antibodies, mepolizumab and reslizumab, have both shown a significant reduction of NP size in 50–60% of patients, specifically in the subpopulation with elevated IL-5 levels in nasal secretions [15, 16]. Similarly, anti-TSLP antibodies used in allergic asthma may also control type 2 inflammation in NPs, and anti-TSLP may be a future therapeutic agent for AERD. Given the role of PGD_2 and its receptor CRTH2 in the

AERD pathophysiology, CRTH2 antagonists could be another potential treatment option. The IL-4/IL-13 pathway and other type 2 inflammatory pathways have also shown potential as targets for CRSwNP, but all require further investigation.

The role of allergen immunotherapy (AIT) is unclear, since a causal relationship between atopy and AERD appears unlikely. Among AERD patients on AIT, 62% did not find it effective in one survey [17]. Nevertheless, in subjects with significant and likely relevant allergic sensitization, use of AIT at the maintenance doses proven to be effective may be beneficial in improving mucosal edema attributed to allergic rhinitis leading to improved airflow in an airway already compromised by nasal polyps. Patients without obvious aeroallergen sensitization still may benefit from omalizumab, a monoclonal IgE-binding antibody. This anti-IgE strategy has shown therapeutic potential in nonatopic patients with NPs and asthma [18]. The administration of omalizumab to AERD patients also sharply decreased the urinary levels of PGD2 metabolites and LTE4 [19].

Platelet-targeted therapies are also being investigated as potential treatment for patients with AERD, including a P2Y12-receptor antagonist and a thromboxane-receptor (TP) antagonist. The administration of a TP receptor antagonist in a murine model was shown to completely block ASA reactions [20].

Despite several promising agents on the horizon, a limited number of therapeutic options are currently available to address AERD. In the present case scenario, the patient should be encouraged to undergo ASA desensitization under the umbrella of GI prophylaxis. The development of GI symptoms during long-term ASA therapy appears to be prevented by H2 blockers or proton pump inhibitors [21]. Further investigations to decipher disease mechanism and trials of targeted therapies are imperative to expand other treatment avenues.

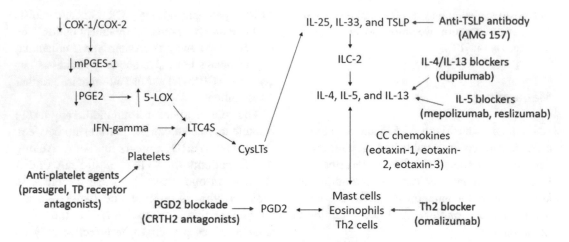

Fig. 14.1 Investigational targeted therapies for AERD based on disease mechanism

Clinical Pearls and Pitfalls

- AERD is defined by mucosal infiltration by eosinophils that suggests a Th2 cytokine milieu.
- CysLT overproduction and hyperresponsiveness are hallmarks of AERD.
- New biologic therapies used in eosinophilic asthma may reduce polyp size and improve sinonasal outcomes, by targeting common pathways of Th2 inflammation.

Case Presentation 2

A 15-year-old female patient presents for the evaluation of episodic shortness of breath and wheeze ongoing for the past 3 years. In addition, she had symptoms for the past 10 years of perennial clear rhinorrhea, postnasal drip, nasal pruritus, and sneezing with occasional ocular pruritus. Symptoms are perennial without obvious seasonal exacerbation, although she thinks they might be worse in the fall.

Her daily regimen consists of montelukast 10 mg daily and inhaled beclomethasone 80 mcg two puffs twice daily. She requires albuterol for rescue several times a week for daytime symptoms triggered by exercise, and once a week for nocturnal awakenings. There is no prior history of hospitalization or systemic corticosteroid use for asthma flares. She has been prescribed fluticasone nasal spray that she uses once a week as needed, along with oral antihistamines for exacerbated nasal congestion.

The patient has no other medical problems. She endorses a history of asthma and allergies in both parents and her siblings.

Her physical examination demonstrates pale and boggy inferior turbinates, and erythema of the posterior pharyngeal wall, but is otherwise normal.

Previous skin testing revealed a positive response (wheal diameter >15 mm) to both house dust mite (HDM) species, *Dermatophagoides pteronyssinus* (DP) and *Dermatophagoides farinae* (DF). Her total IgE level was 147 KU/L, and her fraction of exhaled nitric oxide (FeNO) was 65 parts per billion (normal <20 ppb). Pulmonary function tests showed a FEV1-to-forced vital capacity ratio (FEV1/FVC) of 86%, FEV1 of 3.70 L (90% predicted), FVC of 3.57 L (91% predicted), and a 12% (440 cm^3) improvement in FEV1 after the inhalation of four puffs of inhaled albuterol.

Efforts at allergen avoidance have been undertaken, with dust mite covers on her mattress and pillow, vacuuming the carpets twice a week, and weekly washing of linens in hot water. However, these interventions have had little effect on her symptoms. She presents to discuss allergy shots, but is concerned about the time investment and potential for anaphylactic reactions. She asks about other possible interventions to control her symptoms.

Discussion

The above clinical vignette highlights a common scenario encountered by allergists. HDM is the most common cause worldwide of allergen-induced respiratory disease and is implicated in both allergic rhinitis (AR) and asthma. In one cross-sectional study of 628 AR patients, 56% of patients were sensitized to HDM [22]. The prevalence of HDM sensitization varies between 21 and 85% in asthma populations [23–25].

AR and asthma share a common inflammatory background, which is generally referred to as united airway disease. The relevance of this "unified airway" concept for rhinitis in asthma has long been established [26]. This strong correlation between comorbid allergic asthma and AR often reflects underlying HDM sensitization. Several pediatric cohort studies suggest that sensitization to HDM in children less than 5 years of age is a significant risk factor for asthma later in childhood [23, 27]. The Manchester Asthma and Allergy Study followed children from birth to delineate atopic phenotypes. At age 8 years, sensitization to HDM, both independently and as part of multi-allergen sensitization, increased the risk of respiratory disease in 87% of the cohort [28]. Sensitization to HDM is also a risk factor for asthma development in 20- to 44-year-old patients with AR [29].

HDM allergens are especially virulent since in addition to triggering Th2 cells that drive the IgE-dependent allergic response, they can also activate the innate immune response. They contain proteases and LPS, which are recognized by protease-activated receptors [PARs] and Toll-like receptors [TLRs], respectively, and contribute to allergic inflammation [30].

Der p 1 and Der p 2 are the most frequently recognized clinically relevant HDM allergens. The relationship between IgE antibody titers to HDM allergens and asthma shows that disease is uncommon in subjects with concentrations below about 3.5 IU/mL [31]. Recently, in a cohort of 235 children labeled with dual-HDM sensitization—recognition of specific IgE against both Der p 1 and Der p 2 allergens—a higher risk was noted for recurrent and more severe asthma exacerbations [32].

In this case, uncontrolled AR could be exacerbating the patient's underlying asthma symptoms. The presence of AR is known to be associated with poor asthma control. A cross-sectional study involving 203 children with asthma found that asthma control questionnaire (ACQ) scores were significantly worse in children with AR than in those without ($p = 0.012$). Interestingly, after adjustment for nasal corticosteroid therapy, AR was no longer associated with incomplete asthma control (OR 0.72, $p = 0.150$), suggesting that addressing AR with nasal corticosteroids may improve asthma control [33].

However, it is still a matter of debate whether the treatment of AR helps to improve asthma control. Some studies evaluating the effect of intranasal corticosteroids (INS) on asthma outcomes have shown significant improvements in FEV1 [34, 35], asthma symptom scores [35, 36], and FeNO [37]. In a retrospective evaluation of a cohort with AR and asthma [38], the risk of asthma-related hospitalizations and emergency department visits in the group treated for AR was 1.3% compared to 6.6% in the untreated group. Conversely, a recent trial of intranasal mometasone treatment of the upper airways to improve control of inadequately controlled asthma did not achieve the primary outcome of improvement in Asthma Control Test (ACT) scores in adults or children [39].

The patient in this vignette is mono-sensitized to HDM and would benefit from therapies aimed at ameliorating HDM allergy. This would be a worthwhile investment regardless of whether HDM sensitization exists independently or in the setting of other allergen sensitizations.

According to a recent Cochrane meta-analysis on HDM avoidance, the use of environmental control measures has been found to be of little benefit in reducing rhinitis symptoms with no effect on asthma symptoms [40]. This lack of effect may be due to the inability of these interventions to reduce mite antigen levels low enough to reduce allergen-driven inflammation.

Pharmacotherapy with topical corticosteroids is effective in the control of AR and asthma symptoms, but it does not modify the natural history of the disease. The efficacy of omalizumab has been proven for the treatment of moderate-to-severe, therapy-resistant, uncontrolled allergic asthma, in children down to 6 years of age, particularly also in children with dust mite allergy. However, allergen immunotherapy (AIT), involving the administration of gradually increasing concentrations of allergen extract, is the only treatment modality that has the potential to modify disease course.

Subcutaneous immunotherapy (SCIT) and sublingual immunotherapy (SLIT) are both effective in reducing symptoms of HDM-induced AR and asthma. While a substantial body of evidence supports the efficacy of SCIT [41–44], there remain several deficiencies in the literature. A review of HDM IT articles published through 2013 for AR and asthma found no consensus on basic treatment parameters [45]. The authors highlighted that many of the commercially available HDM extracts have not been investigated in large, multicenter trials, and only scant pediatric studies exist.

The advent of HDM SLIT has added a new dimension to the management of the HDM allergic patient. However, trials to evaluate HDM AIT with SLIT have yielded varying results.

Treatment with HDM SLIT in a cohort of North American adolescent and adult subjects resulted in a 17% improvement in total combined rhinitis score (TCRS) relative to placebo [46]. This is in contrast to a 49% improvement in symptoms observed with the same preparation in a HDM environmental exposure chamber trial [47]. Furthermore, improvement in mild-to-moderate asthma patients with HDM SLIT has been demonstrated [48, 49] as well as a significant decrease in the risk of moderate or severe asthma exacerbations [50].

Overall, based on the currently published literature on HDM AIT, there is good evidence demonstrating the clinical effectiveness and safety of HDM SCIT and SLIT in treating HDM allergic subjects with AR and mild-to-moderate asthma.

Previous studies also suggest that early institution of AIT for AR may have potentially prevented the development of asthma in this patient. Forty-four patients with AR monosensitized to HDM were randomized to AIT versus placebo [51]. The AIT group had decreased airway hyperreactivity, and none developed asthma, compared with 9% patients in the placebo group. More recently, a large retrospective cohort study evaluated AIT for allergic rhinitis in preventing asthma [52]. The risk of asthma was significantly attenuated in patients receiving AIT (relative risk, 0.60; 95% CI, 0.42–0.84); there was also a significant preventive effect of asthma using SCIT (relative risk, 0.54; 95% CI, 0.38–0.84) compared with nontreated control subjects.

In addition, in a recent research review, Demoly et al. highlighted evidence that AIT can assist in stepping down asthma treatment and improve control [53]. Of note, moderate asthmatics rather than mild cases appear to benefit more from this intervention.

A pilot study recently evaluated HDM AIT for primary prevention of allergic disease. In a prospective study, 111 high-risk infants were randomized to a high-dose HDM extract or placebo for 12 months. The study showed a significant reduction in sensitization to any common allergen in the active (9%) compared with placebo (25%) treatment groups [54].

In this case, suboptimal control of AR may be contributing to persistent asthma, and compliance with daily INS should be emphasized. Asthma treatment should be stepped up to an ICS/LABA combination. Omalizumab is yet another option for symptom control, but given the low severity of her disease and the high cost of this treatment is not really appropriate at this juncture to initiate. Finally, HDM AIT should be strongly considered as a disease-modifying intervention due to clinical effectiveness in AR and mild-moderate asthma once her asthma is under good control.

Clinical Pearls and Pitfalls

- A high proportion of allergic asthma patients are sensitized to HDMs, which are the most common allergens worldwide.
- Rhinitis is not just associated with asthma, but is also a risk factor for its development.
- Management of rhinitis and asthma must be jointly carried out, leading to better control of both diseases.
- Allergen immunotherapy for AR may prevent progression to asthma by several potential pathways, and may improve control in established cases of asthma.

References

1. Moore WC, Meyers DA, Wenzel SE, Teague WG, Li H, Li X, et al. Identification of asthma phenotypes using cluster analysis in the severe asthma research program. Am J Respir Crit Care Med. 2010;181:315–23.
2. Gudziol V, Michel M, Sonnefeld C, Koschel D, Hummel T. Olfaction and sinonasal symptoms in patients with CRSwNP and AERD and without AERD: a cross-sectional and longitudinal study. Eur Arch Otorhinolaryngol. 2017;274(3):1487–93.
3. Picado C, Fernandez-Morata JC, Juan M, Roca-Ferrer J, Fuentes M, Xaubet A, et al. Cyclooxygenase-2 mRNA is downexpressed in nasal polyps from aspirin-sensitive asthmatics. Am J Respir Crit Care Med. 1999;160(1):291–6.
4. Steinke JW, Liu L, Huyett P, Negri J, Payne SC, Borish L. Prominent role of IFN-γ in patients with aspirin-exacerbated respiratory disease. J Allergy Clin Immunol. 2013;132(4):856–65.
5. Laidlaw TM, Kidder MS, Bhattacharyya N, Xing W, Shen S, Milne GL, et al. Cysteinyl leukotriene overproduction in aspirin-exacerbated respiratory disease is driven by platelet-adherent leukocytes. Blood. 2012;119:3790–8.
6. Divekar R, Hagan J, Rank M, Park M, Volcheck G, O'Brien E, et al. Diagnostic utility of urinary LTE4 in asthma, allergic rhinitis, chronic rhinosinusitis, nasal polyps, and aspirin sensitivity. J Allergy Clin Immunol Pract. 2016;4(4):665–70.
7. Liu T, Kanaoka Y, Barrett NA, Feng C, Garofalo D, Lai J, et al. Aspirin-exacerbated respiratory disease involves a cysteinyl leukotriene-driven IL-33-mediated mast cell activation pathway. J Immunol. 2015;195(8):3537–45.
8. Buchheit KM, Cahill KN, Katz HR, Murphy KC, Feng C, Lee-Sarwar K, et al. Thymic stromal lymphopoietin controls prostaglandin D2 generation in patients with aspirin-exacerbated respiratory disease. J Allergy Clin Immunol. 2016;137(5):1566–1576.e5.
9. Cahill KN, Bensko JC, Boyce JA, Laidlaw TM. Prostaglandin D(2): a dominant mediator of aspirin-exacerbated respiratory disease. J Allergy Clin Immunol. 2015;135:245–52.
10. Feng X, Ramsden MK, Negri J, Baker MG, Payne SC, Borish L, et al. Eosinophil production of prostaglandin D2 in patients with aspirin-exacerbated respiratory disease. J Allergy Clin Immunol. 2016;138(4):1089–97.
11. Williams AN. Diagnostic evaluation in aspirin-exacerbated respiratory disease. Immunol Allergy Clin N Am. 2016;36(4):657–68.
12. Dursun AB, Woessner KA, Simon RA, Karasoy D, Stevenson DD. Predicting outcomes of oral aspirin challenges in patients with asthma, nasal polyps, and chronic sinusitis. Ann Allergy Asthma Immunol. 2008;100(5):420–5.
13. Berges-Gimeno MP, Simon RA, Stevenson DD. Long-term treatment with aspirin desensitization in asthmatic patients with aspirin exacerbated respiratory disease. J Allergy Clin Immunol. 2003;111:180–6.
14. Esmaeilzadeh H, Nabavi M, Aryan Z, Arshi S, Bemanian MH, Fallahpour M, et al. Aspirin desensitization for patients with aspirin-exacerbated respiratory disease: a randomized double-blind placebo-controlled trial. Clin Immunol. 2015;160(2):349–57.
15. Gevaert P, Lang-Loidolt D, Lackner A, Stammberger H, Staudinger H, Van Zele T, et al. Nasal IL-5 levels determine the response to anti-IL-5 treatment in patients with nasal polyps. J Allergy Clin Immunol. 2006;118(5):1133–41.
16. Gevaert P, Van Bruaene N, Cattaert T, Van Steen K, Van Zele T, Acke F, et al. Mepolizumab, a humanized anti-IL-5 mAb, as a treatment option for severe nasal polyposis. J Allergy Clin Immunol. 2011;128(5):989–95.
17. Ta V, White AA. Survey-defined patient experiences with aspirin-exacerbated respiratory disease. J Allergy Clin Immunol Pract. 2015;3(5):711–8.
18. Gevaert P, Calus L, Van Zele T, Blomme K, De Ruyck N, Bauters W, et al. Omalizumab is effective in allergic and nonallergic patients with nasal polyps and asthma. J Allergy Clin Immunol. 2013;131(1):110–6.
19. Hayashi H, Mitsui C, Nakatani E, Fukutomi Y, Kajiwara K, Watai K, et al. Omalizumab reduces cysteinyl leukotriene and 9alpha,11beta-prostaglandin F2 overproduction in aspirin-exacerbated respiratory disease. J Allergy Clin Immunol. 2016;137:1585–7.
20. Liu T, Laidlaw TM, Katz HR, Boyce JA. Prostaglandin E2 deficiency causes a phenotype of aspirin sensitivity that depends on platelets and cysteinyl leukotrienes. Proc Natl Acad Sci U S A. 2013;110(42):16987–92.
21. Kowalski ML, Wardzyńska A, Makowska JS. Clinical trials of aspirin treatment after desensitization in aspirin-exacerbated respiratory disease. Immunol Allergy Clin N Am. 2016;36(4):705–17.

22. Larenas-Linnemann D, Michels A, Dinger H, Shah-Hosseini K, Mösges R, Arias-Cruz A, et al. Allergen sensitization linked to climate and age, not to intermittent-persistent rhinitis in a cross-sectional cohort study in the (sub)tropics. Clin Transl Allergy. 2014;4:20.

23. Lodge CJ, Lowe AJ, Gurrin LC, Hill DJ, Hosking CS, Khalafzai RU, et al. House dust mite sensitization in toddlers predicts current wheeze at age 12 years. J Allergy Clin Immunol. 2011;128(4):782–8.

24. Peat JK, Tovey E, Toelle BG, Haby MM, Gray EJ, Mahmic A, et al. House dust mite allergens. A major risk factor for childhood asthma in Australia. Am J Respir Crit Care Med. 1996;153(1):141–6.

25. Sunyer J, Jarvis D, Pekkanen J, Chinn S, Janson C, Leynaert B, et al. Geographic variations in the effect of atopy on asthma in the European Community Respiratory Health Study. J Allergy Clin Immunol. 2004;114:1033–9.

26. Bousquet J, Van Cauwenberge P, Khaltaev N, ARIA Workshop Group, and World Health Organization. Allergic rhinitis and its impact on asthma. J Allergy Clin Immunol. 2001;108:S147–334.

27. Holt PG, Rowe J, Kusel M, Parsons F, Hollams EM, Bosco A, et al. Toward improved prediction of risk for atopy and asthma among preschoolers: a prospective cohort study. J Allergy Clin Immunol. 2010;125:653–9.

28. Simpson A, Tan VY, Winn J, Svensen M, Bishop CM, Heckerman DE, et al. Beyond atopy: multiple patterns of sensitization in relation to asthma in a birth cohort study. Am J Respir Crit Care Med. 2010;181:1200–6.

29. Shaaban R, Zureik M, Soussan D, Neukirch C, Heinrich J, Sunyer J, et al. Rhinitis and onset of asthma: a longitudinal population-based study. Lancet. 2008;372:1049–57.

30. Wang JY. The innate immune response in house dust mite-induced allergic inflammation. Allergy Asthma Immunol Res. 2013;5:68–74.

31. Simpson A, Soderstrom L, Ahlstedt S, Murray CS, Woodcock A, Custovic A. IgE antibody quantification and the probability of wheeze in preschool children. J Allergy Clin Immunol. 2005;116:744–9.

32. Custovic A, Sonntag HJ, Buchan IE, Belgrave D, Simpson A, Prosperi MC. Evolution pathways of IgE responses to grass and mite allergens throughout childhood. J Allergy Clin Immunol. 2015;136:1645–52.

33. de Groot EP, Nijkamp A, Duiverman EJ, Brand PL. Allergic rhinitis is associated with poor asthma control in children with asthma. Thorax. 2012;67(7):582.

34. Nair A, Vaidyanathan S, Clearie K, Williamson P, Meldrum K, Lipworth BJ. Steroid sparing effects of intranasal corticosteroids in asthma and allergic rhinitis. Allergy. 2010;65:359–67.

35. Sandrini A, Ferreira IM, Jardim JR, Zamel N, Chapman KR. Effect of nasal triamcinolone acetonide on lower airway inflammatory markers in patients with allergic rhinitis. J Allergy Clin Immunol. 2003;111:313–20.

36. Stelmach R, do Patrocinio TNM, Ribeiro M, Cukier A. Effect of treating allergic rhinitis with corticosteroids in patients with mild-to-moderate persistent asthma. Chest. 2005;128:3140–7.

37. Ribeiro de Andrade C, Chatkin JM, Fiterman J, Scaglia N, Camargos PA. Unified disease, unified management: treating allergic rhinitis and asthma with nasally inhaled corticosteroid. Respir Med. 2010;104(10):1577–80.

38. Crystal-Peters J, Neslusan C, Crown WH, Torres A. Treating allergic rhinitis in patients with comorbid asthma: the risk of asthma-related hospitalizations and emergency department visits. J Allergy Clin Immunol. 2002;109(1):57–62.

39. Dixon AE, Castro M, Cohen RI, Gerald LB, Holbrook JT, Irvin CG, et al. Efficacy of nasal mometasone for the treatment of chronic sinonasal disease in patients with inadequately controlled asthma. J Allergy Clin Immunol. 2015;135:701–9.

40. Nurmatov U, van Schayck CP, Hurwitz B, Sheikh A. House dust mite avoidance measures for perennial allergic rhinitis: an updated Cochrane systematic review. Allergy. 2012;67(2):158–65.

41. Ameal A, Vega-Chicote JM, Fernández S, Miranda A, Carmona MJ, Rondón MC, et al. Double-blind and placebo-controlled study to assess efficacy and safety of a modified allergen extract of Dermatophagoides pteronyssinus in allergic asthma. Allergy. 2005;60(9):1178–83.

42. Pichler CE, Marquardsen A, Sparholt S, Løwenstein H, Bircher A, Bischof M, et al. Specific immunotherapy with Dermatophagoides pteronyssinus and D. farinae results in decreased bronchial hyperreactivity. Allergy. 1997;52(3):274–83.

43. Varney VA, Tabbah K, Mavroleon G, Frew AJ. Usefulness of specific immunotherapy in patients with severe perennial allergic rhinitis induced by house dust mite: a double-blind, randomized, placebo-controlled trial. Clin Exp Allergy. 2003;33:1076–82.

44. Garcia-Robaina JC, Sanchez I, de la Torre F, Fernandez-Caldas E, Casanovas M. Successful management of mite-allergic asthma with modified extracts of Dermatophagoides pteronyssinus and Dermatophagoides farinae in a double-blind, placebo-controlled study. J Allergy Clin Immunol. 2006;118:1026–32.

45. Calderon MA, Casale TB, Nelson HS, Demoly P. An evidence-based analysis of house dust mite allergen immunotherapy: a call for more rigorous clinical studies. J Allergy Clin Immunol. 2013;132(6):1322–36.

46. Nolte H, Bernstein DI, Nelson HS, Kleine-Tebbe J, Sussman GL, Seitzberg D, et al. Efficacy of house dust mite sublingual immunotherapy tablet in North American adolescents and adults in a randomized, placebo-controlled trial. J Allergy Clin Immunol. 2016;138(6):1631–8.

47. Nolte H, Maloney J, Nelson HS, Bernstein DI, Lu S, Li Z, et al. Onset and dose-related efficacy of house dust mite sublingual immunotherapy tablets in an environmental exposure chamber. J Allergy Clin Immunol. 2015;135:1494–501.

48. Mosbech H, Deckelmann R, de Blay F, Pastorello EA, Trebas-Pietras E, Andres LP, et al. Standardized quality (SQ) house dust mite sublingual immunotherapy tablet (ALK) reduces inhaled corticosteroid use while maintaining asthma control: a randomized, double-blind, placebo-controlled trial. J Allergy Clin Immunol. 2014;134(3):568–75.

49. Mosbech H, Canonica GW, Backer V, de Blay F, Klimek L, Broge L, et al. SQ house dust mite sublingually administered immunotherapy tablet (ALK) improves allergic rhinitis in patients with house dust mite allergic asthma and rhinitis symptoms. Ann Allergy Asthma Immunol. 2015;114(2):134–40.

50. Virchow JC, Backer V, Kuna P, Prieto L, Nolte H, Villesen HH, et al. Efficacy of a house dust mite sublingual allergen immunotherapy tablet in adults with allergic asthma. JAMA. 2016;315(16):1715–25.

51. Grembiale RD, Camporota L, Naty S, Tranfa CME, Djukanovic R, Marsico SA. Effects of specific immunotherapy in allergic rhinitic individuals with bronchial hyperresponsiveness. Am J Respir Crit Care Med. 2000;162:2048–52.

52. Schmitt J, Schwarz K, Stadler E, Wüstenberg EG. Allergy immunotherapy for allergic rhinitis effectively prevents asthma: results from a large retrospective cohort study. J Allergy Clin Immunol. 2015;136:1511–6.

53. Demoly P, Makatsori M, Casale TB, Calderon MA. The potential role of allergen immunotherapy in stepping down asthma treatment. J Allergy Clin Immunol. 2017;5(3):640–8.

54. Zolkipli Z, Roberts G, Cornelius V, Clayton B, Pearson S, Michaelis L, et al. Randomized controlled trial of primary prevention of atopy using house dust mite allergen oral immunotherapy in early childhood. J Allergy Clin Immunol. 2015;136:1541–7.

Pediatric Rhinitis

Fuad M. Baroody

Case Presentation 1

A 6-year-old male presents to the office with complaints of a consistent stuffy nose with intermittent clear rhinorrhea. He also complains of episodes of sneezing and itching that occur frequently. He does have intermittent snoring, especially on days when he is significantly congested. His symptoms are present all year long with exacerbations during spring and fall, especially when he is playing outside. His symptoms seem to affect his quality of life as he is often tired on days when his symptoms are prevalent. He has been treated with diphenhydramine, which seems to help the symptoms to a certain extent but, on the other hand, makes him sleepy and worsens his school performance. Review of systems shows asthma treated with an inhaled corticosteroid for control and, as needed, bronchodilators for rescue. He is otherwise healthy and lives at home with mother, father (who are both allergic), and a younger sister. They have no pets in the house.

On physical exam, the notable physical findings are nasal congestion with hypertrophied inferior turbinates that have a pale mucosa and are covered by thin clear secretions. His mouth and throat exam are normal with small, nonobstructive tonsils. His chest is clear without wheezing on auscultation. Because of the history, his nose was decongested and anesthetized topically and a nasal endoscopy was performed. His septum was straight and his inferior turbinates responded well to decongestant with improvement of his airway. His adenoids were present but not obstructive. There was no purulent drainage in his osteomeatal areas. Immunocap testing was performed that showed him to be sensitive to trees, grasses, ragweed, and dust mites.

The working diagnosis of this child is that of perennial allergic rhinitis (PAR) with a seasonal component (SAR), which is the most common chronic disease in children, and has significant signs and symptoms that affect their quality of life as well as their ability to concentrate and learn effectively in school. It is a manifestation of a hypersensitivity response in the nasal mucosa to environmental allergens that elicit an IgE-mediated antibody response. It usually manifests with a spectrum of symptoms including sneezing; runny nose; stuffy nose; itching of the nose, throat, and ears; as well as eye tearing, redness, and itching. Because eye manifestations are often present, the disease is more commonly referred to as allergic rhinoconjunctivitis. Allergic rhinitis is estimated to affect anywhere between 25 and 40% of the pediatric population in the Western world [1]. Allergic rhinitis increases with age from early childhood to the beginning of adolescence.

F. M. Baroody (✉)
Section of Otolaryngology, The University of Chicago Medicine and The Comer Children's Hospital, Chicago, IL, USA
e-mail: fbaroody@surgery.bsd.uchicago.edu

© Springer International Publishing AG, part of Springer Nature 2018
J. A. Bernstein (ed.), *Rhinitis and Related Upper Respiratory Conditions*,
https://doi.org/10.1007/978-3-319-75370-6_15

Although AR is a benign disease, as mentioned above, it has negative effects on quality of life of children and their parents, and negatively affects school performance and sleep. The rhinoconjunctivitis quality-of-life questionnaires for children and adolescents developed by Juniper and colleagues are the most commonly used tools to measure quality of life in children and demonstrate the negative impact of the disease [2, 3]. A survey of 35,757 US households, the "Pediatric Allergies in America" survey, focused on children with nasal allergy between 4 and 17 years of age and showed a significantly lower percentage of allergic children being rated as having excellent health by their parents (43%) as compared to children without allergies (59%) [1]. Similarly, a lower proportion of children with allergies were described as "happy," "calm and peaceful," having "lots of energy" and being "full of life" as compared to children without allergies. Moreover, the proportion of children with diminished performance while at school as assessed by the parents was significantly higher in children with nasal allergies (40%) as compared to their nonallergic peers (11%).

In the Allergic Rhinitis and Its Influence on Asthma (ARIA, an international working group) guidelines, allergic rhinitis is classified based on duration: *as intermittent* (symptoms occurring less than 4 days a week *or* less than 4 weeks a year) or *as persistent* (symptoms occurring more than 4 days per week *and* for more than 4 weeks in a year) [4]. Additionally, AR is classified based on the impact on quality of life: *as mild* (the patient has normal sleep, daily activities, sport, leisure, work and school, and no troublesome symptoms) or *as moderate to severe* (the patient has abnormal sleep, impairment of daily activities, sport, leisure, problems caused at work or school, and troublesome symptoms). Other classifications include *seasonal* (symptoms only during specific allergen seasons), *perennial* (symptoms all year long), or *episodic* (symptoms only upon exposure to a certain allergen, such as exposure to a pet occasionally) [5]. Our patient would qualify as persistent or perennial with seasonal exacerbations depending on which classification terminology is used. His disease would be moderate to severe as it negatively affects his quality of life.

The pathophysiologic mechanisms in AR can be synthesized in the following scenario: sensitization of the nasal mucosa to a certain allergen begins with its breakdown to specific peptides by antigen-presenting cells and presentation of the specific peptide to co-stimulatory molecules on T and B lymphocytes. The release of Th2 cytokines by these cells and differentiation of B cells to plasma cells promote production of allergen peptide-specific IgE antibodies, which then localize to high-affinity IgE receptors (FcER1) on mast cells and basophils. Subsequent exposure to the relevant allergen leads to recognition and cross-linking of specific IgE receptors on mast cells and basophils that results in exocytosis of preformed and newly formed bioactive mediators that result in physiologic responses manifested as AR symptoms. The proinflammatory substances generated after antigen exposure are largely eosinophil-derived enzymes and cellular toxins as well as cytokines that promote the allergic response (IL-4, IL-13) and eosinophilic inflammation (IL-5). These and other cytokines and chemokines are generated in part by lymphocytes, which are abundant in resting and allergen-stimulated nasal mucosa. Mast cells also have an important role in the storage, production, and secretion of cytokines. Cytokines upregulate adhesion molecules on the vascular endothelium, and possibly on marginating leukocytes, leading to the migration of these inflammatory cells into the site of tissue inflammation. Various cytokines also promote the chemotaxis and survival of these recruited inflammatory cells, leading to a secondary immune response by virtue of their capability to promote IgE synthesis by B cells. Also important is the nervous system, which amplifies the allergic reaction by central and peripheral reflexes (orthodromic and antidromic) that result in changes at sites distant from those of antigen deposition, such as the eye, sinuses, and lower airway. These inflammatory changes lower the threshold of mucosal responsiveness to various specific and nonspecific stimuli, making allergic patients more responsive to stimuli to which they are exposed every day [6].

Diagnosis

The basis of the diagnosis of allergic rhinoconjunctivitis in children is the medical history. The most common symptoms of AR are recurrent episodes of sneezing, pruritus, rhinorrhea, nasal congestion, and watery eyes. Less common symptoms include itchy throat, itchy ears, and postnasal drip. The clinician should establish the pattern and timing of allergic symptoms as well as assess severity and interference with daily activities. Timing of symptoms during different seasons, or after exposure to certain pets, gives the physician an idea of the potential sensitizations of each particular patient. Perennial sensitization is a little more difficult to detect from history taking, but chronicity of symptoms may indicate perennial/persistent AR. History should also be elicited about home and school environmental exposures, as well as the effectiveness of any prior allergy therapy. Allergic children have a high likelihood of a history of asthma, eczema, chronic sinusitis, and otitis media with effusion [7]. Other causes of chronic nasal symptoms are adenoid hypertrophy (especially in the younger child) and chronic rhinosinusitis (more in the older child). In unilateral disease, uncommon causes like unilateral choanal atresia, unnoticed foreign bodies, and tumors must be taken into account.

A complete ear, nose, and throat examination is required for children suspected of AR. Classic findings of AR in children include watery rhinorrhea; allergic shiners" (darkening of the lower eyelids as a result of suborbital edema); "allergic salute" (the upward rubbing of the nose with the palm of the hand to relieve nasal itching); "allergic crease" (a transverse white line across the nasal bridge caused by the allergic salute); and red, watery eyes, a sign of conjunctivitis. Anterior rhinoscopy using the largest speculum of the otoscope or a nasal speculum is very useful in evaluating the inferior and the middle turbinates. A pale nasal mucosal color is often very suggestive, though not pathognomonic, of AR, and children with allergies typically have clear, thin nasal drainage. Nasal endoscopy can also be performed in the cooperative and willing child/adolescent. This exam allows the appreciation of all the changes seen with anterior rhinoscopy and adds a thorough evaluation of the middle meatus for signs of sinusitis or nasal polyposis, an appreciation of possible posterior septal abnormalities, and a good look at both posterior choanae and adenoids. Mouth breathing is a common symptom, especially in children who also have concomitant adenoid hypertrophy.

Sensitization can be evaluated by measuring specific IgE in the serum or by skin prick tests. Both tests are equally reliable but measurement of serum-specific IgE is sometimes better tolerated in young children (involves only one blood draw) and is not affected by medication intake, or skin conditions. However, in vitro testing can take 1–2 weeks to obtain results whereas for skin testing, in addition to being more sensitive than serologic testing, results are readily apparent within 15 min. It is important to realize that not all patients who have positive skin tests or elevated serum-specific IgE levels are considered to have AR. To establish the diagnosis of AR it is necessary to exhibit both sensitization and a relevant clinical history of symptoms after exposure to the specific allergen.

Comorbidities

Allergic rhinitis is part of an allergic syndrome that also consists of conjunctivitis, asthma, atopic dermatitis, and food allergy. The sequential development of allergic disease manifestations during early childhood is often referred to as the atopic march [8]. Children most often develop atopic dermatitis and food allergy first and asthma and rhinitis later. A number of respiratory and airway conditions can affect children with AR. In the Pediatric Allergies in America survey, the children with nasal allergies were 2.8-fold more likely to have headaches, 7-fold more likely to have face pain/pressure, 11-fold more likely to report sinus problems, and 2.5- to 3-fold more likely to snore every day or on most days [1]. Furthermore, children with AR were threefold more likely to have an asthma diagnosis and four times more likely to have had asthma in the last 12 months compared to their nonallergic counterparts.

Other studies have supported these findings. In fact, asthma is far more common in patients with AR than in those without, with as many as 50% of AR patients having asthma [9]. Sinusitis and rhinitis also often coexist and are usually referred to as rhinosinusitis. Allergic rhinitis is a risk factor for acute rhinosinusitis across all age groups. The inflammatory response associated with allergic rhinitis contributes to edema and impairment of sinus drainage and may be a contributing factor in as many as 30% of young adult patients with acute rhinosinusitis [10]. Allergic rhinitis also commonly coexists with recurrent or chronic rhinosinusitis with 25–84% of patients with rhinosinusitis having concomitant allergic rhinitis [11].

Acute otitis media and otitis media with effusion (OME) are among the most common problems of childhood. A number of clinical studies have evaluated the association between allergic rhinitis and OME, with one series demonstrating a 21% prevalence of OME in unselected schoolchildren with allergic rhinitis [12] and another finding a 50% prevalence of allergic rhinitis in children with OME [13]. In one study of 209 children with a history of chronic or recurrent otitis media who had been referred to a multidisciplinary "glue ear/allergy" clinic, AR was confirmed in 89%, asthma in 36%, and eczema in 24% [14]. Skin tests were positive to one or more of eight common inhalant allergens in 57% of children, and, among those undergoing serum testing, peripheral eosinophilia was documented in 40% and an elevated serum IgE in 28%. Although there is a clear possibility of referral bias in this specialty population, the high frequency of allergy is notable. Furthermore, analysis of middle-ear effusions and mucosal biopsies from atopic subjects with allergic rhinitis has demonstrated a pattern of inflammatory mediators not seen in non-atopic children, with significantly higher levels of eosinophil activity markers, mast cell products, and cytokines [15].

A link has also been postulated between adenoid hypertrophy and allergy stemming from inflammation of the nasal mucosa, which is in direct proximity to the adenoids [16]. A study found that the incidence of adenoid hypertrophy was almost twofold higher in children with allergic disease (AR, bronchial asthma, or atopic dermatitis) when compared with nonallergic controls (40% vs. 22%) [17]. Among those children with allergic disease, the incidence of adenoid hypertrophy was higher in children with AR, alone or coexisting with bronchial asthma (71%), compared with those children who had bronchial asthma alone (25%). The authors speculate that ongoing nasal inflammation from allergy could contribute to adenoid hypertrophy. Patients with allergic disorders of the upper airway often have significant sleep disturbances. While the mechanisms are not fully understood, congestion in the nose is presumed to be a key factor. Several epidemiologic studies have shown that AR is a risk factor for obstructive sleep apnea syndrome (OSAS) in children [18]. In a group of children presenting to the sleep laboratory for the evaluation of symptoms of OSAS by polysomnogram, 36% had positive serum-specific IgE testing. Furthermore, a significantly higher proportion of allergic children had an abnormal polysomnogram (57%) compared to nonallergic children (40%) [19]. It is therefore clear from these descriptive studies that allergic inflammation of the nose seems to be associated with similar inflammatory processes in other parts of the upper and lower airways. The effects that link these disease processes have been speculated to be related to multiple mechanisms including direct contiguity of the involved organs, systemic allergic inflammation, and neural reflexes.

Management

Management includes education of the patient and parent(s), avoidance of allergens and secondary tobacco smoke, and pharmacotherapy. A stepwise approach is recommended, which depends on the severity of the disorder, the patient's preferences and adherence to treatment, and the presence of comorbidities such as asthma. Although immunotherapy is an effective therapy for AR in properly selected subjects it is typically reserved for those who have symptoms several months out of the year, have incomplete relief with maximal pharmacotherapy, or wish to be less dependent on pharmacotherapy throughout the year. Regardless of whether allergen immunotherapy is implemented, avoidance and pharmacotherapy are the recommended initial therapies for AR.

Avoidance

Few studies are available on the effect of allergen avoidance in children with allergic rhinoconjunctivitis. A Cochrane review on house dust mite avoidance measures for PAR in adults and children found that acaricides and extensive bedroom-based environmental control programs might reduce AR symptoms for some people, but the evidence is not strong [20]. Only two small studies examined the effects of avoidance of pet allergens in children with allergic rhinoconjunctivitis. One found no effect, and the other showed some effect for interventions directed towards controlling dust mites and pets. It seems prudent to avoid owning a pet if the household includes a child with documented pet allergies. However, as pets are an integral part of many families, keeping them out of the bedrooms and main activity rooms and placing HEPA filtration units in these rooms and impermeable but breathable encasements over the pillow, mattress, and box spring in conjunction with frequent vacuuming if there are carpets have been found to reduce indoor animal allergen levels. It is also reasonable and inexpensive to avoid upholstered furniture, curtains, and soft toys that tend to be reservoirs for indoor animal and dust mite allergens, in the bedroom of an allergic child.

Antihistamines

Antihistamines block the action of released histamine and are known to effectively control sneezing, itching, rhinorrhea, and eye symptoms. These agents are not as effective in helping nasal congestion. First-generation antihistamines (diphenhydramine, hydroxyzine, chlorpheniramine, brompheniramine, and clemastine) are lipophilic and cross the blood–brain barrier, thus leading to the notable side effect of sedation. They also have anticholinergic side effects which can lead to drying of secretions. Indeed in a study evaluating learning scores in school children, allergic children receiving placebo were found to have lower scores than normal nonallergic children, suggesting a deleterious effect of allergic rhinitis on learning ability [21]. When the allergic children received diphenhydramine, loratadine, or placebo for 2 weeks, their learning scores became even worse than the group on placebo and were significantly lower than nonallergic controls when receiving diphenhydramine, the sedating antihistamine. In contrast, loratadine, a non-sedating agent, resulted in an improvement of learning scores which were not different from those of the control nonallergic group. To avoid such side effects, second-generation antihistamines were developed. They have reduced or absent anticholinergic side effects and do not lead to significant sedation, as they do not cross the blood–brain barrier [22, 23]. These agents are available in liquid form, and many are approved for use in children as young as 6 months of age. They have relatively rapid absorption and onset of action (within hours) and the longer half-life of the second-generation drugs allows once-daily administration. Multiple clinical studies in children have documented efficacy and safety of second-generation non-sedating H1-antihistamines in AR.

Intranasal H1 antihistamines are also available for use in children. An example of these agents is azelastine, a phthalazinone derivative, approved for the treatment of AR. Its efficacy is comparable to other antihistamines, and it might be more effective than oral antihistamines for nasal congestion. It is usually given twice daily, and in the original seasonal AR studies was noted to cause somnolence which was not consistently found in subsequent studies. Taste alteration may occur immediately after use with an incidence as high as 20%. Olopatadine hydrochloride (0.6%) has been shown to be safe and effective for the treatment of SAR and is usually administered twice daily. A recent study has shown it to be effective for the control of both nasal and ocular symptoms in a group of children over age 6 years [24]. The incidence of bitter taste in this study ranged from 3 to 4%. The incidence of somnolence is minimally higher than placebo vehicle.

Decongestants

Topical as well as systemic decongestants act to cause vascular constriction and reduce the nasal blood supply by alpha-adrenergic stimulation. Prolonged use of topical decongestant agents can lead to rebound nasal congestion, also known as rhinitis medicamentosa. Therefore, their use should be limited to situations where severe allergic nasal congestion precludes the administration of other intranasal medications. In these cases, a short 3- to 5-day course of intranasal decongestants is used in conjunction with other intranasal agents (corticosteroids, antihistamines) to facilitate access to the nasal mucosa. Oral decongestants are less effective than their intranasal counterparts. Pseudoephedrine hydrochloride and phenylephrine are the most commonly used. Pseudoephedrine-containing decongestant products are now sold behind the counter in US pharmacies because of the use of this medication in the illicit manufacture of methamphetamine. They are used most frequently in combination preparations with antihistamines (pseudoephedrine), or over the counter in cough and cold products in combination with analgesics and antitussives. Phenylephrine is another over-the-counter decongestant, also used in combination products. A recent meta-analysis showed lack of efficacy of phenylephrine on both objective and subjective measures of nasal congestion compared to placebo [25]. In addition their most common side effects are insomnia and irritability which can be seen in as many as 25% of patients.

Anticholinergics

These agents are useful in the control of rhinorrhea associated with allergic rhinitis and have no therapeutic efficacy on any of the other symptoms of the disease. Ipratropium bromide is available for intranasal administration and lacks the systemic effects of atropine. It is used in patients with AR who continue to have significant symptoms of rhinorrhea despite maximal therapy with other agents.

Cromolyn Sodium

Cromolyn sodium is a mast cell stabilizer and is available over the counter as a 4% solution for intranasal use in AR. It has been shown to be helpful for sneezing, itching, and rhinorrhea but not as effective for nasal obstruction. It does not cross the blood–brain barrier and is unlikely to

cause sedation. It has a short half-life and therefore needs to be dosed more frequently. It is noted to be very safe in children and pregnant women, but the need for frequent dosing reduces compliance and makes this agent less attractive as a therapeutic choice.

Leukotriene Modifiers

Because leukotrienes are generated in AR, the effects of inhibitors of the 5-lipoxygenase pathway and leukotriene receptor antagonists have been investigated. By far, the most commonly used agent in this category is montelukast which is approved in the United States for the treatment of seasonal and perennial AR in children as young as 6 months of age. Montelukast has repeatedly been shown to be more effective than placebo and equally effective as antihistamines for all ocular and nasal symptoms of allergic rhinitis including congestion, rhinorrhea, and sneezing. Some, but not all, studies examining the combination of montelukast with an antihistamine (loratadine, desloratadine, cetirizine) have shown synergistic benefit [26, 27]. Recent guidelines do not recommend the use of leukotriene modifiers as routine therapy for allergic rhinitis AR but they might have a role in the patient who has both AR and asthma [28].

Intranasal Corticosteroids

Intranasal corticosteroids are considered the most effective treatment for AR, based, in large part, on their potent anti-inflammatory effects. In natural exposure as well as nasal allergen challenge studies, treatment with intranasal corticosteroids inhibit symptoms, mediator release, Th2 cytokine expression, inflammatory cellular influx (notably eosinophils) into nasal secretions and nasal mucosa, as well as hyperresponsiveness to allergen and nonspecific stimuli. These agents have been shown to be superior to both antihistamines and leukotriene receptor antagonists in the control of the symptoms of AR [29, 30]. Most guidelines suggest the use of these agents as first line in moderate-to-severe AR and even in some milder cases. Efficacy begins at 7–8 h after administration and starting these agents a few days before the start of the season has been recommended.

The principal side effect of intranasal corticosteroids is local nasal irritation and epistaxis, which occur in 5–10% of patients. Septal perforations, although rare, have also been reported. Whereas oral candidiasis is a commonly reported side effect of inhaled corticosteroids used for asthma, nasal candidiasis secondary to intranasal corticosteroids has not been commonly reported. Biopsy specimens from the nasal mucosa of patients with perennial allergic rhinitis who had been treated with such agents for 1 year showed no evidence of atrophy or epithelial injury. In the pediatric age group, studies looking at objective reproducible measures of growth (stadiometry or knemometry) and hypothalamic pituitary axis suppression after administration of intranasal corticosteroids for periods up to 1 year failed to show any adverse effects of the newer agents compared to placebo [31, 32]. Studies following intraocular pressure in patients on long-term intranasal corticosteroids have failed to show a significant increase in intraocular pressure or the incidence of glaucoma compared to placebo [33]. Based on these reassuring results, mometasone furoate and fluticasone furoate are approved by the FDA for use starting at 2 years of age and fluticasone propionate starting at 4 years of age.

Most of the intranasal corticosteroids available for clinical use are distributed via aqueous preparations and some patients find the aftertaste or runoff in the form of postnasal drip to be bothersome, thus reducing compliance and adherence to therapy [34]. To this end, two intranasal corticosteroids are now available in nonaqueous preparations. Beclomethasone dipropionate HFA (hydrofluoroalkane) and ciclesonide nasal aerosol are both delivered via HFA propellant and both are approved for use in children ≥12 years of age.

Systemic Corticosteroids

The role of systemic corticosteroids for treatment of AR is limited. Corticosteroid pulses may be useful to help wean patients from topical decongestant use in cases of rhinitis medicamentosa. They can also be useful in cases of severe nasal congestion, given as a 3- to 5-day course, to

enhance the penetration of concomitantly administered intranasal corticosteroids.

Combination Therapy

Despite the efficacy of intranasal corticosteroids, several studies in perennial and seasonal allergic rhinitis in adults report lack of complete relief of symptoms in significant proportions of the subjects studied. In one trial of subjects with PAR taking an intranasal corticosteroid, only 63% achieved symptom suppression defined as ≥75% decrease in total nasal symptoms from baseline [35]. When subjects in seasonal allergic rhinitis trials were asked to report their overall response to therapy at the end of the trials, 33–58% reported only mild improvement, no change, or worsening in the relief of AR symptoms [36, 37]. In an attempt to address this need, combination treatments have been used in clinical practice. Most recently such a combination consisting of fluticasone propionate and azelastine hydrochloride administered intranasally has been approved for clinical use in the United States for patients ≥12 years of age with seasonal allergic rhinitis. To account for the duration of action of the antihistamine component, the medication is administered twice daily as opposed to the once-daily administration used for most intranasal corticosteroids. A meta-analysis was performed in three trials comparing the combination therapy to each of its individual components and placebo, in a total of 3398 patients 12 years and older [38]. The results showed consistent superior efficacy of the combination to placebo and each of the individual components. There is insufficient evidence to support adding an oral antihistamine to an intranasal corticosteroid if that therapy alone is not effective. Thus, recent guidelines recommend the addition of an intranasal antihistamine, not an oral preparation, if the need arises [28].

Case 1 Answers and Commentary

The most obvious diagnosis in the presented case is that of allergic rhinitis. The child has typical symptoms consistent with sensitization to perennial and seasonal allergens, and physical exam supports the diagnosis as there was no purulent drainage to suggest rhinosinusitis. The typical findings of a child with a nasal foreign body are unilateral foul smelling nasal discharge and a physical exam that shows the object.

In this particular instance, AR seems to be at least moderate as it affects the child's quality of life. Although a non-sedating antihistamine would be a reasonable option, most current evidence would support using an intranasal corticosteroid for maximal benefit. Leukotriene modifiers are not recommended by recent guidelines as first-line treatment of AR, and cromolyn requires administration several times a day reducing compliance [28]. Although oxymetazoline would be helpful with nasal congestion, its prolonged use as mandated by the child's consistent symptoms would not be justified secondary to concern with rhinitis medicamentosa.

As mentioned in the management section above, when symptom control is not optimal using an intranasal corticosteroid, the best next step is addition of an intranasal antihistamine, not an oral one. Clearly, if one uses maximal medical therapy and still fails to see significant improvement, then other causes of rhinitis and the potential for rhinosinusitis should be eliminated. Once they are, consideration should be given to specific allergic immunotherapy.

Case Presentation 2

A 5-year-old female presents to the office with complaints of bilateral nasal congestion, postnasal drainage, and nighttime cough of 3-month duration. The symptoms started with an upper respiratory tract infection but never subsided and have become ongoing. She has seen her pediatrician, who attempted treatment with an intranasal corticosteroid with no improvement. Albuterol was administered with only partial relief of the cough. On review of systems, she seems to have symptoms of AR during the spring season but does not usually cough during the season. She has exercise-induced bronchoconstriction relieved by pre-exercise albuterol inhalation. There is no his-

tory of frequent pneumonias or ear infections. On physical exam, she is a healthy young girl in no distress. The ears looked normal and the nasal exam by anterior rhinoscopy showed congested turbinates with red, inflamed mucosa and bilateral purulent nasal drainage emanating from the area lateral to the middle turbinate. She had evidence of postnasal drainage also and small tonsils on mouth and throat exam.

The most likely diagnosis in the child presented in the scenario above is chronic rhinosinusitis (CRS). CRS is defined as the presence of the symptoms of discolored nasal discharge and/or nasal blockage/obstruction/congestion, combined with cough at daytime and nighttime or facial pain for at least 12 weeks [39]. The four most common clinical symptoms are cough, rhinorrhea, nasal congestion, and postnasal drip, with a slightly higher predominance of chronic cough [40, 41]. Although some of the symptoms above could also apply to AR, cough in the absence of asthma and gastroesophageal reflux and discolored nasal drainage are not prominent in allergic disease and sneezing and itching are not common in CRS. Because of the close association of the two entities, questions on allergic symptoms (i.e., sneezing, watery rhinorrhea, nasal itching, and itchy watery eyes) should therefore be included when taking a history. In a study of children with chronic and recurrent rhinosinusitis failing medical treatment and requiring surgical intervention, Cunningham and colleagues showed significant impairment of generic quality-of-life measures compared to children with other common chronic diseases such as asthma, attention-deficit hyperactivity disorder, juvenile rheumatoid arthritis, and epilepsy [42].

Although CRS is a commonly encountered problem, the exact prevalence in children is difficult to determine. Many studies that address prevalence have been performed in children who also have nonspecific upper respiratory complaints. In one such study, CT scans were obtained in 196 children 3–14 years of age presenting with chronic rhinorrhea, nasal congestion, and cough [43]. Maxillary involvement was noted in 63%, ethmoid involvement in 58%, and sphenoidal sinus involvement in 29% of the children of the youngest age groups, and the incidence of abnormalities decreased in the 13- to 14-year-old age group. In a prospective study, all new patients (ages 2–18 years) presenting to two allergy practices with upper respiratory tract symptoms for at least 3 months were investigated with a CT scan [44]. In 91 eligible patients, 63% had CRS with clinical signs and positive CT findings, and 36% had no sinus disease. Age was the single most important risk factor associated with chronic sinusitis, with 73% of 2–6-year-olds, and 74% of 6–10-year-olds having sinus CT abnormalities as opposed to the low incidence of only 38% detected in children over 10 years of age. There is evidence to suggest that children with a family history of atopy or asthma who attend daycare in the first year of life have 2.2 times higher odds of having doctor-diagnosed sinusitis than children who do not attend daycare [45].

Pathogenesis of CRS in Children

Anatomical Factors
Similar to adults, the ostiomeatal complex (OMC) is believed to be the critical anatomic structure in rhinosinusitis and is entirely present, though not at full size, in newborns. Studies in children and adults suggest that despite the common occurrence of anatomical variations such as pneumatized middle turbinate, Haller cell, and agger nasi cell, these do not seem to correlate with the degree and existence of CRS and most likely do not play a role in the pathophysiology of CRS [46].

Bacteriology
The pathogens in CRS are difficult to identify due to low bacterial concentration rates and inconsistent data, and because most cultures are obtained at the time of surgery after patients have had antibiotic therapy. The most common bacterial species recovered during surgery are alpha-hemolytic streptococci, *S. pneumoniae*, *H. influenza*, *M. catarrhalis*, and *Staphylococcus aureus* [47]. Anaerobic organisms are grown from <10% of specimens [48].

Biofilms
Biofilms are complex aggregations of bacteria distinguished by a protective and adhesive matrix. It is hypothesized that biofilms may provide a reservoir for bacteria and may be responsible for the resistance to antibiotics seen in patients with CRS. Sanclement and colleagues demonstrated the presence of biofilms in 80% of sinus surgical specimens obtained from a mixed adult/pediatric population [49]. More research is needed to clearly characterize the contribution of biofilms to the pathophysiology of CRS in children.

The Role of Adenoids
The adenoids are in close proximity to the paranasal sinuses. When comparing middle meatal swabs and adenoid core cultures in children with hypertrophied adenoids and chronic or recurrent sinusitis, very similar bacteria can be found in both locations suggesting that the bacterial reservoir in the adenoids mirrors the bacteriology isolated close to the paranasal sinuses in children [50]. Zuliani et al. found that a large percentage (88–99%) of the mucosal surface area of adenoidectomy specimens from children with CRS was covered with a dense biofilm, compared to a much more modest percentage (0–6.5%) of specimen surface area in the adenoids of patients with obstructive sleep apnea [51]. These studies help explain the reported efficacy of adenoidectomy in resolving the symptoms in a proportion of children with CRS (see below). Other studies suggest a role for the adenoids in patients with CRS, both from a bacteriologic and immunologic perspective. Most of these studies however do not really shed light on the relative contribution of adenoiditis proper vs. CRS in chronic nasal symptomatology in children. Furthermore, the success of adenoidectomy in patients with CRS could be related to improvement of adenoiditis proper (which has identical symptoms to that of CRS) or a beneficial effect by eliminating the nasopharyngeal bacterial reservoir on sinus disease proper.

Cellular Studies
Studies of the cellular response in younger children with CRS showed that pediatric maxillary sinus mucosa had more neutrophils and

significantly more lymphocytes than adult mucosa, but fewer eosinophils and major basic protein-positive cells, with less epithelial disruption and less basement membrane thickening [52].

Comorbidities

Interdisciplinary specialty consultations are useful in evaluating the pediatric patient with medically refractory CRS and may include allergy-immunology, infectious disease, gastroenterology, pulmonary, or genetics to aid in further workup.

Allergic Rhinitis

Although there are several small studies suggesting a positive relationship between CRS and AR based on associations between positive CT scans and allergy testing [53, 54], two recent studies looking at large numbers of children with chronic respiratory complaints or an ICD9 diagnosis of CRS suggest no difference in prevalence of AR in patients with CRS compared to the general population [55, 56]. Thus, the causal relationship between allergies and CRS in children remains controversial. When symptoms of AR are prominent, allergy testing should be considered in the older child.

Asthma

Asthma is another disease that is commonly associated with CRS in the pediatric age group. However, most available studies exploring this relationship have limitations which include the lack of good controls, lack of objective documentation of asthma, or randomization to different treatment modalities; therefore, the relationship between CRS and asthma in children remains largely descriptive.

Gastroesophageal Reflux Disease (GERD)

Gastroesophageal reflux disease has also been associated with rhinosinusitis in several studies [57, 58]. A retrospective study that lacked a placebo control showed that treatment for GERD in patients with CRS allowed many patients to improve and avoid surgery [59]. However, routine anti-reflux treatment

of children with CRS is not warranted, as additional controlled studies are required to confirm and validate this association [60].

Immunodeficiency

Several small studies have demonstrated various abnormalities in humoral immune function including low IgG subclasses, low IgA, and poor response to pneumococcal antigens in varying proportions of the patients [61–63]. It therefore seems prudent to evaluate immune function in the child with chronic/recurrent rhinosinusitis with immunoglobulin isotype quantitation and titers to tetanus, diphtheria, and pneumococcus. If responses are abnormal, a repeat set of titers post-pneumococcal vaccination is appropriate.

Primary Ciliary Dyskinesia

The most common cause of ciliary dysfunction is primary ciliary dyskinesia (PCD) , an autosomal recessive disorder involving dysfunction of cilia, which affects 1 of 15,000 individuals [64]. Approximately 50% of children with PCD also have Kartagener's syndrome (situs inversus, bronchiectasis, and CRS). The diagnosis should be suspected in a child with atypical asthma, bronchiectasis, chronic wet cough and mucus production, chronic rhinosinusitis, and severe otitis media [39]. Specific diagnosis may require evaluation at a specialized center that can perform examination of cilia in mucosal biopsies by light and electron microscopy.

Cystic Fibrosis

Cystic fibrosis (CF) is an autosomal recessive disease caused by mutations in the *CFTR* gene. The incidence of CF is approximately 1 in 3500 newborns. Disruption in cAMP-mediated chloride secretion in epithelial cells and exocrine glands leads to increased viscosity of secretions resulting in bronchiectasis, pancreatic insufficiency, CRS, and nasal polyposis. CF is one of the few causes of nasal polyposis in children, with polyps occurring in 7–50%, and the prevalence of chronic sinusitis is very high. In CF, the histology of nasal polyposis is largely neutrophilic, in contrast to nasal polyposis associated with CRS, which has more prominent eosinophilic infiltrates.

Clinical Evaluation

A complete physical exam should follow a careful medical and family history. The nasal exam in children should begin with anterior rhinoscopy and examination of the middle meatus and the inferior turbinates, noting the mucosal character and the presence of purulent drainage. This is often feasible in younger children using the otoscope fitted with the largest speculum. Topical decongestion may improve the view but may not always be tolerated in younger children.

Nasal endoscopy which will allow superior visualization of the middle meatus, adenoid bed, and nasopharynx is strongly recommended in children who are able to tolerate the examination. An oral cavity exam may reveal purulent drainage, cobblestoning of the posterior pharyngeal wall, or tonsillar hypertrophy. The finding of nasal polyps in children is unusual and, if seen on exam, should raise suspicion for cystic fibrosis or allergic fungal sinusitis. Obviously, antrochoanal polyps occur in children but those are usually unilateral and the rest of the sinuses are clear, which would help differentiate that entity from bilateral nasal polyposis with or without CF.

Following the history and physical examination, appropriate diagnostic tests should be considered including allergy testing, immunologic evaluation, and ciliary assessment if indicated.

Imaging

While the diagnosis of CRS in the pediatric population is generally made on clinical grounds, if imaging is necessary, computed tomography (CT) is the modality of choice. Findings on plain radiographs have been shown not to correlate well with those from CT scans in the context of chronic/recurrent sinus disease. In uncomplicated CRS, scanning is reserved to evaluate for residual disease and anatomic abnormalities after maximal medical therapy proves ineffective. Abnormalities in the CT scan are assessed in the context of their severity and correlation with the clinical picture and guide the

plan for further management, which might include surgical intervention. In children with the clinical diagnosis of rhinosinusitis, the most commonly involved sinus is the maxillary sinus (99%) followed by the ethmoid sinus (91%). Using the Lund-Mackay system (a commonly used CT staging system that quantitates sinus disease based on opacification of the sinuses and occlusion of the osteomeatal units and generates a score range from zero for normal paranasal sinuses to 24 for pansinus opacification and occlusion of the ostiomeatal units) a cutoff score for diseased vs. non-diseased patients of five offers a sensitivity and specificity of 86% and 85%, respectively, in making an appropriate diagnosis [65]. Lund scores of two or less have an excellent negative predictive value, whereas scores of five or more have an excellent positive predictive value. CT scans provide an anatomic road map for surgical treatment and are also useful for identifying areas of bony erosion or attenuation. Magnetic resonance (MR) imaging of the sinuses, orbits, and brain should be performed whenever complications of rhinosinusitis are suspected or invasive disease leads to changes in proximity of the brain and the orbit. As mentioned above, the diagnosis of CRS is made primarily on clinical grounds and CT scans are only obtained after failure of maximal medical therapy or in special circumstances. Repeated CT scanning in children is avoided to minimize the risk of radiation.

Physical exam and history alone do not help in differentiating between adenoiditis and CRS, especially in the younger child. As detailed above, a high Lund-Mackay score on the CT scan (>5) might be more suggestive of CRS than adenoiditis but further studies are clearly required to help distinguish these two entities.

Medical Treatment of Chronic Rhinosinusitis in Children

Nasal Corticosteroids

There are no randomized controlled trials evaluating the effect of intranasal corticosteroids in children with CRS. However the combination of proven efficacy of intranasal corticosteroids in CRS with and without nasal polyps in adults and proven efficacy and safety of intranasal corticosteroids in AR in children makes intranasal corticosteroid the first line of treatment in CRS with or without nasal polyps [39].

Antibiotics

Despite the absence of randomized controlled studies evaluating the role of antibiotics and treatment duration in patients with pediatric CRS, the use of antibiotics for this disease is widespread. The published guidelines also vary in their recommendations as the EPOS (European Position Paper on Rhinosinusitis and Nasal Polyps) document does not recommend antibiotics, whereas the American Academy of Otolaryngology-Head and Neck Surgery consensus statement endorses a 21-day course of antibiotics [39, 60]. The choice of antibiotics hinges on coverage of the typical flora in upper respiratory tract infections and includes amoxicillin-clavulanate, third-generation cephalosporins, and clindamycin in cases of significant drug allergies to the prior two choices. It is difficult to ascertain whether what is actually being treated is CRS or acute exacerbations on top of preexisting chronic disease. Intravenous antibiotic therapy for CRS resistant to maximal medical treatment has been studied as an alternative to endoscopic sinus surgery. In retrospective studies intravenous antibiotics have been claimed to be successful in the treatment of CRS usually in combination with other treatments such as irrigation/aspiration of the sinus and adenoidectomy. Study design issues and considerable side effects of this treatment do not justify the use of intravenous antibiotics alone for the treatment of CRS in children.

Nasal Saline Irrigation

A Cochrane review analyzed randomized controlled trials in which saline was evaluated in comparison with either no treatment, a placebo, as an adjunct to other treatments, or against other treatments [66]. A total of eight trials satisfied inclusion criteria of which three were conducted in children. Overall there was evidence that saline is beneficial in the treatment of the symptoms of CRS when used as the sole modality of treatment. A well-conducted randomized controlled trial in children with

quality-of-life measures and CT scan severity evaluated before and after nasal saline irrigation with and without gentamicin showed benefit of this therapy irrespective of the presence of the antibiotic as part of the irrigation [67]. Therefore, saline irrigation (without antibiotics) is now part of the routine care for children with CRS.

Surgery for Chronic Rhinosinusitis in Children

Surgical intervention for rhinosinusitis is usually considered for patients with CRS (confirmed by CT imaging) who have failed maximal medical therapy. This is hard to define but usually includes a course of antibiotics, nasal saline irrigation, and intranasal and/or systemic corticosteroids. Adenoidectomy with or without antral irrigation and balloon sinus dilation and functional endoscopic sinus surgery (FESS) are the most commonly used modalities.

Adenoidectomy

The rationale behind removal of the adenoids in patients with CRS stems from the hypothesis that the adenoids are a nasopharyngeal bacterial reservoir and the possibility that many of the symptoms might be related to adenoiditis proper. The benefit of adenoidectomy alone in the treatment of children with CRS was recently evaluated by a meta-analysis [68]. All studies in the meta-analysis showed that sinusitis symptoms or outcomes improved in 50% or more of patients after adenoidectomy. The summary estimate of the proportion of patients who significantly improved after adenoidectomy was 69.3%. In a more recent report, Ramadan and colleagues evaluated the hypothesis that CT score can better differentiate between CRS proper and adenoiditis [69]. They therefore retrospectively reviewed their experience with success of adenoidectomy in CRS based on severity of disease on the CT scan. They show that the patients with the lower Lund-Mackay score on CT scan (<5) which would be more likely to suggest adenoiditis as the etiology of the symptoms had a better success rate after adenoidectomy (65%) compared to the children whose CT scores were >5 indicating true sinus disease where the success rate was only 43%.

Maxillary Antral Irrigation

Maxillary antral irrigation is frequently performed in conjunction with adenoidectomy. It has been suggested that antral irrigation adds to the efficacy of adenoidectomy [70]. Balloon sinuplasty was approved by the FDA for use in children in the United States in 2006, and a preliminary study in children has shown the procedure to be safe and feasible when addressing the maxillary sinus. Whether or not balloon maxillary sinuplasty imparts additional benefit to irrigation alone, or in combination with adenoidectomy, cannot be established with available data to date.

Functional Endoscopic Sinus Surgery

A meta-analysis of FESS results in the pediatric population has shown that this surgical modality is effective in reducing symptoms with an 88% success rate and a low complication rate [71]. Initial concerns about possible adverse effects of FESS on facial growth have been allayed by a long-term follow-up study by Bothwell and colleagues that showed no impact of FESS on qualitative and quantitative parameters of pediatric facial growth, evaluated up to 10 years postoperatively [72]. Many advocate a limited approach to FESS in children consisting of removal of any obvious obstruction (such as polyps and concha bullosa), as well as anterior bulla ethmoidectomy and maxillary antrostomy.

Case 2 Answers and Commentary

The child in this clinical scenario, as opposed to the one described in case 1, has postnasal drainage and coughing for 3 months or longer and, most importantly, has purulent drainage on nasal examination. These findings are strongly suggestive of chronic rhinosinusitis. As mentioned above, nasal foreign body typically presents as short-lasting unilateral foul-smelling nasal drainage. Foreign-body aspiration is usually preceded by a choking event and will not include nasal

symptoms or findings as part of the cough clinical presentation.

Current best practice for CRS in children includes a course of antibiotics, nasal saline rinses, and intranasal corticosteroids. There is no data to support the use of antihistamines or leukotriene modifiers. As the presentation does not seem to include any imminent acute complications such as a periorbital abscess or a brain abscess, immediate CT scanning is not recommended and is best reserved to evaluate for persistent/residual disease after maximal medical therapy. The surgical options mentioned are appropriate but would be reserved for cases that fail maximal medical therapy and showed evidence of disease on CT after therapy.

As mentioned above CT scan without contrast is the procedure of choice to evaluate the paranasal sinuses radiographically. It should be performed if there are persistent symptoms after medical therapy to evaluate the need for possible surgical intervention. Intravenous antibiotics have not been found to be beneficial in these cases unless there are concerns about acute complications involving the orbit or brain. CT with contrast is useful when evaluating for a possible orbital abscess as it helps delineate abscess cavities which will be characterized by central lucency surrounded by rim enhancement. MRI of the sinuses is not the standard radiographic modality to evaluate the paranasal sinuses but is very useful in cases of concern with extension of the sinus process to the brain. Finally, imaging is a minimal requirement before considering any surgical options.

References

1. Meltzer EO, Blaiss MS, Derebery J, Mahr TA, Gordon BR, Sheth KK, et al. Burden of allergic rhinitis: results from the pediatric allergies in America survey. J Allergy Clin Immunol. 2009;124:S43–70.
2. Juniper EF, Guyatt GH, Dolovich J. Assessment of quality of life in adolescents with allergic rhinoconjunctivitis: development and testing of a questionnaire for clinical trials. J Allergy Clin Immunol. 1994;93(2):413–23.

3. Juniper EF, Howland WC, Roberts NB, Thompson AK, King DR. Measuring quality of life in children with rhinoconjunctivitis. J Allergy Clin Immunol. 1998;101(2 Pt 1):163–70.

4. Brozek JL, Bousquet J, Baena-Cagnani CE, Bonini S, Canonica GW, Casale TB, et al. Allergic rhinitis and its impact on asthma (ARIA) guidelines: 2010 revision. J Allergy Clin Immunol. 2010;126(3):466–76.

5. Wallace DV, Dykewicz MS, Bernstein DI, Blessing-Moore J, Cox L, Khan DA, et al. The diagnosis and management of rhinitis: an updated practice parameter. J Allergy Clin Immunol. 2008;122(2 Suppl):S1–84.

6. Naclerio RM. Allergic rhinitis. N Engl J Med. 1991;325(12):860–9.

7. Lack G. Pediatric allergic rhinitis and comorbid disorders. J Allergy Clin Immunol. 2001;108(1):S9–S15.

8. Shaker M. New insights into the allergic march. Curr Opin Pediatr. 2014 Aug;26(4):516–20.

9. Meltzer EO. The relationships of rhinitis and asthma. Allergy Asthma Proc. 2005;26(5):336–40.

10. Savolainen S. Allergy in patients with acute maxillary sinusitis. Allergy. 1989;44(2):1116–22.

11. Steinke JW, Borish L. The role of allergy in chronic rhinosinusitis. Immunol Allergy Clin N Am. 2004;24(1):45–57.

12. Luong A, Roland PS. The link between allergic rhinitis and chronic otitis media with effusion in atopic patients. Otolaryngol Clin N Am. 2008;41(2):311–23.

13. Tomonaga K, Kurono Y, Mogi G. The role of nasal allergy in otitis media with effusion. A clinical study. Acta Otolaryngol Suppl. 1988;458:41–7.

14. Alles R, Parikh A, Hawk L, Darby Y, Romero JN, Scadding G. The prevalence of atopic disorders in children with chronic otitis media with effusion. Pediatr Allergy Immunol. 2001;12(2):102–6.

15. Nguyen LHP, Manoukian JJ, Sobol SE, Tewfik TL, Mazer BD, Schloss MD, et al. Similar allergic inflammation in the middle ear and the upper airway: evidence linking otitis media with effusion to the united airways concept. J Allergy Clin Immunol. 2004;114(5):1110.

16. Hellings PW, Fokkens WJ. Allergic rhinitis and its impact on otorhinolaryngology. Allergy. 2006;61:656–64.

17. Modrzynski M, Zawisza E. An analysis of the incidence of adenoid hypertrophy in allergic children. Int J Pediatr Otorhinolaryngol. 2007;71(5):713–9.

18. Ng DK, Chan CC, Hwang GY, Chow P, Kwok K. A review of the roles of allergic rhinitis in childhood obstructive sleep apnea syndrome. Allergy Asthma Proc. 2006;27(3):240–2.

19. McColley SA, Carroll JL, Curtis S, Loughlin GM, Sampson HA. High prevalence of allergic sensitization in children with habitual snoring and obstructive sleep apnea. Chest. 1997;111(1):170–3.

20. Sheikh A, Hurwitz B, Nurmatov U, van Schayck CP. House dust mite avoidance measures for perennial allergic rhinitis. Cochrane Database Syst Rev. 2010;7:CD001563.

21. Vuurman EF, van Veggel LM, Uiterwijk MM, Leutner D, O'Hanlon JF. Seasonal allergic rhinitis and antihistamine effects on children's learning. Ann Allergy. 1993;71(2):121–6.

22. Montoro J, Bartra J, Sastre J, Dávila I, Ferrer M, Mullol J, del Cuvillo A, Jáuregui I, Valero A. H1 antihistamines and benzodiazepines. Pharmacological interactions and their impact on cerebral function. J Investig Allergol Clin Immunol. 2013;23(Suppl 1):17–26.

23. Fitzsimons R, van der Poel LA, Thornhill W, du Toit G, Shah N, Brough HA. Antihistamine use in children. Arch Dis Child Educ Pract Ed. 2015;100(3):122–31.

24. Berger WE, Ratner PH, Casale TB, Meltzer EO, Wall GM. Safety and efficacy of olopatadine hydrochloride nasal spray 0.6% in pediatric subjects with allergic rhinitis. Allergy Asthma Proc. 2009;30(6):612–23.

25. Hatton RC, Winterstein AG, McKelvey RP, Shuster J, Hendeles L. Efficacy and safety of oral phenylephrine: systematic review and meta-analysis. Ann Pharmacother. 2007;41(3):381–90.

26. Meltzer EO, Malmstrom K, Lu S, Prenner BM, Wei LX, Weinstein SF, et al. Concomitant montelukast and loratadine as treatment for seasonal allergic rhinitis: a randomized, placebo-controlled clinical trial. J Allergy Clin Immunol. 2000;105(5):917–22.

27. Ciebiada M, Gorska-Ciebiada M, LM DB, Gorski P. Montelukast with desloratadine or levocetirizine for the treatment of persistent allergic rhinitis. Ann Allergy Asthma Immunol. 2006;97:664–71.

28. Seidman MD, Gurgel RK, Lin SY, Schwartz SR, Baroody FM, Bonner JR, et al. Clinical practice guideline: allergic rhinitis. Otolaryngol Head Neck Surg. 2015;152(1S):S1–S43.

29. Weiner JM, Abramson MJ, Puy RM. Intranasal corticosteroids versus oral H1 receptor antagonists in allergic rhinitis: systematic review of randomized controlled trials. Br Med J. 1998;317(7173):1624–9.

30. Wilson AM, O'Byrne PM, Parameswaran K. Leukotriene receptor antagonists for allergic rhinitis: asystematic review and meta-analysis. Am J Med. 2004;116:338–44.

31. Allen DB, Meltzer EO, Lemanske RF Jr, Philpot EE, Faris MA, Kral KM, et al. No growth suppression in children treated with the maximum recommended dose of fluticasone propionate aqueous nasal spray for one year. Allergy Asthma Proc. 2002;23(6):407–13.

32. Schenkel EJ, Skoner DP, Bronsky EA, Miller SD, Pearlman DS, Rooklin A, et al. Absence of growth retardation in children with perennial allergic rhinitis after one year of treatment with mometasone furoate aqueous nasal spray. Pediatrics. 2000;105(2):E22.

33. Ozkaya E, Ozsutcu M, Mete F. Lack of ocular side effects after 2 years of topical steroids for allergic rhinitis. J Pediatr Ophthalmol Strabismus. 2011;48(5):311–7.

34. Luskin AT, Blaiss MS, Farrar JR, Settipane R, Hayden ML, Stoloff S, et al. Is there a role for

aerosol nasal sprays in the treatment of allergic rhinitis: a white paper. Allergy Asthma Proc. 2011;32:168–77.

35. Clement P, Gates D. Symptom suppression in subjects with perennial allergic rhinitis treated with mometasone furoate nasal spray. Int Arch Allergy Immunol. 2012;157:387–90.

36. Fokkens WJ, Jogi R, Reinartz S, Sidorenko I, Sitkauskiene B, van Oene C, et al. Once daily fluticasone furoate nasal spray is effective in seasonal allergic rhinitis caused by grass pollen. Allergy. 2007;62:1078–84.

37. Kaiser HB, Naclerio RM, Given J, Toler TN, Ellsworth A, Philpot EE. Fluticasone furoate nasal spray: a single treatment option for the symptoms of seasonal allergic rhinitis. J Allergy Clin Immunol. 2007;119:1430–7.

38. Carr W, Bernstein J, Lieberman P, Meltzer E, Bachert C, Proce D, Munzel U, Bousquet J. A novel intranasal therapy of azelastine with fluticasone for the treatment of allergic rhinitis. J Allergy Clin Immunol. 2012;129(5):1282–9.

39. Fokkens WJ, Lund VJ, Mullol J, Bachert C, Alobid I, Baroody F, et al. The European position paper on rhinosinusitis and nasal polyps 2012. Rhinology. 2012;Suppl 23:1–299.

40. Rachelefsky GS, Goldberg M, Katz RM, Boris G, Gyepes MT, Shapiro MJ, et al. Sinus disease in children with respiratory allergy. J Allergy Clin Immunol. 1978;61:310–4.

41. Rachelefsky GS, Shapiro GG. Diseases of paranasal sinuses in children. In: Bierman W, Pearlman D, editors. Management of upper respiratory tract disease. Philadelphia: WB Saunders; 1980.

42. Cunningham MJ, Chiu EJ, Landgraf JM, Gliklich RE. The health impact of chronic recurrent rhinosinusitis in children. Arch Otolaryngol Head Neck Surg. 2000;126:1363–8.

43. Van der Veken P, Clement PA, Buisseret T, Desprechins B, Kaufman L, Derde MP. CAT-scan study of the prevalence of sinus disorders and anatomical variations in 196 children. Acta Otorhinolaryngol Belg. 1989;43(1):51–8.

44. Nguyen KL, Corbett ML, Garcia DP, Eberly SM, Massey EN, Le HT, et al. Chronic sinusitis among pediatric patients with chronic respiratory complaints. J Allergy Clin Immunol. 1993;92:824–30.

45. Celedon JC, Litonjua AA, Weiss ST, Gold DR. Day care attendance in the first year of life and illnesses of the upper and lower respiratory tract in children with a familial history of atopy. Pediatrics. 1999;104:495–500.

46. Al-Qudah M. The relationship between anatomical variations of the sinonasal region and chronic sinusitis extension in children. Int J Pediatr Otorhinolaryngol. 2008;72:817–21.

47. Hsin CH, Su MC, Tsao CH, Chuang CY, Liu CM. Bacteriology and antimicrobial susceptibility of pediatric chronic rhinosinusitis: a 6-year result

of maxillary sinus punctures. Am J Otolaryngol. 2010;31:145–9.

48. Brook I. Bacteriologic features of chronic sinusitis in children. JAMA. 1981;246:967–9.

49. Sanclement JA, Webster P, Thomas J, Ramadan HH. Bacterial biofilms in surgical specimens of patients with chronic rhinosinusitis. Laryngoscope. 2005;115:578–82.

50. Elwany S, El-Dine AN, El-Medany A, Omran A, Mandour Z, El-Salam AA. Relationship between bacteriology of the adenoid core and middle meatus in children with sinusitis. J Laryngol Otol. 2011;125(3):279–81.

51. Zuliani G, Carron M, Gurrola J, Coleman C, Haupert M, Berk R, et al. Identification of adenoid biofilms in chronic rhinosinusitis. Int J Pediatr Otorhinolaryngol. 2006;70(9):1613–6.

52. Chan KH, Abzug MJ, Coffinet L, Simoes EA, Cool C, Liu AH. Chronic rhinosinusitis in young children differs from adults: a histopathology study. J Pediatr. 2004;144(2):206–12.

53. Ramadan HH, Fornelli R, Ortiz AO, Rodman S. Correlation of allergy and severity of sinus disease. Am J Rhinol. 1999;13(5):345–7.

54. Tantimongkolsuk C, Pornrattanarungsee S, Chiewvit P, Visitsunthorn N, Ungkanont K, Vichyanond P. Pediatric sinusitis: symptom profiles with associated atopic condition. J Med Assoc Thail. 2005;88:S149–55.

55. Leo G, Piacentini E, Incorvaia C, Consonni D, Frati F. Chronic rhinosinusitis and allergy. Ped Allergy Immunol. 2007;18:19–21.

56. Sedaghat AR, Phipatanakul W, Cunningham MJ. Prevalence of and associations with allergic rhinitis in children with chronic rhinosinusitis. Int J Pediatr Otorhinolaryngol. 2014;78:343–7.

57. Phipps CD, Wood WE, Bigson WWS, Cohran WJ. Gastroesophageal reflux contributing to chronic sinus disease in children: a prospective analysis. Arch Otolaryngol Head Neck Surg. 2000;126:831–6.

58. El-Serag HB, Gilger M, Kuebeler M, Rabeneck L. Extraesophageal associations of gastroesophageal reflux disease in children without neurological defects. Gasteroenterology. 2001;121:1294–9.

59. Bothwell MR, Parsons DS, Talbot A, Barbero GJ, Wilder B. Outcome of reflux therapy on pediatric chronic sinusitis. Otolaryngol Head Neck Surg. 1999;121:255–62.

60. Brietzke SE, Shin JJ, Choi S, Lee JT, Parikh SR, Pena M, et al. Clinical consensus statement: pediatric chronic rhinosinusitis. Otolaryngol Head Neck Surg. 2014;151(4):542–53.

61. Shapiro GC, Virant FS, Furukawa CT, Pierson WE, Bierman CW. Immune defects in patients with refractory sinusitis. Pediatrics. 1991;89:311.

62. Sethi DS, Winklestein JA, Lederman H. Immunologic deficits in patients with chronic recurrent sinusitis: diagnosis and management. Otolaryngol Head Neck Surg. 1995;112:242–7.

63. Costa Carvalho BT, Nagao AT, Arslanian C, Carneiro Sampaio MMS, Naspitz CK, Sorensen RU, et al. Immunological evaluation of allergic respiratory children with recurrent sinusitis. Pediatr Allergy Immunol. 2005;16:534–8.

64. Sleigh MA. Primary ciliary dyskinesia. Lancet. 1981;2(8244):476.

65. Bhattacharyya N, Jones DT, Hill M, Shapiro NL. The diagnostic accuracy of computed tomography in pediatric chronic rhinosinusitis. Arch Otolaryngol Head Neck Surg. 2004;130(9):1029–32.

66. Harvey R, Hannan SA, Badia L, Scadding G. Nasal saline irrigations for the symptoms of chronic rhinosinusitis. Cochrane Database Syst Rev. 2007;3:CD006394.

67. Wei JL, Sykes KJ, Johnson P, He J, Mayo MS. Safety and efficacy of once-daily nasal irrigation for the treatment of pediatric chronic rhinosinusitis. Laryngoscope. 2011;121:1989–2000.

68. Brietzke SE, Brigger MT. Adenoidectomy outcomes in pediatric rhinosinusitis: a meta-analysis. Int J Pediatr Otorhinolaryngol. 2008;72(10): 1541–5.

69. Ramadan HH, Makary CA. Can computed tomography score predict outcome of adenoidectomy for chronic rhinosinusitis in children. Am J Rhinol Allergy. 2014;28(1):e80–2.

70. Ramadan HH, Cost JL. Outcome of adenoidectomy versus adenoidectomy with maxillary sinus wash for chronic rhinosinusitis in children. Laryngoscope. 2008;118(5):871–3.

71. Hebert RL 2nd, Bent JP 3rd. Meta-analysis of outcomes of pediatric functional endoscopic sinus surgery. Laryngoscope. 1998;108(6):796–9.

72. Bothwell MR, Piccirillo JF, Lusk RP, Ridenour BD. Long-term outcome of facial growth after functional endoscopic sinus surgery. Otolaryngol Head Neck Surg. 2002;126(6):628–34.

Allergic Rhinoconjunctivitis

16

Leonard Bielory and Preeti Wagle

Case Presentation 1

A 35-year-old male patient was referred to the allergist with persistent asthma, atopic dermatitis, rhinitis, and chronic conjunctivitis. The patient complains of symptoms related to eyes that include soreness and excessive tearing, which have been getting progressively worse over the last 10 years: yellowish mucoid discharge upon wakening for the last 5 years and photophobia for the last 9 months. In addition, for the past 6 months, he has had increased ocular discomfort, has started to squint constantly, and has had mild blurring of vision and worsening sensitivity to light without pain. He has been treated for these symptoms by many ophthalmologists over the years and has been prescribed various eye drops and oral medications. The patient's ophthalmologist noted increased curvature of the left cornea with mild keratitis.

His allergic rhinitis has been treated for the past several years with an intranasal corticosteroid. He chronically uses oral over-the-counter second-generation H1-antihistamines to control his sneezing.

The patient's asthma has been well controlled with an inhaled corticosteroid/long-acting beta-agonist therapy. He has had multiple courses of oral corticosteroids, but was never admitted to the hospital.

His atopic dermatitis is being treated with topically applied tacrolimus cream, and his symptoms of itching, redness, and scaling are under control.

His current medications include systemic prednisone (60 mg daily), topically applied (skin) tacrolimus cream, and triamcinolone. He also uses Lotemax™ (loteprednol), Alrex™ (loteprednol), and Vigamox™ (moxifloxacin) eye drops in the right eye four times daily; Restasis™ (cyclosporine) in the left eye twice daily; and Celluvisc™ (carboxymethylcellulose) in both eyes as needed.

His family history is significant for his father having had a myocardial infarction and colorectal cancer and his mother having ovarian cancer.

The patient works as an administrator of an international accounting firm. His job requires extensive use of computer work in excess of 10 h per day. He was stationed in the Middle East for the past 7 years and just relocated to the United States. While in the Middle East he experienced seasonal exacerbations of chronic red eyes, tearing, droopy upper eyelids at times with a glassy appearance, as well as nasal congestion and a runny nose that never completely resolved.

The patient is a nonsmoker and occasionally drinks alcohol. He has also been a contact lens wearer for the last 20 years.

L. Bielory (✉)
Department of Medicine, RWJ Barnabas Robert Wood Johnson University Hospital, Springfield, NJ, USA

P. Wagle
University Asthma and Allergy Associates, Springfield, NJ, USA

© Springer International Publishing AG, part of Springer Nature 2018
J. A. Bernstein (ed.), *Rhinitis and Related Upper Respiratory Conditions*,
https://doi.org/10.1007/978-3-319-75370-6_16

He is allergic to Dovonex™ (calcipotriol), a synthetic derivative of vitamin D cream, and has a history of intolerance to systemic cyclosporine (hypertension and nephropathy).

On physical examination, there is redness and swelling present around both eyes and cheeks, with increased creases below his eyes and a peculiar absence of the lateral eyebrows with eyelids that are slightly asymmetrical. There is thickening of both lids with redness, fissuring, and swelling. There are diffuse fine areas of pinhead-shaped and -sized lesions of the upper and lower tarsal conjunctiva, diffuse multiple blood vessels and increased thickness of the clear portions of the conjunctiva, and a white stringy semisolid thread of white mucus in the inferior fornix. The upper right eyelid touches the iris, with the left upper eyelid touching the pupil.

Discussion

The patient has extensive atopic conditions affecting the nose, skin, and lungs that are commonly treated by the allergists. However, with the assistance of the ophthalmologists it is apparent that the patient also has ocular involvement of his atopic condition, consistent with the diagnosis of atopic keratoconjunctivitis (AKC) with keratoconus.

Atopic keratoconjunctivitis (AKC) is a chronic allergic ocular disease that occurs most often in patients with a history of atopic dermatitis. The exact prevalence is unknown, but appears to be present to some degree in 5% of the atopic dermatitis patients. Thus, AKC is a relatively common disorder with varying degrees of severity. Its severity can be highly asymmetric even though the involvement in this case is bilateral. The periocular skin demonstrated scaling of the upper and lower eyelids with induration of the lower eyelid from the chronic allergic response and the topical application of a preservative-based ophthalmic medication resulting in chronic blepharoconjunctivitis.

Ocular allergy (OA) or AC (allergic conjunctivitis) is a term that refers to a collection of disorders that affect the eyelid and conjunctiva. The IgE-mast cell and non-IgE-mediated hypersensitivity disorders include seasonal and perennial allergic conjunctivitis (SAC and PAC), vernal and atopic keratoconjunctivitis (VKC and AKC), and blepharoconjunctivitis (contact and other variants) [1]. The use of in vivo and in vitro tests assists in identifying the specific allergic trigger(s). Although clinical characteristics support the diagnosis of OA, errors in the final diagnosis are not uncommon due to changing features of the initial or chronic presentations and the overlap with pseudo-allergic forms that present with clinical manifestations similar to allergy but with a nonallergic equivocal pathogenesis. Ocular allergy is easily mimicked and often overlaps other anterior ocular surface disorders including tear film dysfunction, blepharitis, infections, and toxic and mechanical forms of conjunctivitis.

Keratoconus is a disease in which the shape of the cornea is progressively distorted. The cornea becomes thin and steep and protrudes anteriorly. The nature of the protrusion may be complete (oval or globus keratoconus) or localized to the center of the cornea (nipple cone). This results in progressive myopia, astigmatism, and increasing requirement for myopic spectacle prescriptions as the condition progresses. There is also intolerance to wearing contact lens as they sometimes fall off or get dislodged.

Management

The treatment choices for AKC include:

1. High-dose systemic corticosteroid therapy
2. Systemic tacrolimus 4 mg/day
3. Intravenous Zenapax (daclizumab), 75 mg/ infusion (determined by his weight)

In the past, management of acute and more chronic forms of ocular allergy has focused on symptomatic relief, but with a better understanding of the mechanisms involved therapeutic strategies are now more focused [2].

The treatment of severe AKC involving the cornea should include involvement of an allergist working in conjunction with an ophthalmologist.

The identification of the allergenic triggers and education about avoidance of triggers are important aspects in the management of atopic disorders. The triggering antigen may be identified in patients by skin or serum-specific IgE testing against a panel of commonly occurring seasonal and perennial allergens.

Tacrolimus is an immunosuppressive drug (calcineurin inhibitor) used after organ transplants to prevent rejection. Severe AKC may be refractory to topical treatment and in these patients low-dose systemic tacrolimus may be used. However, the patient will need to be monitored for side effects such as infection, hypertension, and nephrotoxicity. In addition to systemic tacrolimus, tacrolimus ointment may be used to treat eyelid eczema in AKC patients [3].

Daclizumab is an immunosuppressive, humanized IgG monoclonal antibody produced by recombinant DNA technology that binds specifically to the alpha subunit (~55 alpha, CD25, or Tat subunit) of the human high-affinity interleukin-2 (IL-2) receptor that is expressed on the surface of activated lymphocytes. Daclizumab, approved for relapsing multiple sclerosis and administered 150 mg subcutaneously monthly, has shown to be effective for AKC in reducing concomitant immunosuppressive medications, stabilizing visual acuity, and preventing uveitic flares [4].

The patient's current medications include prednisone, the side effects of which include posterior subcapsular cataracts. Because one of the associated causes of ocular morbidity in patients with AKC is a high incidence of cataracts (mostly anterior or posterior subcapsular), the patient should be monitored for this complication [5].

Case Presentation 2

The patient is a 27-year-old female who has been referred to the allergist for nasal and ocular complaints of tearing, redness and burning sensation, rhinorrhea, and nasal congestion. She complained of redness and burning of both eyes for the past 6 months that has progressed to increased bilateral tearing for the last month. When further questioned she also admitted to bilateral foreign-body sensation and itching. She says that her ocular symptoms seem to increase as the day progresses. She stated that nasal congestion and sneezing developed in a seasonal pattern several years ago, for which oral antihistamines had been used with decreasing impact. She has maintained their use, but was also instructed to use an intranasal corticosteroid over the past year. She was told that it would help both her nasal complaints (especially nasal congestion) and eye symptoms. The patient has had skin prick testing performed 5 years ago after moving from Colorado to New Jersey that was positive for grass and tree pollens, dust mite, and cat allergens.

Her past medical history was remarkable for a laparoscopic appendectomy 8 years ago. Her current medications include cetirizine 10 mg daily and diphenhydramine 25 mg as needed which usually amounts to 2–3 times a week, at night, during the spring and summer. She is also taking Yaz, a combined oral contraceptive pill, daily for the last 4 years.

Her family history is significant for multiple pollen allergies in her mother and sister, whose symptoms are greatest between May and June as well as diabetes and hypertension in her father.

The patient is a nonsmoker and doesn't drink alcohol. She is married for 2 years and her husband smokes one pack of cigarettes daily indoors at home and while in the car. The patient works as a flight attendant; she used to fly on a domestic airline, but has recently switched to flying from New York to London. She notes that her ocular symptoms have worsened since working on longer flights. The patient previously lived in Denver, but moved to northern New Jersey 6 years ago. The patient was not diagnosed as being allergic to grass pollen until she moved to New Jersey. She has been wearing contact lenses 4–5 times a week for the past 13 years.

The patient has a history of a penicillin allergy since the age of 4 during which time she was treated with oral amoxicillin for acute otitis media and subsequently developed "hives" and pruritus within several hours of taking the first dose. Subsequently, skin testing to penicillin was performed by an allergist, which was positive.

Physical examination revealed redness and a stringy discharge in both eyes. There was mild inflammation of the lids bilaterally. Schirmer's test showed 9 mm of moisture after 5 min in both eyes. Fluorescein stained the cornea in numerous punctate regions. The nasal mucosa was bluish grey in color without evidence of swelling. Mild discharge was seen which was clear and watery. Palpation of the paranasal sinuses produced no pain. The oral mucosa was moist and otherwise unremarkable.

Discussion

A diagnosis of dry eye syndrome was made based on both the patient's symptoms of burning, itching, and foreign-body sensation and the physical exam which showed discharge, an abnormal Schirmer's test, and staining of the cornea with fluorescein.

Dry eye syndrome (DES) is a syndrome in which there is a decreased or absent production of tear film. Patients suffer from symptoms such as dryness, itching, redness, and a burning sensation of the eyes.

There is a significant overlap of symptoms between dry eye syndrome and seasonal allergic conjunctivitis. In patients with significant itchiness, there is a high probability that they also have dryness and redness, and the converse is also true. As seen in this patient, it is more common to start with allergic conjunctivitis (AC) and subsequently develop DES which can be exacerbated by the use of oral antihistamines [6]. Dry eye syndrome is also seen as part of the development of chronic forms of anterior surface disorders including ocular allergies [7].

The patient is currently taking both cetirizine and diphenhydramine, both of which are antihistamines, the first line of treatment in allergic rhinoconjunctivitis. However, studies have shown that these drugs also create problems with excessive drying, including the eyes. It appears that all antihistaminic drugs can cause abnormalities in tear film composition with the older formulations (e.g., first-generation H1-antagonists) having the greater anticholinergic activity [8].

Hormonal changes are also associated with various forms of ocular surface disorders. Oral contraceptives especially in those patients wearing contact lenses have been shown to be twice as likely to develop symptoms of dry eye as those patients who were not taking oral contraceptives [9].

Several environmental factors that are known to aggravate anterior surface disorders include cigarette smoke in her home [10], chronic use of extended-wear contact lenses, and occupational issues such as working as a flight attendant due to excessive dry airplane cabin air [11].

Management

Treatment choices for this patient include eye lubricants, lifitegrast, and cyclosporine. The treatment of DES begins with eye lubricants. Guar-based lubricants improve tear film stability. These formulas contain substances such as propylene glycol, hydroxypropylguar, borate, and sorbitol, as well as mineral oil and a phospholipid surfactant, that create an artificial lipid layer over the aqueous component of the tear film [12].

Lifitegrast, marketed as Xiidra™, is another drug being used for treatment of dry eye. It is an antagonist of lymphocyte function-associated antigen-1 that binds to intracellular adhesion molecule 1 (ICAM-1), which is overexpressed in dry eye, thereby potently inhibiting T-cell activation, adhesion, migration, proliferation, and cytokine release. It has been shown in trials to improve dryness and ocular discomfort. However, there was no difference in clinical findings such as light sensitivity and foreign-body sensation or tear breakup time. There was also no statistical difference in the Schirmer's test. Adverse effects include eye irritation and blurred vision [7, 13].

Restasis™, or cyclosporine, has been long recognized for its use in dry eye syndrome. It is an inhibitor of T-cell activation and has been shown to decrease activated T-cells. It also prevents the release of various cytokines. Cyclosporine emulsion has been shown in studies to increase goblet cell density and production of the immunoregulatory factor TGF-beta 2 in the bulbar conjunctiva [14].

Table 16.1 shows the signs and symptoms to be used in the differential diagnosis of ocular allergy. Conjunctival redness is seen with various

Table 16.1 Differential diagnosis of ocular allergy

	AKC	VKC	SAC	PAC	GPC	CBC	VC	BC	Dry Eye	Sjögren's Syndrome	KCS
Conjunctival redness											
Photophobia											
Conjunctival giant papillae											
Limbal inflammation											
Chemosis											
Mucoid discharge											
Watery discharge/ Tearing											
Lid eczema											
Itching											
Burning			-	-							
Blepharitis											
Conjunctival papillae											
Conjunctival follicles											
Superficial punctate keratopathy, corneal scars, pannus											
Corneal shield ulcer or plaque											
Pain											
Nasal Symptoms											
Dry oral mucosa											
Foreign body sensation											

Symptoms present

Symptoms especially present

Symptoms may or may not be present

Symptoms are severe

Abbreviations: *AKC* atopic keratoconjunctivitis, *VKC* vernal keratoconjunctivitis, *SAC* seasonal allergic conjunctivitis, *PAC* perennial allergic conjunctivitis, *GPC* giant papillary conjunctivitis, *CBC* contact blepharoconjunctivitis, *VC* viral conjunctivitis, *BC* bacterial conjunctivitis, *KCS* keratoconjunctivitis sicca intensities in all types of anterior surface disorders. Clinical features such as mucoid discharge, conjunctival giant papillae, limbal inflammation, lid eczema, superficial punctate keratopathy, corneal scars, pannus, corneal shield ulcer or plaque, and pain can assist in further differentiating more chronic forms of ocular allergy (e.g., AKC and VKC) versus milder acute forms such as SAC and PAC. When making a diagnosis between AKC and VKC, blepharitis and burning are more commonly seen in AKC than VKC.

Dry eye syndrome can be differentiated from Sjögren's syndrome and keratoconjunctivitis sicca by the severity of symptoms. Patients with non-Sjögren's aqueous tear deficiency do not have symptoms as severe as those with Sjögren's syndrome [15]. Watery discharge is seen in some forms of dry eye syndrome due to increased reflex tearing, but in Sjögren's syndrome and keratoconjunctivitis sicca associated with fibrosis of the lacrimal glands severe dryness ensues. Itching is seen in dry eye syndromes, but not seen in Sjögren's or keratoconjunctivitis sicca. Dry eye syndrome also needs to be differentiated from allergic conjunctivitis as there is significant overlap between the two conditions. Although conjunctival redness, itching, foreign-body sensation, and discharge are seen in both conditions, chemosis is not commonly seen in dry eye syndrome, but is seen in allergic conjunctivitis. Nasal symptoms are seen in 90% of patients with allergic conjunctivitis and not in DES.

References

1. Bielory L. Allergic and immunologic disorders of the eye. Part II: ocular allergy. J Allergy Clin Immunol. 2000;106(6):1019–32.
2. Bielory L. Ocular allergy guidelines: a practical treatment algorithm. Drugs. 2002;62(11):1611–34.
3. Anzaar F, Gallagher MJ, Bhat P, Arif M, Farooqui S, Foster CS. Use of systemic T-lymphocyte signal transduction inhibitors in the treatment of atopic keratoconjunctivitis. Cornea. 2008;27(8):884–8.
4. Wroblewski K, Sen HN, Yeh S, Faia L, Li Z, Sran P, et al. Long-term daclizumab therapy for the treatment of noninfectious ocular inflammatory disease. Can J Ophthalmol. 2011;46(4):322–8.
5. Bielory BP, Perez VL, Bielory L. Treatment of seasonal allergic conjunctivitis with ophthalmic corticosteroids: in search of the perfect ocular corticosteroids in the treatment of allergic conjunctivitis. Curr Opin Allergy Clin Immunol. 2010;10(5):469–77.
6. Hom MM, Nguyen AL, Bielory L. Allergic conjunctivitis and dry eye syndrome. Ann Allergy Asthma Immunol. 2012;108(3):163–6.
7. Bielory BP, Shah SP, O'Brien TP, Perez VL, Bielory L. Emerging therapeutics for ocular surface disease. Curr Opin Allergy Clin Immunol. 2016;16(5):477–86.
8. Bielory L. Ocular toxicity of systemic asthma and allergy treatments. Curr Allergy Asthma Rep. 2006;6(4):299–305.
9. Chen SP, Massaro-Giordano G, Pistilli M, Schreiber CA, Bunya VY. Tear osmolarity and dry eye symptoms in women using oral contraception and contact lenses. Cornea. 2013;32(4):423–8.
10. Thomas J, Jacob GP, Abraham L, Noushad B. The effect of smoking on the ocular surface and the precorneal tear film. Australas Med J. 2012;5(4):221–6.
11. Teson M, González-García MJ, López-Miguel A, Enríquez-de-Salamanca A, Martín-Montañez V, Benito MJ, et al. Influence of a controlled environment simulating an in-flight airplane cabin on dry eye disease. Invest Ophthalmol Vis Sci. 2013;54(3):2093–9.
12. Nye M, Rudner S, Bielory L. Emerging therapies in allergic conjunctivitis and dry eye syndrome. Expert Opin Pharmacother. 2013;14(11):1449–65.
13. Perez VL, Pflugfelder SC, Zhang S, Shojaei A, Haque R. Lifitegrast, a novel integrin antagonist for treatment of dry eye disease. Ocul Surf. 2016;14(2):207–15.
14. Pflugfelder SC, De Paiva CS, Villarreal AL, Stern ME. Effects of sequential artificial tear and cyclosporine emulsion therapy on conjunctival goblet cell density and transforming growth factor-beta2 production. Cornea. 2008;27(1):64–9.
15. Pflugfelder SC. Differential diagnosis of dry eye conditions. Adv Dent Res. 1996;10(1):9–12.

Reece Jones, Geetika Sabharwal, and Timothy Craig

Case Presentation 1

MS is a 20-year-old female who presents to your office for evaluation of nasal congestion and fatigue. Her chief complaint for today's appointmentis "I can't breathe through my nose, and I am tired all the time." Her symptoms began shortly after starting work at the local restaurant where she has worked for the past 2 years since moving from her parents' home in San Diego, CA. Her main complaints are nasal congestion, especially during the night, and daytime somnolence, which have progressed from moderate to severe over the last 6 months. She has tried several over-the-counter medications including intranasal corticosteroids, which initially provided relief, but had to be discontinued due to frequent epistaxis. She currently takes a second-generation antihistamine with little if any relief of symptoms. She cannot identify a trigger or a seasonal pattern to her symptoms. She has used topical nasal decongestants and other over-the-counter cold remedies when she feels she "can't take it anymore."

She notes snoring associated with these symptoms for approximately the past year. She uses the bathroom several times each night despite limiting her fluids prior to bed, which also contributes to her poor sleep. She has not found any way to improve her sleep, and is worried because she fell asleep on her 15-min work break the other day. She also experiences daytime shortness of breath with less exertion than in the past, which she attributes to her weight gain and not exercising.

She has no relevant past medical history. The only medications she is taking other than the oral non-sedating antihistamine are an oral contraceptive pill and a multivitamin. She has no known drug allergies. Her surgical history is remarkable for a tonsillectomy as a child, a cesarean section, and subsequent incisional hernia repair. Her mother had asthma as a child and now has emphysema and her father has seasonal allergies. She denies drug use, is a nonsmoker, and only drinks alcohol socially (four drinks per month). She recently moved to this area 2 years ago but has no recent changes in her environment. She is exposed to second-hand smoke from co-workers. She is up to date on her vaccinations but has not yet received the flu shot. Her review of systems is remarkable for a 30-pound weight gain over the last 2 years, watery eyes, sinus pressure, sore throat, exercise

R. Jones · T. Craig
Department of Medicine, Division of Pulmonary, Allergy and Critical Care Medicine, Penn State Health Hershey Medical Center, Hershey, PA, USA

G. Sabharwal (✉)
Department of Allergy and Immunology, Penn State University, Hershey Medical Center, Hershey, PA, USA
e-mail: gsabharwal@hmc.psu.edu

© Springer International Publishing AG, part of Springer Nature 2018
J. A. Bernstein (ed.), *Rhinitis and Related Upper Respiratory Conditions*,
https://doi.org/10.1007/978-3-319-75370-6_17

Table 17.1 Common etiologies of chronic rhinitis

Allergic rhinitis					
Seasonal			Perennial		

Nonallergic rhinitis					
Vasomotor		Gustatory		Nonallergic rhinitis with eosinophils	

Systemic diseases					
Hypothyroidism	Wegener's	Sarcoidosis	Cystic fibrosis	Immotile cilia	Midline granuloma

Medications known to cause rhinitis	
Medication class	Examples
Alpha-blockers	Clonidine, methyldopa, guanfacine, prazosin
Antihypertension medications	ACE inhibitors, beta-blockers, calcium channel blockers, hydralazine, hydrochlorothiazide
Erectile dysfunction drugs	Sildenafil tadalafil, etc.
Psychiatric medications	Some antidepressants, benzodiazepines, psychotropics, antiepileptics, gabapentin
Pain medications	NSAIDS if aspirin-exacerbated respiratory disease
Estrogens and progesterone	Mostly in the form of birth control

Other causes of chronic rhinitis
Mixed (both allergic and nonallergic components)
CPAP-induced rhinitis
Occupational rhinitis
Rhinitis medicamentosa
Pregnancy
Atrophic rhinitis

intolerance, acid reflux, poor sleep, poor memory, and daytime hypersomnolence.

On physical exam, her vital signs revealed that a temperature was 36.8 C (98.2 F), blood pressure 130/88 mmHg, pulse 88 BPM, respiratory rate 12 breaths/min, SpO2 97%, BMI 38, weight 100 kg (220 lbs.), and height 162 cm (5′4″). Her physical exam was remarkable for significant nasal discharge and swollen inferior nasal turbinates bilaterally. Her posterior throat is barely visible but there is no cobblestoning or postnasal drainage. She has a large neck circumference without cervical lymphadenopathy. Her chest exam was clear to auscultation and her heart exam revealed a pericardial rub. Other than her well-healed surgical scars, and being obese, her abdominal exam was benign. There were no previous labs or imaging tests for review.

Skin testing for a selection of environmental allergens revealed positive results to house dust mite. The rest of the panel, except for the positive control, was negative.

Differential Diagnosis and Assessment

There are various forms of chronic rhinitis, which can generally be divided into three categories: acute (less than 4 weeks' duration), subacute (greater than 4 weeks, but less than 12), and chronic (greater than 12 weeks). Most commonly acute rhinitis is infectious in nature with the majority of cases being caused by viral upper respiratory infections. Subacute and chronic rhinitides have a variety of causes as summarized in Table 17.1.

Of these diagnoses allergic, nonallergic, and mixed rhinitis are the most common conditions. Allergic rhinitis affects 10–30% of the

Table 17.2 ARIA Classification of allergic rhinitis.

Symptoms	
Intermittent	Less than 4 days per week or less than 4 weeks/year
Persistent	Present at least 4 days per week or greater than 4 weeks per year
Severity	
Mild	No impairment of sleep, daily activities, leisure, and/or sport No troublesome symptoms No impairment of school or work
Moderate-severe	One or more of the following: • Impairment in sleep • Impairment of daily activities, leisure, and/or sport • Impairment of school or work • Troublesome symptoms

Table 17.3 Multiple pro-inflammatory factors in allergic rhinitis affect sleep and symptoms[a]

Mediator	Effect on sleep
Histamine	Balance between wakefulness and sleep, arousal; ↑ **nasal obstruction, rhinorrhea, and pruritus**
CysLT	↑ Slow-wave sleep, ↑ sleep-disordered breathing; ↑ nasal obstruction, rhinorrhea
IL-1	↑ latency to REM, and ↓ REM duration
IL-4	
IL-10	
Bradykinin	↑ Sleep apnea; ↑ nasal obstruction, and rhinorrhea
Substance P	↑ Latency to REM, arousal; ↑ nasal obstruction

[a]From Ferguson BJ. Influences of allergic rhinitis on sleep. Otolaryngol Head Neck Surg 2004 May;130(5):617–29. Copyright © 2004, © SAGE Publications

world's population, and up to 40% of children [1]. Its prevalence has continued to climb in the industrialized world for more than 50 years [2]. In some questionnaire-based studies, over 68% of rhinitis patients attributed their symptoms to allergies, either seasonal allergic rhinitis (SAR) or perennial allergic rhinitis (PAR). However, there are data to suggest that about 50% of patients have "mixed" rhinitis, which is a combination of SAR and nonallergic rhinitis (NAR) [3].

The Allergic Rhinitis and Its Impact on Asthma (ARIA) international guideline's classification scheme also assesses severity of allergic symptoms (Table 17.2). Severity by ARIA is based upon the impact on productivity and quality of life, mostly influenced by interference with sleep. The interference of rhinitis on sleep is complex and secondary to multiple processes to include congestion. Passive nasal congestion can cause sleep-disordered breathing, especially arousals, and other allergic symptoms such as ocular pruritus can cause difficulty falling asleep. Finally rhinitis can increase inflammatory mediators that can directly influence the sleep cycle (Table 17.3).

For the case presented many of the above-listed causes of rhinitis could be applicable, but this discussion will focus on allergic and nonallergic rhinitis and its effect on sleep. Age of onset can be a clinical clue as to the type of

rhinitis she is experiencing. In general allergic patients report symptoms at a younger age in childhood or adolescence whereas nonallergic rhinitis (NAR) patients typically present after age 20 in up to 70% of cases [4]. Nonallergic rhinitis also seems to affect females more than males and is typically aggravated by a spectrum of irritants such as smoke, perfumes, and potpourris but also by changes in temperature or barometric pressure [5]. In contrast, allergic rhinitis patients typically report a positive family history, allergic conjunctivitis (as high as 60%), and sneezing if the allergen exposure is intermittent [6, 7]. With continuous exposure the symptoms of congestion and poor sleep become increasingly prominent and are frequently the two most common reasons a patient presents for care.

Physical examination can also be helpful since allergic patients are more likely to have allergic shiners due to venous congestion and edematous/pale boggy nasal mucosa whereas NAR patients may have more erythematous beefy turbinates but can also have normal-appearing nasal mucosa. In either case mucosal congestion is a frequent finding in those experiencing SDB, even though it is the authors' experience that subjective nasal congestion and congestion noted on physical exam correlate minimally.

The skin test findings suggest that mite avoidance intervention is indicated and that allergy vaccine may be indicated, if medical management continues to improve her clinical symptoms.

Treatment

Because of her congestion and SDB initial treatment for this patient is similar regardless as to whether she has NAR or AR, but due to her skin test findings mite avoidance education should also be provided. Multiple data are available confirming that topical intranasal corticosteroids (INCS) have been found to be effective for congestion and can improve the associated SDB. The improvement of the associated SDB can be attributed to reduction of congestion, as well as other symptoms of rhinitis and conjunctivitis through a reduction of inflammatory mediators [8]. It should also be noted that, although most glucocorticoid nasal sprays have some effect after 24–48 h, in order to obtain maximal clinical effect, they should be used consistently for several weeks. It is the author's opinion that a 4-week trial of high-dose INCS, two sprays bid, is an ample trial to determine if the congestion, SDB, and daytime somnolence will be responsive to this approach.

If INCS are not completely effective, the addition of an intranasal antihistamine would be the suggestion by many. Most of the studies investigating combination INCS and intranasal antihistamines have been conducted using intranasal azelastine and have demonstrated a benefit of the combination over the use of either product alone [9]. It should be noted that topical antihistamines are partially absorbed and can lead to sedation, and in this case could further increase her daytime somnolence, and thus attention to this detail is imperative [10].

An alternative if sedation increases with the addition of a topical nasal antihistamine may be the addition of a leukotriene-modifying agent to the INCS, such as montelukast, which has been shown to have modest benefits for congestion and for SDB. This is despite the recommendation by the guidelines [11] that leukotriene-modifying agents add minimally to nasal symptom relief and are not recommended to continue when starting INCS nor being added to INCS. Despite the guideline suggestion, data do exist demonstrating some benefit when montelukast is initiated for congestion and poor sleep [12].

In order to achieve the maximum clinical effect from INCS sprays, patients should be properly instructed so as to achieve the maximum benefit and be spared adverse events. The INCS should be aimed away from the nasal septum, with the head bent forward/down slightly. However, as evident with our patient, even with good technique, epistaxis can occur in up to 12% of patients. If the amount of blood is minimal the nasal spray can be resumed after stopping for a couple days. Nasal saline rinses may help in these situations to remove crusting and mucus that could be interfering with the proper deposition of the nose spray. Some nasal sprays contain alcohol or propylene glycol, which can be irritating to the nasal mucosa, so a trial of an aqueous-based/propylene glycol-free nasal spray may be of benefit in reducing nasal bleeding. Another potential remedy is to use water-based lubricants, which are available as gels or nasal sprays to protect the mucosa from adverse effects of INCS. As a last medical intervention, though controversial and expensive, large-volume lavage, defined as 8 oz. of warm saline, mixed with 0.25, 0.5, or 1.0 mg of budesonide twice daily, may reduce congestion and improve SDB. This approach may not be associated with nasal bleeding despite INCS sprays causing epistaxis. This was the intervention that ultimately benefited our patient. Since starting irrigation with budesonide, she has experienced improved sleep, with infrequent awakenings, and less daytime somnolence and has started a weight loss program. If this intervention fails, other considerations include allergy immunotherapy, as well as a sinus CT scan to assess for structural problems that require a surgical intervention. If the CT scan of the sinuses fails to show surgical pathology and she is unresponsive to aggressive medical management, referral for a polysomnography (PSG) study would be appropriate.

Discussion

There are many studies associating sleep impairment, daytime somnolence, and fatigue with chronic rhinitis. These sleep-related problems include micro-arousals, SDB including snoring, and sleep apnea, as defined as an abnormal amount of apnea/hypopnea episodes per hour of sleep, and are not uncommon in patients with rhinitis. As noted in the case, the sleep disturbance in rhinitis patients is multifactorial and influenced by nasal congestion, other symptoms of rhinitis, and inflammatory mediators. There are many inflammatory mediators, including cytokines, that are increased in AR that may play a role in sleep disturbance which also worsen associated daytime somnolence [13] (see Table 17.3).

Nasal congestion can affect up to 85% of rhinitis patients. Some studies report that 40% of rhinitis patients rate their nasal congestion symptoms as severe. One study found that AR patients with nasal congestion were twice as likely to suffer from moderate-to-severe sleep-disordered breathing (SDB) than AR patients not reporting nasal congestion [14]. In our patient's case, her nasal congestion regardless if it is related to allergic or nonallergic rhinitis is likely predisposing her to snoring and SDB. Early studies by Zwillich et al. demonstrated that passive obstruction of the nasal passage by a clip can induce arousals and increase apneas and hypopneas [15].

Nasal obstruction occurs when the cavernous tissues of the turbinates enlarge from increased blood flow through the capacitance vessels. It is not uncommon for nasal congestion to worsen at night presumably due to postural changes and circadian rhythm. Normal individuals have a protection from increased congestion associated with reclining position; however, this is lost in patients with chronic rhinitis. As discussed, the first step in treatment would be with an INCS, which has been shown to improve sleep quality and decrease daytime somnolence secondary to their anti-inflammatory effect, which decreases nasal congestion [16].

As noted, other symptoms of AR adversely affect sleep mainly by increasing latency from lying down to falling asleep. Ocular itch, postnasal drip, and rhinorrhea all can have this negative impact. Multiple therapies including INCS, topical antihistamines, LTRA, second-generation antihistamines, and immunotherapy may alleviate these symptoms with improvement in sleep. This is different than the symptom of congestion for which INCS have been demonstrated to be superior to other treatments.

Lastly, as noted in the table, inflammatory mediators are increased in rhinitis. These mediators can directly affect sleep by affecting latency to REM sleep, quality of REM sleep, and other stages of sleep. In turn with sleep disruption IL-6, IL-1, and TNF are increased and can further worsen daytime somnolence and fatigue. This effect can reduce tolerance for exercise and increase weight gain, which can further increase SDB.

There is also a significant amount of research into the structure of the upper airway, and its relation to obstructive sleep apnea. This might include septal deviation and turbinate hypertrophy in all ages. Tonsillar/adenoid enlargement would be more commonly implicated in children. There are studies showing improved symptoms posttreatment of these conditions, and surgical correction of an anatomic obstruction should be considered if feasible. Surgical correction can result in increased CPAP compliance in certain patients. Therefore, both surgical and nonsurgical approaches should be considered in our obstructive sleep apnea patients [17, 18].

For the aforementioned reasons, patients with chronic rhinitis with associated SDB should be followed carefully to ensure that sleep, daytime somnolence, and fatigue improve and if refractory to therapy PSG and metabolic causes should be investigated. If there is associated weight gain, it is important to provide education and encouragement for lifestyle modification/weight loss and exercise. Sleep hygiene should be assessed early on in the course of therapy and include an assessment of noise, darkness, and physical stimuli at night. The room should be quiet, dark, and free of external stimuli.

Clinical Pearls and Pitfalls

- Rhinitis-associated congestion is common and can cause sleep-disordered breathing and increased risk of apnea/hypopnea.
- Inflammation associated with chronic rhinitis decreases sleep quality and can also cause daytime somnolence and fatigue. Symptoms other than rhinitis may influence sleep quality.
- Topical nasal corticosteroids can be key in the treatment of congestion and associated SDB.

Case Presentation 2

MJ is a 55-year-old male who presents to your office for nasal congestion, headaches, and fatigue. His past medical history is remarkable for hypertension, asthma, gastroesophageal reflux disease (GERD), obesity, adult-onset diabetes non-insulin dependent and low testosterone, and chronic musculoskeletal issues. His medications include lisinopril, hydro-chlorothiazide, albuterol inhaler as needed, metformin, testosterone shots, cetirizine, and omeprazole. He has a remote history of an amoxicillin rash as a child. He previously underwent an L4/L5 fusion and bilateral total knee replacements. His family history is remarkable for cardiac disease as his father died from MI at age 60 and mother from a stroke at age 62. He has a 20-pack per year history of smoking, but quit 5 years prior, and he is a social drinker. He has had his influenza and pneumonia vaccines. Of note his wife complains of his loud snoring and often has to sleep in another room. She also notes that he often gasps while sleeping, which appears like he ceases to breathe for short periods of time.

On review of systems he complains of fatigue, poor sleep, frequent awakening, nocturia, daytime somnolence, a 10-pound weight gain over the past year, morning headaches with irritability, postnasal drainage with frequent throat clearing, sinus pressure, exercise intolerance, wheezing, cough, shortness of breath on exertion, acid reflux, frequent urination, and back/knee pain.

On physical examination his blood pressure was 155/95 mmHg, weight was 120 kg (265 lbs.), and height was 178 cm (5′10″). His nasal turbinates were enlarged, he had a small posterior pharynx orifice obstructed by a large tongue, and his neck circumference was significantly increased. Otherwise there were no other remarkable findings.

In office spirometry revealed an FVC-95% predicted, and FEV1 90% predicted with an FEV1/FVC ratio of 0.83.

Skin testing was negative in the presence of a positive and negative control.

He was initially tried nasal corticosteroids, but failed to improve. CT scan of the sinuses was ordered and demonstrated enlarged turbinates explaining his nasal congestion, but was otherwise unremarkable. A referral for PSG was made and revealed 35 apneas/hypopneas per hour consistent with severe sleep apnea. CPAP was prescribed, but the patient could not tolerate it secondary to his nasal congestion.

Discussion

In this case, MJ has many significant medical problems, including most of the clinical and physical features suggestive of obstructive sleep apnea (OSA). He snores, and has morning headaches and irritability, hypersomnolence throughout the day, and obesity. More importantly he has many clinical problems that can be caused or worsened by OSA such as hypertension, and is at risk for cardiac disease.

Obstructive sleep apnea (OSA) is a very common subtype of SDB, affecting up to 30% of males and 15% of females in North America. The prevalence for OSA has risen throughout the world largely due to increasing obesity rates. However, even in normal-weight males and females the prevalence is 9% and 3%, respectively [19, 20]. The most common diagnostic criteria used for OSA is greater than or equal to 5 apnea-hypopnea events in 1 h. This is termed the apnea/hypopnea index (AHI) and as noted in adults an AHI below 5 is normal, 5–15 is mild, 15–30 is moderate, and greater than 30 is severe. Though in-home assessment of AHI is possible, polysomnography (PSG) in a sleep laboratory remains the gold standard especially for individuals with more complex concomitant medical

Table 17.4 Classifications of obstructive sleep apnea severity

Classification	AHI for diagnosis	Common clinical manifestations
Mild	5–15	Often asymptomatic or minimal daytime somnolence
Moderate	15–30	Clear daytime somnolence, coexisting hypertension is common
Severe	>30	Daytime somnolence interfering with daily activities, increased cardiovascular disease and mortality

problems. [21]. Table 17.4 summarizes the diagnostic criteria for OSA.

In the case presented, obesity and being a male are significant risk factors for OSA. However, there is also a threefold increased risk of OSA in smokers compared to ex-smokers or nonsmokers. Family history of OSA also increases the risk of OSA. African-Americans and Asians are also at greater risk for OSA secondary to craniofacial structure [22]. Other risk factors for OSA include nasal congestion, menopause, chronic lung disease, stroke, heart failure, renal disease, and pregnancy. Some findings make OSA more likely such as in our patient's case an enlarged neck circumference, crowded oropharynx, and subjective history of nocturnal choking and nocturia.

If OSA is suspected, and an underlying etiology that is correctable is not apparent, a formal sleep study (PSG) is recommended. In some cases, allergy assessment before referral is indicated. If the patient is found to have perennial allergies, it is possible that appropriate exposure reduction may alleviate symptoms and improve SDB. This is unlikely to be effective in our patient since his skin tests are negative. If there is evidence of nasal obstruction, septal deviation or sinusitis than a sinus CT should be obtained before referral for PSG to rule out structural issues. Regardless of whether the patient has allergic or nonallergic rhinitis, if there is a significant history of nasal congestion, then a trial of tailored medical therapy to their condition, as in case one, could be initiated and response to therapy should be assessed before referral for PSG.

Ideally the diagnosis of OSA and ideal pressures for CPAP would be determined during an overnight PSG, usually by a split night with the first part being diagnostic and second used to titrate therapy. However, if acquisition or insurance approval is difficult or impossible based on geographic location or for other reasons, a home sleep apnea test for uncomplicated patients may be appropriate with an auto-titrating continuous positive airway pressure (CPAP) machine. There are several randomized trials demonstrating that in-home titration may be equivalent to polysomnography for most cases [23–25].

Some of the main disadvantages of home sleep studies are that the data collected is not as comprehensive and the combined expertise of a "sleep doctor" and technician is lacking. There are many variations of masks including oral, oronasal, and nasal masks as well as different styles and sizes. For patients who do not require high pressures, nasal pillows may also be an option. Ultimately, it is important to find the apparatus that is most comfortable for the patient to help improve compliance with the CPAP.

Patients with congestive heart failure, COPD, central sleep apnea, and other hypoventilation syndromes (obesity hypoventilation syndrome, opiate use, and neuromuscular disease) are not candidates for auto-titrating CPAP and these patients should have a formal sleep study under the direct care of a sleep specialist.

There are several types of positive airway pressure (PAP) approaches but generally they can be divided into CPAP (continuous positive airway pressure) and BPAP (bi-level positive airway pressure). Either of these types can be "fixed" or "auto-titrating." As the name implies the auto-titrating machines can adjust to give more or less pressure, in order to maintain a patent airway and prevent upper airway collapse. The BPAP approach is generally not indicated as an initial therapy as it is more expensive, less studied, and more difficult to use. It does offer advantages for some patients and it may be better tolerated by those who can't tolerate CPAP.

Due to increased airway resistance seen in patients with nasal congestion, higher pressures are required if nasal masks are used. This may lead to patient discomfort and decreased compliance. In general, a mask that covers the face (and not just the nose) will usually be better tolerated [26]. As mentioned previously, treatment of underlying nasal congestion with individual or combination of therapies such as INCS, nasal irrigation with saline, nasal antihistamines, or anticholinergic sprays may enhance compliance and effectiveness of PAP [27]. Auto-titrating CPAP may also be more effective than standard PAP in patients with chronic rhinitis, as it can adjust to variation in nasal obstruction. Even in patients without preexisting chronic rhinitis there is a condition termed "CPAP-rhinitis," which is likely caused by the dry pressurized air contacting the nasal mucosa. This condition can be treated with a small amount of intranasal water-based lubricant, nasal saline, and heated humidification of the air used for PAP. Heated humidity alone can decrease nasal resistance by approximately 50% in some studies [28]. It should also be noted that oil-based lubricants can be aspirated into the lung and cause exogenous lipoid pneumonia and therefore should be avoided [29–31].

Current guidelines suggest that 5–20 cm H_2O is generally a good starting parameter for auto-titrating CPAP. In general, pressures greater than 20 cm H_2O may be better treated with BPAP. Another general guideline is that pressures above 12 cm H_2O are not well tolerated with the use of nasal pillows, and will likely require a mask. Optimally PAP should be titrated to reduce events to less than 5 per hour with few or no spontaneous arousals [32, 33]. The pressure that eliminates all obstruction for more than 90–95% of the time would be used as the constant pressure if fixed CPAP is desired. This information can be obtained by an auto-titrating CPAP at home or by a PSG.

Oral devices are available which can be effective in reducing obstruction without the use of PAP. Not all patients are suitable or tolerate oral devices, but in those unable to tolerate CPAP assessment and fitting for a mouth device may be an effective therapeutic intervention. In fact, some studies show that they can be equally effective in mild-moderate OSA due to increased patient compliance, fewer side effects, and greater patient satisfaction [34, 35]. One disadvantage of oral devices is that they are expensive and often not covered by insurance.

Long-term treatment of OSA requires a multidisciplinary specialty approach to address the many comorbidities associated with this disorder. This includes optimal management of blood pressure and other underlying cardiac problems, weight reduction, chronic rhinitis, asthma, and GERD.

Management/Outcome

Given the multiple comorbidities that this patient presented with, a formal polysomnography would be recommended. In the meantime, recommendations should be made for aggressive lifestyle modification including a medically monitored weight reduction program which could include a surgical approach to control obesity.

Since he is at high risk for OSA and has no contraindications for home sleep apnea testing, a self-titrating CPAP may be an option if there is a delay in obtaining a formal sleep study. This patient should have close follow-up in the office over time given his significant cardiac risk factors.

As discussed briefly earlier, congestion often interferes with CPAP. In cases such as this medication interventions as outlined in case one of this chapter are indicated, in addition to warm humidification during CPAP treatment. A trial of INCS at usual doses and if necessary high doses can be attempted. Addition of an intranasal antihistamine may be helpful as studies have found that they have a synergistic effect with INCS. Though providing minimal benefit in population studies, some individuals may be very responsive to LTRA and for this reason an addition to INCS may be warranted. If congestion still is a concern and surgical pathology and allergies are excluded, large-volume sinus rinse with budesonide may be indicated, despite the lack of literature supporting this intervention. Once congestion is optimally controlled re-titration of pressure may be indicated. The anticipated outcome is improved tolerance of CPAP, and thus improved compliance and optimal benefit.

Clinical Pearls and Pitfalls

- Obstructive sleep apnea prevalence is increasing due to obesity, and it is more common in males and smokers, and can be exacerbated by rhinitis/congestion.
- Home sleep studies using auto-titrating CPAP can be effective for some patients.
- Contraindications to in-home CPAP testing include congestive heart failure, COPD, central sleep apnea, and other hypoventilation syndromes.
- Continuous positive airway pressure is the best studied form of PAP and can be used with either fixed pressures or auto-titrating devices.
- Overcoming patient concerns prior to initiating CPAP may improve success.
- In patients with chronic rhinitis with nasal congestion requiring positive airway pressure treatment, INCS and/or other combinations of medications may improve tolerability.
- Heated/humidified air also reduces chronic rhinitis symptoms and increases compliance.
- Patients with chronic rhinitis with congestion who require PAP may benefit from a full facemask.
- For those patients who cannot tolerate CPAP an oral device may be effective.
- Most patients with sleep apnea benefit from a multidisciplinary management approach.

References

1. Meltzer EO, Nathan R, Derebery J, Stang PE, Campbell UB, Yeh WS, et al. Sleep, quality of life, and productivity impact of nasal symptoms in the United States: findings from the burden of rhinitis in America survey. Allergy Asthma Proc. 2009;30:244.
2. Schiller JS, Lucas JW, Ward BW, Peregory JA. Summary health statistics for U.S. adults: National Health Interview Survey, 2010. Vital Health Stat. 2012;252:1–207. http://www.aaaai.org/about-aaaai/newsroom/allergy-statistics
3. Dykewicz MS, Fineman S, Skoner DP, Nicklas R, Lee R, Blessing-Moore J, et al. Diagnosis and management of rhinitis: complete guidelines of the joint task force on practice parameters in allergy, asthma and immunology. Ann Allergy Asthma Immunol. 1998;81:478.
4. Togias AK. Nonallergic rhinitis. In: Mygine N, Naclerio RM, editors. Allergic and nonallergic rhinitis: clinical aspects. Copenhagen: Munksgaard; 1993. p. 159.
5. Enber RN. Perennial nonallergic rhinitis: a retrospective review. Ann Allergy. 1989;63:513.
6. Bielory L. Allergic and immunologic disorders of the eye. Part II: ocular allergy. J Allergy Clin Immunol. 2000;106:1019.
7. Rolla G, Guida G, Heffler E, Badiu I, Bommarito L, De Stefani A, et al. Diagnostic classification of persistent rhinitis and its relationship to exhaled nitric oxide and asthma: a clinical study of a consecutive series of patients. Chest. 2007;131:1345.
8. Craig TJ, Teets S, Lehman EB, Chinchilli VM, Zwillich C. Nasal congestion secondary to allergic rhinitis as a cause of sleep disturbance and daytime fatigue and the response to topical nasal corticosteroids. J Allergy Clin Immunol. 1998;101:633.
9. Carr W, Bernstein J, Lieberman P, Meltzer E, Bachert C, Price D, et al. A novel intranasal therapy ofazelastine withfluticasonefor the treatment of allergic rhinitis. J Allergy Clin Immunol. 2012;5·1282 9.
10. Liberman PL, Settipane RA. Azelastine nasal spray: a review of pharmacology and clinical efficacy I allergic and nonallergic rhinitis. Allergy Asthma Proc. 2003;24(2):95–105.
11. Epstein L, Kristo D, Strollo PJ Jr, Friedman N, Malhotra A, Patil SP, et al. Clinical guideline for evaluation, management and long-term care of obstructive sleep apnea in adults. J Clin Sleep Med. 2009;5(3):263–76.
12. Santos C, Hanks C, McCann J, Lehman EB, Pratt E, Craig TJ. The role of Montelukast on perennial allergic rhinitis, and associated sleep disturbances and daytime somnolence. Allergy Asthma Proc. 2008;29(2):140–5.
13. Krouse HJ, Davis JE, Krouse JH. Immune mediators in allergic rhinitis and sleep. Otolaryngol Head Neck Surg. 2002;126:607.
14. Zwillich CW, Pickett C, Hanson FN, Weil JV. Disturbed sleep and prolonged apnea during nasal obstruction in normal men. Am Rev Respir Dis. 1981;124(2):158–60.
15. Mintz M, Garcia J, Diener P, Liao Y, Dupclay L, Georges G. Triamcinolone acetonide aqueous nasal spray improves nocturnal rhinitis-related quality of life in patients treated in a primary care setting: the quality of sleep in allergic rhinitis study. Ann Allergy Asthma Immunol. 2004;92(2):255–61.
16. Powell NB, Zonato AL, Weaver EM, Li K, Troell R, Riley RW, et al. Radiofrequency treatment of turbinate hypertrophy in subjects using continuous positive airway pressure: a randomized, double blind, placebo-controlled clinical pilot trial. Laryngoscope. 2001;111(10):1783–90.
17. Kempfle JS, BuSaba NY, Dobrowski JM, Westover MB, Bianchi MT. A cost-effectiveness analysis of nasal surgery to increase continuous positive airway pressure adherence in sleep apnea patients with nasal obstruction. Laryngoscope. 2017;127(4):977–83. Epub 2016 Sep 22.

18. Young T, Skatrud J, Peppard PE. Risk factors for obstructive sleep apnea in adults. JAMA. 2004;291:2013.
19. Young T, Palta M, Dempsey J, Peppard PE, Nieto FJ, Hla KM. Burden of sleep apnea: rationale, design, and major findings of the Wisconsin sleep cohort study. WMJ. 2009;108:246.
20. Peppard PE, Young T, Barnet JH, Palta M, Hagen EW, Hla KM. Increased prevalence of sleep-disordered breathing in adults. Am J Epidemiol. 2013;177:1006.
21. Indications and standards for use of nasal continuous positive airway pressure (CPAP) in sleep apnea syndromes. American Thoracic Society. Official statement adopted march 1994. Am J Respir Crit Care Med. 1994;150:1738.
22. Dempsey JA, Veasey SC, Morgan BJ, O'Donnell CP. Pathophysiology of sleep apnea. Physiol Rev. 2010;90:47.
23. Skomro RP, Gjevre J, Reid J, McNab B, Ghosh S, Stiles M, et al. Outcomes of home-based diagnosis and treatment of obstructive sleep apnea. Chest. 2010;138:257.
24. Masa JF, Jimenez A, Duran J, Capote F, Monasterio C, Mayos M, et al. Alternative methods of titrating continuous positive airway pressure: a large multicenter study. Am J Respir Crit Care Med. 2004;170:1218.
25. Cross MD, Vennelle M, Engleman HM, White S, Mackay TW, Twaddle S, et al. Comparison of CPAP titration at home or the sleep laboratory in sleep apnea hypopnea syndrome. Sleep. 2006;29(11):1451.
26. Prosise GL, Berry RB. Oral-nasal continuous positive airway pressure as a treatment for obstructive sleep apnea. Chest. 1994;106:180.
27. Strollo PJ, Sanders MH, Stiller RA. Continuous and bi-level positive airway pressure therapy in sleep-disordered breathing. Atlas Oral Maxillofac Surg Clin North Am. 1995;7:221.
28. Gorospe L, Gallego-Rivera JI, Hervás-Morón A. Exogenous lipoid pneumonia secondary to Vaseline application to the tracheostomy in a laryngectomy patient: PET/CT and MR imaging findings. Clin Imaging. 2013;37(1):163–6.
29. Brown AC, Slocum PC, Putthoff SL, Wallace WE, Foresman BH. Exogenous lipoid pneumonia due to nasal application of petroleum jelly. Chest. 1994;105(3):968–9.
30. Khilnani GC, Hadda V. Lipoid pneumonia: an uncommon entity. Indian J Med Sci. 2009;63(10):474–80.
31. Richards GN, Cistulli PA, Ungar RG, Berthon-Jones M, Sullivan CE. Mouth leak with nasal continuous positive airway pressure increased nasal airway resistance. Am J Respir Crit Care Med. 1996;154:182.
32. Kushida CA, Chediak A, Berry RB, Brown LK, Gozal D, Iber C, et al. Clinical guidelines for the manual titration of positive airway pressure in patients with obstructive sleep apnea. J Clin Sleep Med. 2008;4:157.
33. Hishkowitz M, Sharafkhaneh A. Positive airway pressure therapy of OSA. Semin Respir Crit Care Med. 2005;26:68.
34. Ferguson KA, Ono T. A randomized crossover study of an oral appliance vs. nasal continuous positive airway pressure in the treatment of mild-moderate obstructive sleep apnea. Chest. 1996;109(5):1269–75.
35. Phillips C, Grunstein R. Health outcomes of continuous positive airway pressure versus oral appliance treatment for obstructive sleep apnea a randomized controlled trial. Am J Respir Crit Care Med. 2013;187(8):879–87.

Drug-Induced Rhinitis

18

Benjamin T. Prince and Deepa D. Patadia

Introduction

Drug-induced rhinitis is a rhinitis subtype that occurs as a direct result of inflammatory, neurogenic, or undefined properties of an implicated drug. Many different classes of drugs, including topical decongestants, antihypertensives, nonsteroidal anti-inflammatory drugs (NSAIDs), psychotropic drugs, and drugs for erectile dysfunction, have been implicated in drug-induced rhinitis (Table 18.1) [1]. The mechanism by which rhinitis occurs varies by the drug responsible for inducing symptoms. The following two cases will illustrate the presentation, diagnosis, and management of drug-induced rhinitis. The discussion sections include an overview of the natural history, pathophysiology, and treatment of the specific etiologies of drug-induced rhinitis that should be considered in each case. General principles important in the evaluation and management of drug-induced rhinitis along with clinical pearls and pitfalls are reviewed at the end of the chapter.

B. T. Prince (✉)
Division of Allergy and Immunology, Department of Pediatrics, Nationwide Children's Hospital, The Ohio State University College of Medicine,
Columbus, OH, USA
e-mail: Benjamin.Prince@nationwidechildrens.org

D. D. Patadia
Department of Allergy and Clinical Immunology, Respiratory Institute, Cleveland Clinic, Cleveland, OH, USA

Case Presentation 1

A 45-year-old man presents to the clinic for evaluation of a 5-year history of rhinitis symptoms, which have worsened in the past month. He reports chronic nasal congestion, runny nose, and anosmia. He has had frequent sinus infections, averaging five to six episodes per year. He was prescribed a daily intranasal corticosteroid, but forgets to take it 3 days per week. Two years ago, he was diagnosed with asthma. His asthma is generally well controlled on a moderate dose of inhaled corticosteroid. However, he was hospitalized 2 weeks ago for an asthma exacerbation, requiring systemic corticosteroids. Two months ago, he had an upper respiratory tract infection and used over-the-counter oxymetazoline for 3 days. He has otherwise been healthy, except for a knee injury sustained while playing tennis 1 month ago, for which he has been taking ibuprofen as needed. He has a remote history of cocaine abuse, in his early 20s. He is a former smoker, with a seven-pack-year history. He quit smoking 20 years ago. Physical examination is remarkable for pale masses near the middle turbinates that have a cluster-of-grapes appearance. He has no wheezing on lung examination, but does demonstrate a mildly prolonged expiratory phase of respiration. Skin prick testing for aeroallergens was previously negative. Office spirometry today demonstrates a mild obstructive defect.

© Springer International Publishing AG, part of Springer Nature 2018
J. A. Bernstein (ed.), *Rhinitis and Related Upper Respiratory Conditions*,
https://doi.org/10.1007/978-3-319-75370-6_18

Table 18.1 Medications associated with drug-induced rhinitis

Medication category	Examples
Nonsteroidal anti-inflammatory drugs (NSAIDs)	Aspirin
	Ibuprofen
	Ketorolac
Antihypertensive medications	Beta-blockers
	ACE inhibitors
	Calcium channel blockers
	Prazosin
	Clonidine
	Hydralazine
	Amiloride
	Hydrochlorothiazide (HCTZ)
Erectile dysfunction medications (phosphodiesterase-5 inhibitors)	Sildenafil
	Tadalafil
	Vardenafil
Psychotropic medications	Risperidone
	Chlorpromazine
	Amitriptyline
Other	Local nasal decongestants
	Gabapentin

Discussion

Aspirin-Exacerbated Respiratory Disease

Aspirin-exacerbated respiratory disease (AERD) is an acquired inflammatory condition characterized by chronic, eosinophilic airway inflammation, and underlying arachidonic acid metabolism dysregulation [2]. Patients experience pathognomonic exacerbations of asthma and rhinosinusitis within minutes to hours of exposure to aspirin or other COX-1-inhibiting nonsteroidal anti-inflammatory drugs (NSAIDs), on a background of underlying upper and lower respiratory inflammation [3]. AERD, also referred to as aspirin triad or Samter's triad, was first described in 1922 by Widal et al. and commonly presents with the triad of chronic sinusitis with nasal polyps, asthma, and aspirin intolerance [4]. It occurs more commonly in adults than in children, and it does not follow a Mendelian pattern of inheritance. Studies have identified several candidate genes involved in the arachidonic acid pathway, airway remodeling, and immune response that may be associated with AERD.

Epigenetic factors, such as DNA methylation, may also be involved [5, 6]. Environmental factors, such as viral infections, are thought to play a role in AERD. Although a subset of AERD patients have allergic sensitization to aeroallergens, it is important to emphasize that atopy is not believed to be an underlying cause of nasal polyps or AERD [7, 8]. The prevalence of AERD varies depending on the study population and methods. A recent meta-analysis estimated the prevalence of AERD in asthmatics to be 7% with an even higher rate of 14% in patients with severe asthma. Additionally, 10% of patient with nasal polyps and 9% with chronic rhinosinusitis were found to have AERD [9].

The natural history of AERD includes a specific sequence of symptoms, beginning with rhinitis onset around age 30. Symptoms include rhinorrhea, nasal obstruction, and sneezing, often following an upper respiratory tract infection. Nasal polyposis develops over time and anosmia can occur. Asthma symptoms begin about 2 years after rhinitis onset. Aspirin or NSAID reactions are typically noted about 6 years after rhinitis onset; however, many patients may be unaware of their intolerance to these medications at the time of diagnosis [8]. Patients with AERD have respiratory disease even in the absence of NSAID exposure. At baseline, their asthma and sinus disease may be difficult to control. Their asthma is persistent and severe, with an increased medication requirement and a greater risk for near-fatal asthma [10]. Interestingly, most patients with AERD also experience respiratory symptoms with alcohol ingestion. In one study, 83% of AERD patients reported alcohol-induced respiratory symptoms, with 75% of patients having upper respiratory symptoms and 51% of patients having lower respiratory symptoms after alcohol ingestion [11]. Their rhinosinusitis is generally chronic and severe, and the nasal polyps tend to recur [10]. Patients with AERD undergo more frequent sinus surgeries and have more sinus infections compared to patients with chronic rhinosinusitis without polyps. The average AERD patient typically receives three sinus surgeries over his or her lifetime and is diagnosed with 5.5 sinus infections per year [12].

The pathogenesis of AERD is related to underlying abnormalities in arachidonic acid metabolism that result in chronic elevations of eosinophils and mast cells in the mucosa and peripheral blood [7] (Fig. 18.1). Patients with AERD have a baseline deficiency of prostaglandins and an overproduction of cysteinyl leukotrienes. An unknowing or accidental ingestion of aspirin or NSAIDs results in a complete block of prostaglandin production as a result of inhibiting the cyclooxygenase-1 (COX-1) enzyme. An absence of prostaglandin E2 (PGE2), which is an anti-inflammatory prostaglandin important for inhibiting 5-lipoxygenase, leads to overproduction of cysteinyl leukotrienes, upregulation of leukotriene receptors, and increased Th2 cytokine production. This ultimately results in an influx of eosinophils and mast cells in the upper and lower respiratory tissue that is characteristic of the disease [13, 14]. As a result, within 30–180 min after exposure to an NSAID or aspirin, patients develop respiratory symptoms typical of an asthma exacerbation. They may also concomitantly experience anterior or posterior rhinorrhea, nasal congestion, ocular symptoms, flushing, urticaria, angioedema, or GI symptoms. In some cases, increased nasal and ocular symptoms may be the primary clinical symptoms without asthma exacerbation. As such, patients should strictly avoid aspirin and other COX-1-inhibiting NSAIDs. However, avoidance of NSAIDs or aspirin does not improve the patient's underlying respiratory or sinus disease [15].

A diagnosis of AERD is suggested if there is a history of typical symptoms with NSAID or aspirin use. History alone, however, is not reliable in making the diagnosis and can lead to over- or under-diagnosis of this condition. In one study, 15% of patients with AERD did not recognize their NSAID intolerance prior to an aspirin provocation challenge [8]. Another study of patients with asthma, sinusitis, and nasal polyps, who were referred for aspirin challenge, demonstrated that 42% of patients who had no recollection of respiratory reactions to NSAIDs or who had not used NSAIDs had a positive aspirin challenge [16]. Furthermore, although most patients with AERD have reactions with all COX-1 inhibitors, Lee-Sarwar and colleagues identified seven patients with chronic rhinosinusitis who tolerated 81 mg of aspirin daily immediately prior to failing a formal aspirin challenge [17].

Aspirin-provocation challenge is the gold standard for the diagnosis of AERD as there are no validated in vitro tests. If the diagnosis is not clear based on the patient's history or if a definitive diagnosis is required, an aspirin challenge can be performed in an outpatient setting by experienced personnel with

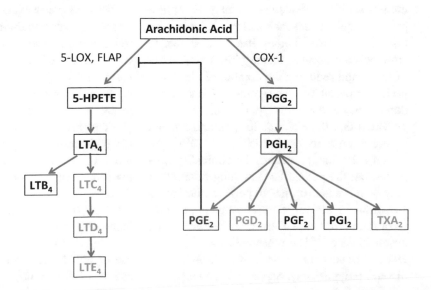

Fig. 18.1 Abnormalities in arachidonic acid metabolism underlie the pathophysiology of AERD. Substances that are produced in excess in AERD are shown in green; substances that are deficient are shown in red

resuscitative equipment immediately available, provided that the patient's lung function is not severely compromised (FEV1 < 70% predicted). During the challenge, the patient is given escalating doses of aspirin over 1–2 days depending on the protocol used. The challenge is positive if there is a significant drop in FEV1 of at least 20% from baseline or if symptoms occur, confirming the diagnosis [7]. Recently, a cohort of AERD patients was described who underwent an aspirin challenge without eliciting symptoms, and the diagnosis was only made after a positive repeat challenge [18]. Although this phenomenon appears to be rare, it is important to consider this scenario, particularly in a patient with a convincing clinical history.

The initial management of AERD requires strict avoidance of strong COX-1 inhibitors. Selective COX-2 inhibitors (e.g., celecoxib) are generally tolerated and may be used as needed. Chronic rhinosinusitis and asthma are treated per standard practice guidelines with the addition of leukotriene-modifying agents, which include 5-lipoxygenase inhibitors or LT receptor antagonists. In some cases, a short course of oral corticosteroids may be necessary. Polypectomy can be helpful in the short term, but polyps typically recur [19]. For patients with a strong medical indication for aspirin or NSAID therapy or for those whose AERD is not well controlled with other treatments, aspirin desensitization may be appropriate. Aspirin desensitization followed by high-dose aspirin therapy has been shown to slow polyp regrowth, thereby improving sense of smell and reducing the number of sinus surgeries required for management. This procedure can be done in the outpatient setting provided that the patient's lung function is not severely compromised (FEV1 < 70% predicted). If this procedure is clinically warranted but the patient has low lung function, it may be more appropriate to perform the desensitization in the inpatient setting. It has also been found that patients respond better to ASA desensitization if it is preceded by a surgical or medical (a sufficient course of high-dose prednisone) polypectomy. Aspirin therapy has been

shown to improve asthma symptoms and quality of life in AERD patients [20, 21]. Following desensitization, patients are continued on a dose of 650 mg of aspirin twice daily, which can subsequently be decreased to 325 mg twice daily after 1–6 months. However, some patients will have a return of their symptoms on the lower dose and need to be increased back to 650 mg twice daily [22]. Aspirin desensitization is contraindicated in patients with gastric ulcers, uncontrolled asthma, significant renal or liver disease, and planned pregnancy [23].

Rhinitis Medicamentosa

Rhinitis medicamentosa is characterized by nasal congestion and rebound rhinitis that occurs after prolonged use of topical nasal decongestants. It was first described in 1944 by Feinberg and Friedlaender with the use of the local nasal decongestant naphazoline [24]. It commonly occurs following an acute viral illness for which a nasal decongestant was initiated. Nasal congestion develops with persistent use and as it worsens causes the patient to increase the frequency and quantity of the nasal decongestant [25]. The need for continued decongestant use can be intense, and a psychological dependence has even been described [26]. Although the precise duration of use that results in rhinitis medicamentosa is not clear, it is recommended that nasal decongestants should be used for short durations only.

Nasal decongestants are divided into two classes: sympathomimetic amines and imidazolines. The sympathomimetic amines cause release of norepinephrine in sympathetic nerves, resulting in vasoconstriction via binding of norepinephrine to the postsynaptic alpha-receptors. The sympathomimetic amines include pseudoephedrine, ephedrine, phenylephrine, phenylpropanolamine, and amphetamines. The imidazolines act as alpha-receptor agonists, resulting in vasoconstriction and nasal decongestion. They also decrease endogenous norepinephrine production. The imidazolines include oxymetazoline, xylometazoline, clonidine, and naphazoline [25, 27]. Persistent use of either class of decongestant can lead to rhinitis medicamentosa.

The pathophysiology of rhinitis medicamentosa is not well understood. One proposed mechanism is that intense vasoconstriction from the stimulation of alpha-receptors leads to ischemia and development of interstitial edema. Another possible explanation is that continued stimulation of alpha-receptors causes their downregulation along with a decrease in endogenous noradrenaline production secondary to presynaptic, negative feedback. This leads to the dilation of submucosal venous plexuses resulting in congestion. Alpha-receptors may also become refractory to nasal decongestants leading to tachyphylaxis or tolerance [28, 29]. Tissue samples from the inferior turbinates of patients with rhinitis medicamentosa show damage to the nasal epithelium, cilia, and vascular endothelium [30]. On physical examination, the nasal mucosa commonly appears beefy red, with punctate bleeding and scant mucous. This finding is variable, however, and with continued decongestant use the mucosa can appear atrophic [29].

The treatment of rhinitis medicamentosa begins with discontinuation of the topical decongestant. The rebound congestion resolves over time without further treatment; however, intranasal corticosteroids have been shown to improve nasal congestion more rapidly [31]. Intranasal antihistamines may also be helpful in weaning patients off of nasal decongestants. In some cases, a short course of oral corticosteroids may be necessary [29].

Recently, several studies have reported that topical nasal decongestants can be used for extended periods of time without developing rhinitis medicamentosa if they are used in conjunction with a nasal corticosteroid which is believed to upregulate or prevent downregulation of the alpha-adrenergic receptors. Thus for patients with severe refractory nasal congestion, which is more typical of nonallergic and mixed rhinitis conditions, this approach may be an option to improve their short- and long-term clinical outcomes [32–34].

Diagnosis and Conclusion

This patient most likely has AERD, based on his clinical presentation. He has a long history of chronic rhinitis, which preceded his diagnosis of adult-onset asthma by several years. His respiratory disease was under good control until he started taking ibuprofen, an over-the-counter NSAID, for knee pain. This likely contributed to his recent asthma exacerbation and current abnormal spirometry. His chronic rhinosinusitis continues to be problematic, and is likely also driven by continued NSAID use. His exam shows evidence of nasal polyps, which likely explains his anosmia.

This patient's presentation is classic for AERD, and he likely does not need a provocation challenge to confirm the diagnosis. He should be advised to strictly avoid aspirin and all COX-1 inhibitors. Instead, he can be started on a selective COX-2 inhibitor for his knee pain. His rhinitis should be treated aggressively with a daily intranasal corticosteroid. Due to the presence of multiple nasal polyps and significant rhinitis symptoms, he may benefit from evaluation by an otolaryngologist. However, he should be counseled that polypectomy generally results in only temporary symptom relief, with a high likelihood of polyp recurrence and that most studies demonstrate that medical and surgical interventions have similar outcomes. He may benefit from starting a daily leukotriene-modifying agent for treatment of his AERD. His asthma symptoms should be closely monitored off NSAIDs. Therapy may be stepped up or stepped down as per usual asthma management guidelines.

At this time, the patient does not have a compelling medical reason to be on aspirin or NSAIDs. If his AERD symptoms fail to improve with the therapies above, he may benefit from referral to an allergist-immunologist for aspirin desensitization and high-dose aspirin therapy.

The patient in this case is unlikely to have rhinitis medicamentosa as a cause for his current rhinitis symptoms. While he did use oxymetazoline for an upper respiratory infection, the event was 2 months ago and the medication was discontinued after 3 days. The short duration of use makes it unlikely that he developed rhinitis medicamentosa. Although cocaine abuse has also been implicated as a cause of rhinitis medicamentosa by inhibiting reuptake of norepinephrine, the patient has not used this drug in over 20 years. Additionally, the appearance of his nasal turbinates was not consistent with rhinitis medicamentosa. While the absence of physical findings does not exclude the possibility in the correct clinical scenario, in this case, it suggests an alternate diagnosis.

Case Presentation 2

A 62-year-old man with a history of hypertension presents for evaluation of new-onset nasal congestion for the past 2 months. His current medications include antihypertensives, but he does not remember the names of the drugs and has forgotten to bring his medication list to his appointment. He reports that his blood pressure has been well controlled on the same regimen for several years. A few months ago, he was started on vardenafil for treatment of erectile dysfunction. He has no other complaints. He denies any prior history of rhinitis. He tried using over-the-counter antihistamines for his rhinitis but had no improvement so discontinued them 2 weeks prior to his visit. His physical examination, including the nasal mucosa, is unremarkable. He requests allergy testing at his appointment. Skin prick testing for aeroallergens is negative.

Discussion

Antihypertensives

Antihypertensive medications have been associated with nasal congestion and rhinitis through their blockade of nicotinic, alpha-adrenergic, or beta-adrenergic receptors, resulting in increased parasympathetic activity [35]. Among commonly used antihypertensive agents, beta-blockers are known to cause rhinitis as a side effect. The incidence of beta-blocker-induced rhinitis was reported to range between 1 and 7% in patients

taking nebivolol [36]. Rhinitis has also been a reported adverse effect of labetalol [37]. In addition, ACE inhibitors are known to induce rhinitis in some individuals [29]. Intranasal corticosteroids have been shown to be an effective treatment for reducing nasal congestion associated with these medications [35].

Phosphodiesterase-5 Inhibitors

Rhinitis is a common side effect of phosphodiesterase-5 (PDE-5) inhibitors that are typically used for the treatment of erectile dysfunction. Rhinitis occurs with a frequency of 9.2% with vardenafil (vs. 2.9% with placebo) in studies of drug safety and tolerability [38]. Rhinitis incidence increased with increasing doses of vardenafil. At low doses, rhinitis improved over time with continued use, but at higher doses it tended to persist [39].

The nasal turbinates contain erectile tissue and are thought to be affected by PDE-5 inhibitors through an increase in nitric oxide within the nasal mucosa that results in venous engorgement and rhinitis [40]. Sexual activity, in the absence of PDE-5 inhibitor use, can also induce rhinitis symptoms by an unknown mechanism in some patients [41]. If used infrequently, short-term nasal decongestants can be useful in treating PDE-5 inhibitor-induced rhinitis. In patients with more frequent symptoms, intranasal corticosteroids should be utilized as monotherapy or in conjunction with nasal decongestants to prevent the development of rhinitis medicamentosa [35].

Diagnosis and Conclusion

This patient's rhinitis is most likely due to his PDE-5 inhibitor. While some antihypertensives have been implicated in rhinitis cases, the onset of this patient's symptoms suggests that his PDE-5 inhibitor is responsible for his symptoms. The patient has been on antihypertensive medications without any change in therapy for years, without symptoms. The onset of his symptoms correlates with starting vardenafil.

At low doses, the rhinitis associated with vardenafil may improve over time, with continued use. At higher doses, the rhinitis is expected to persist. Based on the patient's preferences and perception of how bothersome the rhinitis is, he may either continue or discontinue the medication. Joint decision-making with the patient is appropriate in this case. Depending on symptom frequency, symptomatic management with a nasal decongestant or a daily intranasal corticosteroid could be offered if the patient chooses to continue the vardenafil.

General Principles in the Evaluation and Management of Drug-Induced Rhinitis

Evaluation of a patient with rhinitis requires obtaining a detailed history, including symptoms, onset, patterns, triggers, and associated features. A complete medication history is particularly important, as many commonly used medications are known to cause rhinitis. The physical examination should focus on the upper respiratory tract, with additional attention to signs of other atopic diseases [28]. Allergy skin prick testing for aeroallergens is useful for characterizing the patient's allergic status as treatment and outcomes of allergic versus nonallergic rhinitis vary significantly. In addition to considering other causes of rhinitis, conditions that can mimic rhinitis should also be considered including nasal polyps, benign or malignant nasal masses, illicit drug use, anatomic abnormalities, and laryngopharyngeal reflux.

The mainstay of management for drug-induced rhinitis is discontinuation of the offending drug. If this is not feasible, treatment of rhinitis symptoms is appropriate. In these cases, a daily intranasal corticosteroid can be started. Intranasal antihistamines can be added if adequate symptom relief is not achieved with intranasal corticosteroids alone. The management of rhinitis medicamentosa and AERD requires special considerations, as discussed above.

Clinical Pearls and Pitfalls

- Drug-induced rhinitis has been associated with multiple classes of commonly encountered drugs.
- When evaluating a patient for rhinitis, it is important to consider medications as a potential cause.
- Other etiologies of rhinitis, including allergic rhinitis, should be considered as a cause or comorbidity in patients presenting with rhinitis.
- Obtaining a detailed history, including symptoms, onset, and triggers, is an important component to rhinitis evaluation.
- The mainstay of treatment for drug-induced rhinitis is avoidance of the offending drug where possible. In cases where the drug is necessary and cannot be avoided, symptomatic management of the rhinitis is appropriate.
- Rhinitis medicamentosa and aspirin-exacerbated respiratory disease are special cases of drug-induced rhinitis, which require specific management.

References

1. Corren JBF, Pawankar R. Allergic and nonallergic rhinitis. In: Adkinson NF, Bochner BS, Burks AW, Busse WW, Holgate ST, Lemanske RF, et al., editors. Middleton's allergy: principles and practice. Philadelphia, PA: Elsevier Saunders; 2014. p. 664–85.
2. Steinke JW, Bradley D, Arango P, Crouse CD, Frierson H, Kountakis SE, et al. Cysteinyl leukotriene expression in chronic hyperplastic sinusitis-nasal polyposis: importance to eosinophilia and asthma. J Allergy Clin Immunol. 2003;111(2):342–9.
3. Ledford DK, Wenzel SE, Lockey RF. Aspirin or other nonsteroidal inflammatory agent exacerbated asthma. J Allergy Clin Immunol Pract. 2014;2(6):653–7.
4. Widal MF, Abrami P, Lermeyez J. Anaphylaxieet idosyncrasie. Presse Med. 1922;30:189–92.
5. Chang HS, Park JS, Shin HR, Park BL, Shin HD, Park CS. Association analysis of FABP1 gene polymorphisms with aspirin-exacerbated respiratory disease in asthma. Exp Lung Res. 2014;40(10):485–94.
6. Park SM, Park JS, Park HS, Park CS. Unraveling the genetic basis of aspirin hypersensitivity in asthma beyond arachidonate pathways. Allergy Asthma Immunol Res. 2013;5(5):258–76.

7. Park HKM, Sanchez-Borges M. Hypersensitivity to aspirin and other nonsteroidal antiinflammatory drugs. In: Adkinson NF, Burks AW, Busse WW, Holgate ST, Lemanske RF, et al., editors. Middleton's allergy: principles and practice. Philadelphia, PA: Elsevier Saunders; 2014. p. 1296–309.

8. Szczeklik A, Nizankowska E, Duplaga M. Natural history of aspirin-induced asthma. AIANE investigators. European network on aspirin-induced asthma. Eur Respir J. 2000;16(3):432–6.

9. Rajan JP, Wineinger NE, Stevenson DD, White AA. Prevalence of aspirin-exacerbated respiratory disease among asthmatic patients: a meta-analysis of the literature. J Allergy Clin Immunol. 2015;135(3):676–81 e1.

10. Kowalski ML, Makowska JS, Blanca M, Bavbek S, Bochenek G, Bousquet J, et al. Hypersensitivity to nonsteroidal anti-inflammatory drugs (NSAIDs)—classification, diagnosis and management: review of the EAACI/ENDA(#) and GA2LEN/HANNA*. Allergy. 2011;66(7):818–29.

11. Cardet JC, White AA, Barrett NA, Feldweg AM, Wickner PG, Savage J, et al. Alcohol-induced respiratory symptoms are common in patients with aspirin exacerbated respiratory disease. J Allergy Clin Immunol Pract. 2014;2(2):208–13.

12. Berges-Gimeno MP, Simon RA, Stevenson DD. The natural history and clinical characteristics of aspirin-exacerbated respiratory disease. Ann Allergy Asthma Immunol. 2002;89(5):474–8.

13. Stevenson DD, Szczeklik A. Clinical and pathologic perspectives on aspirin sensitivity and asthma. J Allergy Clin Immunol. 2006;118(4):773–86.

14. Stevens W, Buchheit K, Cahill KN. Aspirin-exacerbated diseases: advances in asthma with nasal polyposis, urticaria, angioedema, and anaphylaxis. Curr Allergy Asthma Rep. 2015;15(12):69.

15. Kowalski ML, Asero R, Bavbek S, Blanca M, Blanca-Lopez N, Bochenek G, et al. Classification and practical approach to the diagnosis and management of hypersensitivity to nonsteroidal anti-inflammatory drugs. Allergy. 2013;68(10):1219–32.

16. Dursun AB, Woessner KA, Simon RA, Karasoy D, Stevenson DD. Predicting outcomes of oral aspirin challenges in patients with asthma, nasal polyps, and chronic sinusitis. Ann Allergy Asthma Immunol. 2008;100(5):420–5.

17. Lee-Sarwar K, Johns C, Laidlaw TM, Cahill KN. Tolerance of daily low-dose aspirin does not preclude aspirin-exacerbated respiratory disease. J Allergy Clin Immunol Pract. 2015;3(3):449–51.

18. White AA, Bosso JV, Stevenson DD. The clinical dilemma of "silent desensitization" in aspirin-exacerbated respiratory disease. Allergy Asthma Proc. 2013;34(4):378–82.

19. Ledford DK, Lockey RF. Aspirin or nonsteroidal anti-inflammatory drug-exacerbated chronic rhinosinusitis. J Allergy Clin Immunol Pract. 2016;4(4):590–8.

20. Cho KS, Soudry E, Psaltis AJ, Nadeau KC, McGhee SA, Nayak JV, et al. Long-term sinonasal outcomes of aspirin desensitization in aspirin exacerbated respiratory disease. Otolaryngol Head Neck Surg. 2014;151(4):575–81.

21. Esmaeilzadeh H, Nabavi M, Aryan Z, Arshi S, Bemanian MH, Fallahpour M, et al. Aspirin desensitization for patients with aspirin-exacerbated respiratory disease: a randomized double-blind placebo-controlled trial. Clin Immunol. 2015;160(2):349–57.

22. Lee JY, Simon RA, Stevenson DD. Selection of aspirin dosages for aspirin desensitization treatment in patients with aspirin-exacerbated respiratory disease. J Allergy Clin Immunol. 2007;119(1):157–64.

23. Woessner KM. Update on aspirin-exacerbated respiratory disease. Curr Allergy Asthma Rep. 2017;17(1):2.

24. Feinberg SM, Friedlaender S. Nasal congestion from frequent use of privine hydrochloride. J Am Med Assoc. 1945;128:1095–6.

25. Ramey JT, Bailen E, Lockey RF. Rhinitis medicamentosa. J Investig Allergol Clin Immunol. 2006;16(3):148–55.

26. Snow SS, Logan TP, Hollender MH. Nasal spray 'addiction' and psychosis: a case report. Br J Psychiatry. 1980;136:297–9.

27. Varghese M, Glaum MC, Lockey RF. Drug-induced rhinitis. Clin Exp Allergy. 2010;40(3):381–4.

28. Graf P. Rhinitis medicamentosa: a review of causes and treatment. Treat Respir Med. 2005;4(1):21–9.

29. Wallace DV, Dykewicz MS, Bernstein DI, Blessing-Moore J, Cox L, Khan DA, et al. The diagnosis and management of rhinitis: an updated practice parameter. J Allergy Clin Immunol. 2008;122(2 Suppl):S1–84.

30. Knipping S, Holzhausen HJ, Goetze G, Riederer A, Bloching MB. Rhinitis medicamentosa: electron microscopic changes of human nasal mucosa. Otolaryngol Head Neck Surg. 2007;136(1):57–61.

31. Hallen H, Enerdal J, Graf P. Fluticasone propionate nasal spray is more effective and has a faster onset of action than placebo in treatment of rhinitis medicamentosa. Clin Exp Allergy. 1997;27(5):552–8.

32. Meltzer EO, Bernstein DI, Prenner BM, Berger WE, Shekar T, Teper AA. Mometasone furoate nasal spray plus oxymetazoline nasal spray: short-term efficacy and safety in seasonal allergic rhinitis. Am J Rhinol Allergy. 2013;27(2):102–8.

33. Vaidyanathan S, Williamson P, Clearie K, Khan F, Lipworth B. Fluticasone reverses oxymetazoline-induced tachyphylaxis of response and rebound congestion. Am J Respir Crit Care Med. 2010;182(1):19–24.

34. Baroody FM, Brown D, Gavanescu L, DeTineo M, Naclerio RM. Oxymetazoline adds to the effectiveness of fluticasone furoate in the treatment of perennial allergic rhinitis. J Allergy Clin Immunol. 2011;127(4):927–34.

35. Cingi C, Ozdoganoglu T, Songu M. Nasal obstruction as a drug side effect. Ther Adv Respir Dis. 2011;5(3):175–82.

36. Cheng JW. Nebivolol: a third-generation beta-blocker for hypertension. Clin Ther. 2009;31(3):447–62.

37. Labetalol and hydrochlorothiazide in hypertension. Labetalol/Hydrochlorothiazide Multicenter Study Group. Clin Pharmacol Ther. 1985;38(1):24–7.

38. Hellstrom WJ. Vardenafil: a new approach to the treatment of erectile dysfunction. Curr Urol Rep. 2003;4(6):479–87.

39. Hellstrom WJ, Gittelman M, Karlin G, Segerson T, Thibonnier M, Taylor T, et al. Sustained efficacy and tolerability of vardenafil, a highly potent selective phosphodiesterase type 5 inhibitor, in men with erectile dysfunction: results of a randomized, double-blind, 26-week placebo-controlled pivotal trial. Urology. 2003;61(4 Suppl 1):8–14.

40. Hicklin LA, Ryan C, Wong DK, Hinton AE. Nosebleeds after sildenafil (Viagra). J R Soc Med. 2002;95(8):402–3.

41. Monteseirin J, Camacho MJ, Bonilla I, Sanchez-Hernandez C, Hernandez M, Conde J. Honeymoon rhinitis. Allergy. 2001;56(4):353–4.

Index

© Springer International Publishing AG, part of Springer Nature 2018
J. A. Bernstein (ed.), *Rhinitis and Related Upper Respiratory Conditions*,
https://doi.org/10.1007/978-3-319-75370-6

Printed in the United States
By Bookmasters